Interdisciplinary Rheumatology

Ask rheumatologists what is one thing that they most desire, and they will say:

"I wish I knew more about nephrology so I could care for patients whose rheumatologic diseases manifest with renal complications. Nephrologists feel just the same, seeking to understand the implications that autoimmune diseases have for their patients."

As part of the *Interdisciplinary Rheumatology* book series, this book will serve as a dialogue between rheumatologists and nephrologists and provide a masterclass from world-renowned experts on these topics, led by a team of international editors with in-depth knowledge and cutting-edge research on topics like vasculitis and systemic lupus erythematous, among others.

Key Features:

- Provides a clinical approach to the patient with nephrological manifestations of rheumatic disease.

- Details cutting-edge research with inputs from the world's leading experts, both nephrologists and rheumatologists.

- Discusses possible future directions for research and advancement.

Interdisciplinary Rheumatology Series

Rheumatology and Gastroenterology
Edited by Reem Jan and Sushila Dalal

Rheumatology and Cardiology
Edited by Vaneet K. Sandhu

Rheumatology and Nephrology
Karina D. Torralba, Duvuru Geetha, and Anisha B. Dua

Interdisciplinary Rheumatology

Rheumatology and Nephrology

Edited by

Karina D. Torralba, Duvuru Geetha, and Anisha B. Dua

CRC Press
Taylor & Francis Group
Boca Raton London New York

CRC Press is an imprint of the
Taylor & Francis Group, an **informa** business

First edition published 2025
by CRC Press
2385 NW Executive Center Drive, Suite 320, Boca Raton FL 33431

and by CRC Press
4 Park Square, Milton Park, Abingdon, Oxon, OX14 4RN

CRC Press is an imprint of Taylor & Francis Group, LLC

© 2025 selection and editorial matter, Karina D. Torralba, Duvuru Geetha, and Anisha B. Dua individual chapters, the contributors

ISBN: 978-1-032-57218-5 (hbk)
ISBN: 978-1-032-57217-8 (pbk)
ISBN: 978-1-003-43837-3 (ebk)

DOI: 10.1201/9781003438373

Typeset in Palatino
by Apex CoVantage, LLC

We dedicate this book to all of our patients with rheumatic diseases who have given us the privilege to participate in their care. We draw inspiration from their strength.

Contents

Preface xv
Karina D. Torralba, Duvuru Geetha, Anisha B. Dua

Foreword xvii
Frédéric A. Houssiau

Editor Biographies xix

List of Contributors xxi

Part I: Approach to the Rheumatic Disease Patient with Renal Disease 1

1. Approach to the Patient with Renal Manifestations of Rheumatic Disease 2
   Meridith Balbach[†], Erin Chew[†], Andreas Kronbichler[‡], and Philipp Gauckler[‡]
   1.1   Introduction 2
   1.2   General Diagnostic Principles 2
        1.2.1   How to Assess Kidney Function and Damage 2
   1.3   Kidney Manifestations of Rheumatologic Disease 7
        1.3.1   Glomerular Disease 7
        1.3.2   Tubulointerstitial Nephritis 9
   1.4   Clinical Approach to Renal Involvement in Rheumatologic Disease 11
        1.4.1   Clinical Features of Rheumatologic Diseases with Kidney Involvement 11
        1.4.2   Non-Rheumatologic Diagnostic Workup of Kidney Disease 13
        1.4.3   Rheumatologic Diagnostic Workup of Kidney Disease 13

2. Dosing and Monitoring of Rheumatologic Medications in Patients with Renal Disease 18
   Jennifer Strouse, M. Lee Sanders, Chelsea McIntire, and Priyanka Iyer
   2.1   Introduction 18
   2.2   Non-Steroidal Anti-Inflammatory Drugs (NSAIDs) 18
   2.3   Conventional Synthetic Disease-Modifying Antirheumatic Drugs (csDMARDs) 18
        2.3.1   Methotrexate 18
        2.3.2   Hydroxychloroquine 20
        2.3.3   Sulfasalazine 20
        2.3.4   Leflunomide 20
        2.3.5   Azathioprine 20
        2.3.6   Mycophenolate Mofetil 20
        2.3.7   Cyclophosphamide 20
        2.3.8   Intravenous Immunoglobulin 20
        2.3.9   Calcineurin Inhibitors 21
   2.4   Biologic Disease-Modifying Antirheumatic Drugs (DMARDs) 21
   2.5   Targeted Synthetic Disease-Modifying Antirheumatic Drugs (tsDMARDs) 21
        2.5.1   Janus Kinase (JAK) Inhibitors 21
   2.6   Pharmacologic Treatment of Gout 22

2.6.1 Colchicine. 22

2.6.2 Xanthine Oxidase Inhibitors 24

2.6.3 Probenecid 24

2.6.4 Pegloticase 24

2.6.5 Other Agents Used to Treat Gout 24

2.7 Other Rheumatologic Medications 24

2.7.1 Apremilast 24

2.8 Conclusion 25

3. Renal Disease in the Pregnant Patient with Rheumatic Disease 26

Lauren He, Namrata Parikh, Silvi Shah, and Cuoghi Edens

3.1 Introduction. 26

3.2 Systemic Lupus Erythematosus 27

3.3 APS/Catastrophic APS 32

3.4 Vasculitis 32

3.5 Inflammatory Arthritides 33

3.6 Sjögren's Disease. 33

3.7 Other Connective Tissue Diseases. 34

3.8 Rheumatic Medications in Pregnancy 34

3.9 Contraception in RD Patients with Kidney Disease 35

3.10 Conclusion 35

4. Considerations for Pediatric Rheumatology Patients with Renal Disease 39

Megan Mariko Perron, Jennifer C. Cooper, and Jerome C. Lane

4.1 Introduction. 39

4.2 Systemic Lupus Erythematosus 39

4.3 Vasculitides 40

4.3.1 ANCA Associated Vasculitis. 40

4.3.2 IgA Vasculitis. 41

4.3.3 Tubulo-Interstitial Nephritis with Uveitis Syndrome. 41

4.3.4 Anti-GBM (Goodpasture's) Disease. 41

4.4 Pediatric Considerations for Drug Toxicities 42

4.4.1 Glucocorticoids 42

4.4.2 Cyclophosphamide. 42

4.5 Kidney Transplant in Pediatric Rheumatologic Disease 42

4.6 Measurement of Kidney Function in Children 43

4.7 Vaccinations. 43

4.8 Supporting Self-Management Efficacy and Transition to Adult Care 44

4.9 Conclusion 45

Part II: Kidney Disease in Specific Rheumatic Diseases 49

5. Lupus Nephritis 50

Brian J. Skaggs, David Kellner, Jose M. Monroy Trujillo, and Maureen McMahon

5.1   Introduction...50

5.2   Epidemiology and Risk Factors 50

    5.2.1   Clinical Presentation and Diagnosis 50

5.3   Pathogenesis of LN...51

    5.3.1   Epidemiology....................................51

    5.3.2   Genetics......................................51

    5.3.3   Immune Cells...................................52

    5.3.4   Endoplasmic Reticulum Stress 52

    5.3.5   Immune Complex Deposition.........................53

5.4   Biopsy Classification and Histopathology 53

5.5   Biomarkers of Lupus Nephritis 54

    5.5.1   Serum Biomarkers................................55

    5.5.2   Urinary Biomarkers 55

5.6   Treatment of LN 56

    5.6.1   Mycophenolate Mofetil............................56

    5.6.2   Cyclophosphamide................................57

    5.6.3   Belimumab.....................................57

    5.6.4   Calcineurin Inhibitors 57

    5.6.5   Rituximab.....................................58

    5.6.6   Novel Therapeutics on the Horizon.....................58

5.7   Guidelines for LN 59

6. Kidney Involvement in Pauci-Immune Anti-Neutrophil Cytoplasmic Antibody-Mediated Small-Vessel Vasculitis 70

Madeline Chung, Zachary Wallace, Ashwin R. Shetty, Alana Dasgupta, Salem Almaani, Duvuru Geetha, and Anisha B. Dua

6.1   ANCA-Associated Vasculitis 70

    6.1.1   Clinical Presentation..............................70

    6.1.2   Epidemiology...................................72

    6.1.3   Pathogenesis....................................72

6.2   Kidney Involvement..72

    6.2.1   Diagnostic Approach 73

    6.2.2   Relationship between Histology and Prognosis 74

6.3   Treatment..75

    6.3.1   Microscopic Polyangiitis (MPA), Granulomatosis with Polyangiitis (GPA), and Renal-Limited Vasculitis (RLV)...........................75

    6.3.2   Eosinophilic Granulomatosis with Polyangiitis (EGPA)......77

    6.3.3   Assessing Treatment Response........................77

6.4   Conclusion...77

7. Renal Involvement in Immune Complex Vasculitides 81

Margaret A. Deoliveira, Desh Nepal, Michael Putman, and Abdallah S. Geara

7.1   Immune Complex Vasculitis...................................81

7.2   Common Features of IC Vasculitis. 81

7.3   Cryoglobulinemic Vasculitis. 81

7.4   IgA Vasculitis 84

7.5   Anti-GBM Vasculitis 85

7.6   Hypocomplementemic Urticarial Vasculitis 85

7.7   Drug-Induced Immune Complex Vasculitis 86

7.8   Vasculitis in Monoclonal Gammopathy 87

7.9   Conclusion 87

8. Large- and Medium-Vessel Vasculitis 90

Raisa Lomanto Silva[†], Zain M. AlShanableh[†], Syeda Behjat Ahmad[†], and Sebastian E. Sattui[‡]

8.1   Introduction 90

8.2   Takayasu Arteritis 90

    8.2.1   Definition and Epidemiology 90

    8.2.2   Pathogenesis. 90

    8.2.3   Clinical Manifestations 90

    8.2.4   Diagnosis 91

    8.2.5   Treatment 92

8.3   Polyarteritis Nodosa. 92

    8.3.1   Definition and Epidemiology 92

    8.3.2   Pathogenesis. 92

    8.3.3   Clinical Manifestations 93

    8.3.4   Diagnosis 94

    8.3.5   Treatment 94

9. Scleroderma Renal Crisis and Other Renal Complications in Scleroderma 99

Brian S. Lee, Marissa Savoie, Andrew Z. Fenves, and Lorinda S. Chung

9.1   Introduction. 99

9.2   Brief Overview of Systemic Sclerosis 99

9.3   Scleroderma Renal Crisis 99

    9.3.1   Epidemiology and Risk Factors 99

    9.3.2   Pathophysiology 99

    9.3.3   Histopathology 101

    9.3.4   Diagnosis 101

    9.3.5   Differential Diagnosis of SRC and Non-SRC Renal Manifestations of SSc 102

    9.3.6   Management and Treatment 102

9.4   Conclusion 104

10. Renal Manifestations of Rheumatoid Arthritis, Spondyloarthropathies, Inflammatory

Myopathies and MCTD. 107

Suguni Loku Galappaththy, Jemima Albayda and Didem Saygin

10.1   Introduction. 107

10.2   Renal Manifestations of Rheumatoid Arthritis. 108

    10.2.1   Glomerulonephritis in RA. 108

10.2.2 Renal Involvement in Rheumatoid Vasculitis 111

10.2.3 Secondary Amyloidosis Due to RA 111

10.3 Renal Manifestation of Spondyloarthropathies. 111

10.3.1 Secondary Amyloidosis Due to SpA 111

10.3.2 NSAID-Induced Renal Injury 111

10.3.3 IgA Nephropathy 112

10.4 Renal Manifestations of Idiopathic Inflammatory Myopathies 112

10.4.1 Rhabdomyolysis-Induced AKI 112

10.4.2 Glomerulonephritis and Other Renal Pathologies Related to IIM 113

10.5 Renal Manifestations of Mixed Connective Tissue Disease 113

11. Kidney Disease in Sarcoidosis, Sjögren's Disease, and IgG4-Related Disease 116

Ellen Romich[†], Maria Jose Zabala Ramirez[†], Vanessa Romero, Dana Direnzo[‡], and Koyal Jain[‡]

11.1 Introduction... 116

11.2 Sarcoidosis... 116

11.2.1 General Diagnostic/Classification Criteria........................... 116

11.2.2 Renal Diagnostic Criteria.. 116

11.2.3 General Treatment Approach 117

11.2.4 Renal Treatment Approach 117

11.3 Sjögren's Disease... 117

11.3.1 Classification Criteria 117

11.3.2 Renal Diagnostic Criteria... 118

11.3.3 General Treatment Approaches 118

11.3.4 Renal Treatment Approach 119

11.4 IGG4-Related Disease 119

11.4.1 General Diagnostic/Classification Criteria........................... 119

11.4.2 Renal Diagnostic Criteria... 119

11.4.3 General Treatment Approaches 120

11.4.4 Renal Treatment Approach 120

11.5 Outcomes.. 120

11.6 Conclusion... 120

12. Renal Disease in Gout 124

Chen Xie and John FitzGerald

12.1 Prevalence of Renal Failure in Patients with Gout 124

12.2 Urate Transport in the Kidney and Gut 124

12.3 Dialysis and Urate Excretion. 125

12.4 Urate Management in CKD. 126

12.4.1 Dose Escalation in Patients with CKD............................. 127

12.5 Anti-Inflammatory Management in CKD 127

12.6 NSAIDs.. 127

12.7 Colchicine.. 127

12.8 Glucocorticoids 128

12.9 IL-1 Inhibitors 128

12.10 Conclusion 128

Part III: Special Considerations 133

13. Bone Health in Rheumatology Patients with Renal Disease 134

    S. Bobo Tanner, Cinduja Nathan, and Sergio Infante

    13.1 Introduction 134

    13.2 Assessing Bone Health in the Rheumatology Patient with CKD. 134

    13.3 Laboratory Evaluation. 134

    13.4 Bone Biopsy. 135

    13.5 Impact Microindentation 135

    13.6 Imaging 135

    13.7 DXA Bone Density Testing. 136

    13.8 Vertebral Fracture Assessment 136

    13.9 Trabecular Bone Score. 136

    13.10 Fracture Risk Assessment Tools in Patients with CKD 136

    13.11 Treatment Approach to Reduce Fracture Risk in the Rheumatology

          Patient with CKD-MBD 137

    13.12 Antiresorptive Agents. 137

    13.13 Anabolic Agents. 138

    13.14 Conclusion. 138

14. Dialysis and Kidney Transplantation Outcomes in Rheumatic Disease Patients 142

    Manal Alotaibi[†], Karina D. Torralba[†], Vaneet K. Sandhu[‡], and Sam Kant[‡]

    14.1 Introduction. 142

    14.2 Considerations for Starting Dialysis 142

        14.2.1 Outcomes in Rheumatic Disease Patients on Dialysis 142

        14.2.2 Treatment Considerations for Rheumatic Disease Patients on Dialysis. 143

    14.3 Renal Transplantation in Rheumatic Disease Patients. 144

        14.3.1 Eligibility Criteria for Renal Transplantation. 144

        14.3.2 Pre-Transplant Assessment of Rheumatic Disease

               Activity and Organ Involvement 146

        14.3.3 Balancing Rheumatic Disease Control and Organ Transplantation

               Outcomes in Rheumatic Disease Transplant Recipients. 147

        14.3.4 Graft Survival and Function, and Recurrence of Autoimmune Disease

               Post-Transplant 147

        14.3.5 Infections Post-Transplant 148

        14.3.6 Long-Term Management and Optimizing Outcomes 148

    14.4 Conclusion. 148

15. Musculoskeletal Complications in Dialysis Patients. 153

    Ana Valle and Shereen N. Mahmood

    15.1 Introduction. 153

    15.2 Generalized Pain and Fatigue 153

15.3 Muscle Disorders 153

15.4 Other Soft Tissue Involvement 154

15.5 Skin Manifestations 155

15.6 Joint Disorders. 155

15.7 Bone Disorders 156

15.8 Musculoskeletal Infections 156

15.9 Conclusion 157

Index 159

†These are co-first authors.
‡These are co-senior authors.

Preface

This book is part of an interdisciplinary rheumatology series that is spearheaded by Dr Philip Seo and Dr Jason Liebowitz. Other books in the series cover other specialty topics such as hematology, pulmonology, and cardiology. There has been no book series of its kind ever published. This is a nod to the fact that rheumatic diseases cut across multiple disciplines and as such there is an ever-increasing demand for rheumatologists and specialists to work hand in hand to take care of these patients.

As rheumatic disease patients present with more complex disease involving multiple organ systems, individuals involved in health systems, be it physicians, advanced practice providers, nurses, and even residents in training, need to also evolve to be able to manage these complications and prevent more from happening. A more wholistic approach to care is needed, frequently requiring one-on-one collaboration between rheumatologists and other organ-specific specialists.

Rheumatic disease patients may present with or develop renal manifestations during their disease course. Additionally, medications used to treat rheumatic disease can impact renal function, and those with abnormal renal function may be at higher risk of developing musculoskeletal complications or treatment-related adverse events. Much needs to be done to identify the main drivers of morbidity and mortality in rheumatic disease patients presenting with multi-organ disease. In many situations, it is the renal involvement that is the foremost problem. It is highly useful to know that there are guidelines that cover conditions that present with renal disease such as lupus nephritis and the pauci-immune glomerulonephritides. However, due to the relative rarity of rheumatic diseases in general and the rarity of renal manifestations in certain rheumatic diseases, there may not be formal and official guidance on how to manage these cases. This textbook offers insights into the complex interplay of renal involvement, evaluation, and management in multiple rheumatic diseases, including crystalline arthropathies, connective tissue diseases, vasculitides, and inflammatory arthritides. We highlight special considerations in rheumatic disease patients who are pediatric, pregnant, and in those undergoing dialysis or considering renal transplantation. In patients with renal disease from any etiology, we discuss overlying complexities related to common musculoskeletal complications, bone health, as well as the dosing and monitoring of immunosuppressive medications.

In 2003, the Institute of Medicine (IOM) published the book *Health Professions Education: A bridge to quality*. It highlighted five core competencies that define what a clinician must possess to provide high-quality care in the 21st century: patient-centered care, interdisciplinary teams, evidence-based practice, quality improvement, and informatics. Just a few years before that, the Accreditation Council of Graduate Medical Education (ACGME) came up with the six core competencies that define the foundational knowledge, skills, and attitudes that every practicing physician should possess: patient care, medical knowledge, interprofessional communication skills, professionalism, systems-based practice, and practice-based learning and improvement. In line with the ACGME's role to oversee post-graduate training programs, these ACGME core competencies have been developed and have been used to guide the education and evaluation of residents and fellows. Both the IOM and ACGME competencies underscore the need for collaboration between physicians and other healthcare providers. It is no longer enough as a healthcare provider to possess patient care and medical knowledge; communication skills, evidence-based practice, and professionalism are also other essential characteristics that define the modern-day physician. We hope that these are all attributes that our readers can take away from engaging with this book.

Dr Karina D. Torralba, Dr Duvuru Geetha, Dr Anisha B. Dua Editors,
Interdisciplinary Rheumatology-Nephrology

Foreword

Few medical specialties have as much in common as rheumatology and nephrology! The kidney is unfortunately the target of many autoimmune rheumatic diseases, which considerably compromises their prognosis. Conversely, chronic kidney disease has a major impact on the musculoskeletal system, particularly on bone. Additionally, some treatments used in rheumatology have deleterious effects on the kidney. Overall, in most hospitals, not a day goes by without a meeting between a rheumatologist and a nephrologist to discuss a complicated case of lupus, vasculitis, or bone mineral disorder. Not a week goes by without looking together in the microscope to look at slides and discuss renal pathology.

As true inheritors of internal medicine, rheumatologists and nephrologists share the same hypothetico-deductive mode of reasoning based on rigorous history-taking, full clinical examination, and appropriate request for additional tests, always duly interpreted with skepticism. We prescribe the same treatments, such as glucocorticoids, immunosuppressants, and, more recently, targeted therapies, some of them already used for years to prevent transplant rejection. We share knowledge of their side effects and have therefore learned together to balance their benefits against their drawbacks, for example, by prescribing as few glucocorticoids as possible. As clinicians dealing with chronic illnesses, we favor a holistic approach to patients, considering also psychological, socio-economic, and cultural aspects. In terms of research, we share the same paradigm, which goes from the bedside to the laboratory. Our approach is mainly pathophysiological. By looking into the diseased tissues themselves (i.e., the kidney, the synovium, or the bone), we try to unmask the mechanisms underlying and driving diseases, especially by applying the full set of recently developed -omics technologies and taking advantage of artificial intelligence and network medicine.

As a rheumatologist and researcher in the field of lupus nephritis for more than three decades, the reader will likely forgive me to use this disease as an example of collaborative work between rheumatologists and nephrologists. Most investigator-initiated or pharma-driven lupus nephritis trials leading to therapeutic advances have been co-designed by physicians belonging to the two specialties. For almost 15 years, rheumatologists and nephrologists with specific expertise in lupus nephritis have gathered on a regular basis to edit recommendations under the joint auspices of the European rheumatology (EULAR) and nephrology (ERA/EDTA) scientific societies. At lupus meetings, on sessions dealing with lupus nephritis, the panel stage is always shared by rheumatologists and nephrologists. When it comes to choosing between therapies at the bedside (for example, between a calcineurin inhibitor and a monoclonal antibody blocking a cytokine), different comfort levels may explain different attitudes. Yet through multidisciplinary case discussions, the best option for the patient will always be selected.

For these very reasons, it is an honor and a privilege to introduce *Interdisciplinary Rheumatology: Rheumatology and Nephrology* edited by Karina D. Torralba (rheumatologist at Loma Linda University and the University of California Riverside), Duvuru Geetha (nephrologist at Johns Hopkins University), and Anisha B. Dua (rheumatologist at Northwestern University). The book, published by Taylor & Francis Group, is part of a series of Interdisciplinary books edited by Philip Seo (Johns Hopkins University) and Jason Liebowitz (Columbia University). Most of the 15 chapters are co-written by a rheumatology and a nephrology lead author. They deal with all possible connections between our two smart specialties. The few of us who still hesitate to bring rheumatologists and nephrologists together for the sake of our patients should read this book. After just a few pages, they will be convinced that we can learn a lot from each other.

—*Frédéric A. Houssiau, MD, PhD*
Head of the Rheumatology Department, Cliniques universitaires Saint-Luc, Bruxelles
Full Professor, Université catholique de Louvain, Belgium

Editor Biographies

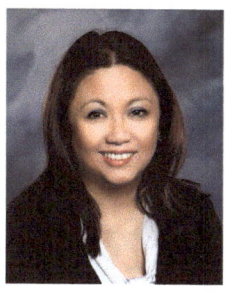

Karina D. Torralba, MD, MACM, CCD, RhMSUS is Professor of Medicine at Loma Linda University (LLU) School of Medicine and at University of California Riverside. As of May 2024, after completion of the writing of this book, she joined Amgen as a Global Development–Clinical Research Medical Director in Inflammation. She obtained a master's in academic medicine (medical education) from the Keck School of Medicine of University of Southern California in 2012. She was Chief (2015–2022) and Fellowship Program Director (2014–2021) for the Division of Rheumatology at Loma Linda University (LLU) in Loma Linda, California, USA. At LLU Medical Center, she served as the Director of Rheumatology Clinical Trials, Co-Director of the Ambulatory Infusion Center, and Director of the Fracture Liaison Service. She is a member of the Alpha Omega Alpha Society. She was Board President of the Ultrasound School of North American Rheumatologists (USSONAR) from 2021–2023 and of the Southern California Rheumatology Society (2022–2023). She received the Clinician Scholar Educator Award (2008–2011) from the Rheumatology Research Foundation. She is an active member of the American College of Rheumatology (ACR) and has chaired the ACR Basic and Advanced Musculoskeletal Ultrasound Courses (January 2023–May 2024, January–December 2019). She is an editor and reviewer for many journals. She is a member of the Lupus, Large-Vessel Vasculitis, and Autoimmune Interstitial Lung Disease ultrasound subgroups for the Outcome Measures in Rheumatoid Arthritis (OMERACT) and was co-lead for the Lupus Ultrasound subgroup. She has authored many publications in clinical, translational, quality-of-life, quality improvement, and educational research. She is also known for her work on psychological safety in clinical medicine.

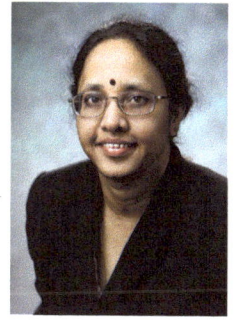

Duvuru Geetha, MD is a Professor of Clinical Medicine in the Divisions of Nephrology and Rheumatology at Johns Hopkins University School of Medicine. A graduate of Madras Medical College, India, she completed internal medicine training in the UK. She did her internal medicine residency in York, PA, and Nephrology fellowship at Johns Hopkins Bayview Medical Center. She has been on the Hopkins faculty since 1998. She is a member of Royal College of Physicians (UK), American Society of Nephrology, and International Society of Nephrology. Dr Geetha served on the post-graduate committee of the American Society of Nephrology and is a consultant for the Vasculitis Foundation. She is a member of the Miller Coulson Academy of Clinical Excellence at Hopkins. Her clinical interests include renal disease in vasculitis patients, with a focus on ANCA-associated vasculitis and Henoch–Schönlein purpura, also called IgA vasculitis. She does clinical and translational research in vasculitis, with a focus on ANCA-associated vasculitis and renal disease. Dr Geetha participates in multi-center clinical trials in vasculitis and other glomerular diseases.

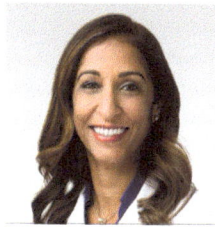

Anisha B. Dua, MD, MPH is an Professor of Medicine in the Division of Rheumatology, Rheumatology Fellowship Program Director, and Director of the Northwestern Vasculitis Center at Northwestern University Feinberg School of Medicine.

Her interests are in rheumatology education and vasculitis. She has completed fellowships in rheumatology at Rush, medical education at The University of Chicago, and integrative medicine at Northwestern. Dr Dua currently leads a multidisciplinary team in the clinical management of vasculitis patients. She assisted in the development of the American College of Rheumatology (ACR) Guideline for the Treatment and Management of Vasculitis, is on the Board of Directors for the Vasculitis Foundation, and is a recipient of the Clinical Scholar Educator award from the Rheumatology Research Foundation. She has served in multiple leadership roles, both locally and nationally, through the American College of Rheumatology, the Vasculitis Foundation, and the ACGME in the areas of education as well as vasculitis.

Contributors

Syeda Behjat Ahmad, MD
Assistant Professor of Medicine
Division of Renal-Electrolyte
University of Pittsburgh
Pittsburgh, Pennsylvania, USA

Jemima Albayda, MD
Associate Professor of Medicine
Division of Rheumatology, Department of
 Medicine
Johns Hopkins University School of Medicine
Baltimore, Maryland, USA

Salem Almaani, MD
Clinical Assistant Professor of Internal Medicine
Division of Nephrology, Department
 of Internal Medicine
The Ohio State University Wexner Medical
 Center
Columbus, Ohio, USA

Manal Alotaibi, MD
Assistant Professor of Nephrology
Division of Internal Medicine
College of Medicine
Umm Al-Qura University
Makkah, Saudi Arabia

Zain M. AlShanableh, MD
Fellow
Division of Renal-Electrolyte
University of Pittsburgh Medical Center
Pittsburgh, Pennsylvania, USA

Meridith Balbach, MD
Resident
Department of Internal Medicine
Vanderbilt University Medical Center
Nashville, Tennessee, USA

Erin Chew, MD
Assistant Professor of Medicine
Division of Rheumatology and Immunology
Department of Internal Medicine
Vanderbilt University Medical Center
Nashville, Tennessee, USA

Lorinda S. Chung, MD
Division of Immunology and Rheumatology
Department of Medicine
Stanford University School of Medicine
Palo Alto, CA, USA

Madeline Chung, MD, MS
Division of Nephrology
Department of Internal Medicine
The Ohio State University Wexner
 Medical Center
Columbus, Ohio, USA

Jennifer C. Cooper, MD, PharmD
Assistant Professor of Pediatrics
Division of Rheumatology
University of Colorado Anschutz School of
 Medicine
Denver, Colorado, USA

Alana Dasgupta, MD
Assistant Clinical Professor
Department of Pathology
The Ohio State University Wexner Medical
 Center
Columbus, Ohio, USA

Margaret A. Deoliveira, MD
Division of Renal, Electrolytes and Hypertension
University of Pennsylvania
Philadelphia, Pennsylvania, USA

Dana DiRenzo, MD
Assistant Professor of Clinical Medicine
Division of Rheumatology
Department of Medicine
University of Pennsylvania, Philadelphia, PA

Anisha B. Dua, MD, MPH
Associate Professor of Medicine
Division of Rheumatology
Northwestern University Feinberg School of
 Medicine
Chicago, Illinois, USA

Cuoghi Edens, MD
Assistant Professor
Sections of Rheumatology and Pediatric
 Rheumatology
University of Chicago Medicine
Chicago, Illinois, USA

Andrew Z. Fenves, MD
Department of Medicine, Division of Nephrology
Massachusetts General Hospital
Harvard Medical School
Boston, Massachusetts, USA

John FitzGerald, MD
Professor of Medicine Division of Rheumatology
Department of Medicine
University of California Los Angeles
Los Angeles, California, USA

Suguni Loku Galappaththy, MD
Fellow
Division of Rheumatology and
 Clinical Immunology
University of Pittsburgh Medical Center
University of Pittsburgh School of Medicine
Pittsburgh, Pennsylvania, USA

Philipp Gauckler, MD
Department of Internal Medicine IV
    (Nephrology and Hypertension)
Medical University Innsbruck
Innsbruck, Austria

Abdallah S. Geara, MD
Division of Renal, Electrolytes and
    Hypertension
University of Pennsylvania
Philadelphia, Pennsylvania, USA
Division of Nephrology
Lebanese American University
Lau, Byblos, Lebanon

Duvuru Geetha, MD
Professor of Clinical Medicine
Division of Nephrology, Division of
    Rheumatology, Department of Medicine
Johns Hopkins University School
    of Medicine
Baltimore, Maryland, USA

Lauren He, MD
Fellow
Division of Rheumatology
University of Michigan
Ann Arbor, Michigan, USA

Sergio Infante, MD
Associate Professor of Medicine
Division of Nephrology
Loma Linda University Medical Center
Loma Linda, California, USA

Priyanka Iyer, MBBS, MPH
Division of Rheumatology
Department of Medicine
University of California Irvine
Irvine, California, USA

Koyal Jain, MD
Assistant Professor of Medicine
UNC Kidney Center
Division of Nephrology and Hypertension
Department of Medicine
University of North Carolina
Chapel Hill, NC, USA

Sam Kant, MD, MRCPI, FASN, FACP
Assistant Professor of Medicine
Comprehensive Transplant Center and Division
    of Nephrology
Department of Medicine
Johns Hopkins University School
    of Medicine
Baltimore, Maryland, USA

David Kellner, MD
Fellow
Division of Rheumatology, Department of
    Medicine
University of California Los Angeles
Los Angeles, California, USA

Andreas Kronbichler, MD
Department of Internal Medicine IV
    (Nephrology and Hypertension)
Medical University Innsbruck
Innsbruck, Austria

Jerome C. Lane, MD
Associate Professor of Pediatrics
Division of Nephrology
Department of Pediatrics
Northwestern University Feinberg School of
    Medicine
Chicago, Illinois, USA

Brian S. Lee, MD
Department of Medicine
Division of Immunology and
    Rheumatology
Stanford University School of Medicine
Palo Alto, CA, USA

Shereen N. Mahmood, MD, RhMSUS
Albert Einstein College of Medicine
Bronx, New York, USA

Chelsea McIntire, PharmD, BCACP
Department of Pharmaceutical Care
University of Iowa Iowa City, Iowa, USA

Maureen McMahon, MD
Professor of Medicine
Division of Rheumatology, Department of
    Medicine
University of California Los Angeles

Cinduja Nathan, MD
Resident
Department of Internal Medicine
Loma Linda University Medical Center
Loma Linda, California, USA

Desh Nepal, MD
Division of Rheumatology
Medical College of Wisconsin
Milwaukee, Wisconsin, USA

Namrata Parikh, MD
Fellow, Kidney/Pancreas Transplantation
Division of Transplantation
Mayo Clinic Jacksonville, Florida, USA

Megan Mariko Perron, MD
Instructor of Pediatrics
Department of Immunology
Harvard Medical School
Boston Children's Hospital
Boston, Massachusetts, USA

Michael Putman, MD/MSci
Assistant Professor of Medicine
Medical College of Wisconsin
Milwaukee, Wisconsin, USA

Maria Jose Zabala Ramirez, MD
Assistant Professor of Medicine
UNC Kidney Center
Division of Nephrology and Hypertension
Department of Medicine
University of North Carolina
Chapel Hill, NC, USA

Vanessa Romero, MD
Clinical Assistant Professor
Director of Nephropathology
University of North Carolina,
Chapel Hill, NC, USA

M. Lee Sanders, MD, PhD
Division of Nephrology
Department of Medicine
University of Iowa
Iowa City, Iowa, USA

Vaneet K. Sandhu, MD, FACR, RhMSUS
Associate Professor of Medicine
Division of Rheumatology, Department of
    Medicine
Loma Linda University School of
    Medicine
Loma Linda, California, USA
Clinical Associate Professor of Medicine
Department of Medicine
University of California Riverside
Riverside, California, USA

Sebastian E. Sattui MD, MS
Assistant Professor of Medicine
Division of Rheumatology and Clinical
    Immunology
University of Pittsburgh
Pittsburgh, Pennsylvania, USA

Marissa Savoie, MD
Department of Medicine
Massachusetts General Hospital
Boston, Massachusetts, USA

Didem Saygin, MD
Assistant Professor of Medicine
Division of Rheumatology
Department of Medicine
Rush University Medical Center
Chicago Illinois, USA

Silvi Shah, MD
Associate Professor
Division of Nephrology and Hypertension
University of Cincinnati College of Medicine
Cincinnati, Ohio, USA

Ashwin R. Shetty, MD
Associate Program Director
Division of Nephrology
Department of Internal Medicine
Swedish Hospital, a part of Endeavor Health
Chicago, Illinois, USA

Raisa Lomanto Silva, MD
Clinical Assistant Professor of Medicine
Division of General Internal Medicine
University of Pittsburgh Medical Center
Pittsburgh, Pennsylvania, USA

Brian J. Skaggs, PhD
Adjunct Associate Professor
Division of Rheumatology
Department of Medicine
University of California Los Angeles
Los Angeles, California, USA

Jennifer Strouse, MD
Division of Immunology
Department of Medicine
University of Iowa
Iowa City, Iowa, USA

S. Bobo Tanner, MD
Assistant Professor of Medicine
Division of Rheumatology and Immunology
Vanderbilt University Medical Center
Nashville, Tennessee, USA

Karina D. Torralba, MD, MACM, RhMSUS
Professor of Medicine
Division of Rheumatology, Department of
    Medicine
Department of Medical Education
Loma Linda University School of Medicine
Loma Linda, California, USA
Clinical Professor of Medicine
University of California Riverside
Riverside, California, USA

Jose M. Monroy Trujillo, MD
Assistant Professor of Medicine
Division of Nephrology,
Department of Medicine
Johns Hopkins University School of Medicine
Baltimore, Maryland, USA

Ana Valle, MD, MHS
Division of Rheumatology, Inflammation, and
Immunity
Department of Medicine
Brigham and Women's Hospital
Boston, Massachusetts, USA

Zachary Wallace, MD
Assistant Professor of Medicine
Division of Rheumatology
Department of Medicine
Harvard Medical School
Boston, Massachusetts, USA

Chen Xie, MD
Assistant Professor
Division of Rheumatology
Department of Medicine
University of California Los Angeles
Los Angeles, California, USA

PART I

APPROACH TO THE RHEUMATIC DISEASE PATIENT WITH RENAL DISEASE

1 Approach to the Patient with Renal Manifestations of Rheumatic Disease

Meridith Balbach[†], Erin Chew[†], Andreas Kronbichler[‡], and Philipp Gauckler[‡]
[†]These are co-first authors.
[‡]These are co-senior authors.

1.1 INTRODUCTION

Rheumatologic and kidney diseases frequently overlap. Oftentimes, kidney involvement represents a highly morbid manifestation of a rheumatologic disorder. Additional challenges arise as many of the treatments for these conditions have the potential to harm the kidneys, leading to acute kidney injury (AKI), chronic kidney disease (CKD), disturbances in electrolyte and acid–base homeostasis, or arterial hypertension. Furthermore, rheumatologic complications frequently develop because of kidney pathology. The early identification of kidney damage, initiation of basic diagnostic assessments, and referral to a nephrologist are key to mitigating a progressive decline in kidney function.

The aim of this chapter is to outline essential diagnostic principles and fundamental patterns of kidney damage. We also present a general diagnostic approach for daily use by the rheumatologist.

1.2 GENERAL DIAGNOSTIC PRINCIPLES

1.2.1 How to Assess Kidney Function and Damage

The kidney is not only the central regulatory organ for electrolyte, acid–base, and fluid homeostasis but is also involved in numerous endocrine functions, including the synthesis of erythropoietin, calcitriol, and renin. A given kidney injury event does not affect all domains to the same extent. However, the determination of the glomerular filtration rate (GFR) has been established as the key parameter to assess excretory kidney function. In conjunction with the degree of albuminuria, the GFR is used as a crucial marker for the diagnosis and staging of kidney disease, as well as appropriate drug dosing (1).

Assessment of Glomerular Filtration Rate

Since the precise measurement of GFR (mGFR) is cumbersome and expensive, formulas to estimate GFR (eGFR) based on serum concentrations of creatinine and/or cystatin C are generally used in daily clinical practice. Although impractical for clinical practice, the gold standard of mGFR remains the determination of the urinary clearance of inulin during continuous intravenous infusion (2). The alternative use of other exogenous markers (iothalamate, iohexol, EDTA, DPTA) is therefore recommended when a confirmatory test for GFR assessment is necessary and should be performed by a nephrologist (1). Measuring the clearance of endogenous markers such as creatinine (mCrCl) is less expensive but not capable of reflecting mGFR correctly. The tubular secretion of creatinine leads to the overestimation of GFR. Moreover, the clinical utility of 24-hour collections is limited by the impracticality of collection and prevalent mistakes leading to imprecise calculation.

Various serum creatinine-based formulas to estimate GFR have been developed and validated over the past decades. Currently, the Chronic Kidney Disease Epidemiology Collaboration (CKD-EPI) equation is recommended to be used for most scenarios and populations (1, 3). However, creatinine is an inaccurate GFR marker if skeletal muscle mass is significantly altered. Such conditions include patients with large limb amputation, spinal cord injury, neuromuscular disease, severe malnutrition, advanced heart failure, and liver disease (1). The use of cystatin C-based equations has been demonstrated to have advantages in such patient cohorts. However, cystatin C is likewise not an ideal marker, and eGFR based on cystatin C may be influenced by other factors, including steroid use and thyroid disease, thus limiting its value in rheumatic disorders. Equations using both creatinine and cystatin C may have the best performance as compared with mGFR (4). Recently, a debate has been carried out regarding the use of the adjustment coefficient for Black patients. Therefore, a new "race-free" CKD-EPI equation for both creatinine and cystatin C has been proposed (5), replacing prior formulas to estimate GFR.

Critically, eGFR can only be determined when endogenous markers (creatinine, cystatin C) are in a steady state and should therefore not be reported in scenarios such as acute kidney injury (AKI), dialysis, or acute edematous states (6).

Not all clinical laboratories routinely provide eGFR values using CKD-EPI equations. However, this can be done using freely available calculators (e.g., National Kidney Foundation eGFR Calculator).

DOI: 10.1201/9781003438373-2

Urine Diagnostics

The basic analysis of urine is readily accessible, inexpensive, and unveils crucial information about the type and location of damage in the kidneys or urinary tract. Therefore, urinalysis—at least in the form of a dipstick test—is an essential part of any nephrological workup and should be performed regularly, commensurate with the frequency of renal involvement in the rheumatologic disease at hand.

Urine Dipstick

Urine dipstick testing provides a cheap and rapid semiquantitative assessment of several urinary characteristics. Typical characteristics included are summarized in Table 1.1.

The rheumatologist should be aware of urinary dipstick testing limitations (see Table 1.1). The persistent detection of heme should always be verified by sediment examination. The detection of albuminuria should always prompt further quantification, as the semiquantitative grading of albuminuria with a urinary dipstick is highly dependent on urinary concentration and therefore often misleading.

Table 1.1: Urinary Dipstick Characteristics and Relevant Caveats for Their Interpretation

Test	Significance	Context/Pitfalls
Specific gravity	Concentration/ osmolality	Specific gravity varies with urinary osmolality. Isosmotic urine (to plasma) is associated with a specific gravity of 1.008–1.009. • *Falsely high gravity*: Large molecules such as glucose or radiocontrast media. • *Falsely low gravity*: No causes. A specific gravity < 1.003 is indicating maximally diluted urine (≤ 100 mOsm/kg).
pH	Acidity	Mostly used to evaluate metabolic acidosis. • Inability to acidify urine (pH > 5) indicates renal tubular acidosis. • *Falsely high pH*: Urease-producing pathogens (e.g., *Proteus* spp.).
Heme	Hematuria	• *Falsely positive*: Free hemoglobin/myoglobin. • *Falsely negative*: Unlikely, as this test has very high sensitivity. • Confirmation by urine sediment examination is required (57, 58).
Leukocyte esterase	Leukocytes	• *Falsely negative*: Concentrated urine (59).
Nitrite	Bacteriuria	• *Falsely negative*: Bacteria with no or low expression of nitrate reductase (e.g., *Enterococcus* spp.).
Protein	Albuminuria	Used to detect albumin only (i.e., does not detect non-albumin proteins such as immunoglobulins or light chains) • Microalbuminuria (< 300 mg/day) may not be detected (especially when urine is diluted). • Semiquantitative results may be misleading, as the degree (1+, 2+, 3+) is highly dependent on urinary concentration. Proteinuria quantification (uPCR, uACR, 24-hour urine collection) should always be performed when proteinuria is detected.
Glucose	Glycosuria	When kidney function is normal, significant glycosuria does not occur until plasma glucose concentration exceeds 180 mg/dL. Glycosuria with euglycemia is indicative of a proximal tubular defect or intake of sodium glucose co-transporter (SGLT2) inhibitors. • *Falsely negative*: Ascorbic acid.

Abbreviations: uPCR, urine protein-to-creatinine ratio; uACR, urine albumin-to-creatinine ratio
Source: Based on Perazella et al. (56)

Urine Sediment Examination

Manual microscopic examination has been increasingly replaced by automated laboratory analysis of the urine sediment in recent years. Still, the diagnostic yield may be substantially greater when performed by trained personnel (7). More details about urine sediment examination with a detailed discussion on manual versus automated microscopy are discussed elsewhere (8).

Urine sediment examination is an indispensable diagnostic technique to complement clinical findings and urine dipstick testing. Typical findings seen on urine microscopy include the presence of cells (red blood cells, leukocytes, epithelial cells), casts, crystals, microorganisms, and lipids.

Hematuria can be grossly visible (macrohematuria) or microscopic (microhematuria). The latter is usually defined as the presence of three or more red blood cells per high power field (9, 10). A comprehensive diagnostic workup of microhematuria is out of the scope of this chapter, though respective guidelines and a clinically useful algorithm are provided by the American Urological Association (10). An overview of common causes of hematuria is illustrated in Figure 1.1.

A differentiation between transient and persistent hematuria is helpful, as transient hematuria is a frequent and mostly benign condition (e.g., following exercise, sexual intercourse, or menstruation). However, in the absence of dysmorphic erythrocytes, urological evaluation should always occur in individuals > 50 years of age to exclude underlying malignancy. Urinary sediment examination is particularly valuable in the evaluation of unexplained hematuria, as it may allow for differentiation between glomerular and non-glomerular causes. The presence of dysmorphic erythrocytes (e.g., acanthocytes) or red blood cell casts is strongly suggestive of underlying glomerular disease, although the latter lacks sensitivity (11). It is important to recognize that the absence of dysmorphic red blood cells or casts does not exclude glomerular hematuria.

White blood cells: White blood cells are mainly associated with bacteriuria. However, when urine culture remains negative ("sterile pyuria"), other entities such as tubulointerstitial nephritis, urolithiasis, and renal tuberculosis need to be considered. White blood cell casts are relatively specific for tubulointerstitial nephritis, especially in the context of tubular proteinuria (see Section 1.2.1.2.3) and other features of tubulointerstitial damage such as Fanconi syndrome. However, all features lack sensitivity, and a renal biopsy is required to make a definitive diagnosis (12).

Evaluation of Proteinuria

The evaluation and quantification of urinary protein excretion are fundamental parts of every nephrological workup. Although protein is physiologically excreted only minimally in the urine,

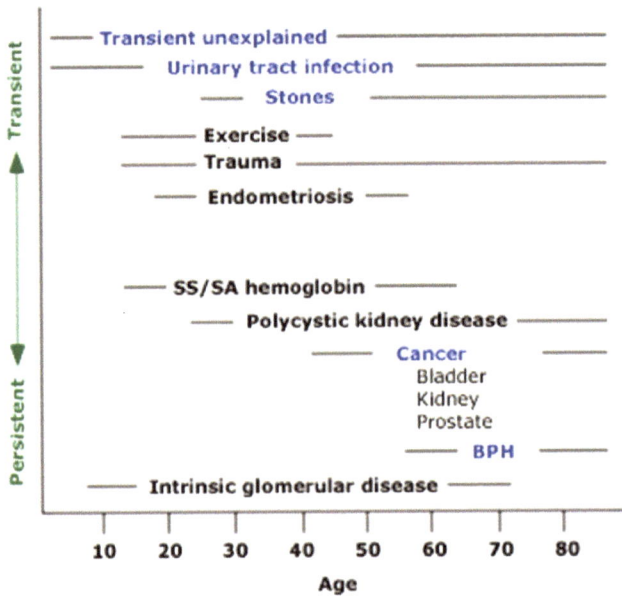

Figure 1.1 Common causes of hematuria by age and duration thereof (transient of persistent). BPH, benign prostate hyperplasia. (Modified from [56]).

certain forms of proteinuria such as transient proteinuria or orthostatic proteinuria in adolescents are benign and need to be distinguished from definitive pathological proteinuria. Albumin excretion in a healthy individual is below 20 mg per day. Albuminuria between 30 mg and 300 mg per day is classified as moderately increased albuminuria (formerly "microalbuminuria") and > 300 mg as severely increased albuminuria ("macroalbuminuria").

Two different methods to quantify urinary protein excretion are used in daily clinical practice. The gold standard is quantitative measurement of protein excretion from a 24-hour urine collection. As discussed earlier, urine collection is error prone, thereby often leading to inaccurate measurements. The consideration of the total amount of creatinine excreted over 24 hours may be helpful to prove the adequacy of the present sample. The total daily creatinine excretion in adults < 50 years of age should be 20–25 mg/kg of lean body weight in males and 15–20 mg/kg of lean body weight in females and declines progressively with age.

Based on the assumption that the daily urinary excretion of creatinine remains roughly stable, approaching about 1 gram per day, the urine protein-to-creatinine ratio (uPCR) or urine albumin-to-creatinine ratio (uACR) measured from a spot urine sample will reasonably correlate with the total amount of protein or albumin excreted in the urine over a 24 hour period. The use of uACR and uPCR from a morning first-void mid-stream sample is therefore recommended as the principal method to evaluate proteinuria in adults and children (13). However, it needs to be emphasized that the accuracy of uACR and uPCR is dependent on the individual creatinine excretion, which may be substantially higher or lower than 1 gram per day. uPCR and uACR should be measured simultaneously at least once. In the case of a significant discrepancy, nonglomerular proteinuria is to be assumed, and an additional measurement of free light chains and beta2 microglobulin in the urine can provide further insights into the origin of the kidney damage.

Evolving Urinary Biomarkers (Perspective)

Several evolving novel biomarkers aim to non-invasively improve early diagnosis and prognostication in the setting of AKI and CKD.

A major unmet need among immune-mediated kidney diseases is the differentiation between ongoing inflammatory activity versus chronic kidney damage with glomerular scarring, tubulointerstitial atrophy, and fibrosis, which may similarly present with progressive GFR decline, proteinuria, and even persistent hematuria. Currently, histopathological evaluation via kidney biopsy is needed to allow for the adequate evaluation of active and chronic lesions, as exemplified in the management of proliferative lupus nephritis (LN) (14). Non-invasive diagnostic tools are therefore urgently needed. A variety of urinary biomarkers improving the localization (e.g., markers of tubular injury: IL-18, KIM-1, NGAL versus endothelial/microvascular injury: TNFR1/2) and type (markers of inflammation: IL-18, TNFR1/2 versus markers of fibrosis: MCP-1, EGF) of kidney injury have been investigated (15). Urinary MCP-1, a marker of monocyte activation in the kidneys, has even been tested in the Phase 2 CLEAR and Phase 3 ADVOCATE trials supporting the approval of avacopan in the management of severe anti-neutrophil cytoplasmic antibody (ANCA)-associated vasculitis (16, 17). Another interesting biomarker candidate is the urine-soluble CD163, which discriminates patients with active LN from patients with nonactive LN or non-renal SLE (18). This marker holds great promise to distinguish active ANCA-glomerulonephritis (GN) from patients in remission and can also identify active GN from other causes of AKI (19). Levels of urinary soluble CD163 increase ahead of disease relapse, and further investigations to refine relapse prediction based on biomarkers in ANCA-GN are ongoing (19). A commercially available kit has been developed and is available to implement urine-soluble CD163 into clinical practice.

Although promising, evidence of the superiority of these experimental biomarkers over easily measurable and currently available markers will be needed before their clinical application, particularly their ability to yield early detection of disease relapse.

Additional Diagnostics

Ultrasound

Kidney ultrasound is a cheap and safe technique offering valuable additional information for the treating physician and should be considered in the workup of every patient with suspected kidney disease (20). Besides classical kidney ultrasound techniques, point-of-care ultrasound (POCUS) is increasingly available to facilitate the bedside detection of structural pathologies (e.g., hydronephrosis, urolithiasis) and gather relevant functional information about the volume status and kidney perfusion (21). Ultrasound is obligatory in the setting of AKI to detect postrenal causes. In CKD, kidney length and cortical thickness correlate with kidney function (22). Ultrasound therefore yields prognostic information that may aid in the decision-making process regarding the necessity for invasive diagnostic procedures such as kidney biopsy or the potential benefits of immunosuppressive treatments.

Kidney Biopsy

Kidney biopsy remains the gold standard and—with very few exceptions—is indispensable for the diagnosis of most kidney diseases. Furthermore, histopathology provides valuable prognostic information. Distinguishing between chronic and active lesions can be of particular importance in the risk–benefit assessment to start (immunosuppressive) therapies.

Historically, most biopsies have been performed with ultrasound guidance by nephrologists. However, the fractions of biopsies performed by radiologists and CT-guided kidney biopsies are increasing. It is crucial that an adequate sample size is obtained, as adequate assessment includes light microscopy (LM), immunofluorescence (IF) or immunohistochemistry (IH), and electron microscopy (EM). For LM assessments, a total number of 8–10 glomeruli is required to adequately assess the severity and distribution of lesions (23). Typical indications to perform a biopsy are summarized in Table 1.2.

However, the native kidney biopsy is an invasive procedure with certain risks and should therefore be avoided when potential harm to the patient exceeds any likely benefit (24). Potential complications include pain at the site of biopsy, hematomas, macroscopic hematuria, blood loss requiring transfusions, and interventions to achieve hemostasis (25). Therefore, the indication for kidney biopsy is always made individually on a case-by-case basis and may vary substantially. In SLE, for example, the indication for kidney biopsy is usually made when uPCR exceeds 0.5 g/g creatinine (26). Contraindications to perform a biopsy include an elevated bleeding risk (e.g., hemophilic diathesis or indication for anticoagulation), uncontrolled hypertension, small/atrophic kidneys on ultrasound, and the patient's desire.

It is important to recognize that generally, neither defined lesions nor histopathological diagnoses are specific for one individual disease. In contrast, a histopathological diagnosis usually demands the exclusion of underlying secondary causes (e.g., underlying malignancy, infection, or systemic autoimmune disease). This applies almost universally with only a few exceptions. As an example, membranous nephropathy is a typical lesion pattern seen on LM that is associated with the clinical phenotype of the nephrotic syndrome. The EM correlates are subepithelial deposits of immune complexes. However, this clinicopathologic constellation may be idiopathic or occur secondarily to an underlying malignancy or SLE (thus denominated membranous LN ISN/RPS Class V).

An overview of clinicopathologic entities is available in the Atlas of Renal Pathology II by the AJKD (available free online).

Table 1.2: Suggested Features Guiding the Decision to Pursue Kidney Biopsy

Clinical Scenario	Indications
Hematuria	• Presence of dysmorphic red blood cells or red blood cell casts ± impaired kidney function ± proteinuria
Proteinuria	• > 1 g/day (confirmed) in absence of overt secondary cause/comorbidity (*consider*) • > 3 g/day in absence of overt secondary cause/comorbidity (*recommended*)
AKI	• If intrinsic/intrarenal cause is suspected • Persistent injury despite reversal of cause or if baseline GFR is not achieved 7–14 days after injury onset • In presumptive acute interstitial nephritis with an unclear trigger or without resolution of injury despite removal of suspected precipitant
CKD	• Rapid GFR loss or new-onset/worsening hematuria or proteinuria
Kidney injury with concomitant rheumatic disease	• Unexplained or progressive loss of kidney function • Proteinuria ≥ 500 mg/day or 500 mg/g uPCR (especially if SLE) • Hematuria with active sediment or with concomitant proteinuria

Abbreviations: GFR, glomerular filtration rate; uPCR, urine protein-to-creatinine ratio
Source: Modified from Luciano et al. (24)

1.3 KIDNEY MANIFESTATIONS OF RHEUMATOLOGIC DISEASE

The rheumatologist often employs the aforementioned renal diagnostics because rheumatologic and kidney diseases frequently co-occur. Most often this occurs in the context of kidney involvement as a direct manifestation of rheumatologic disease, though indirect involvement because of the treatment of rheumatologic disease is well described. Alternatively, rheumatologic disease may arise as a result of long-standing primary renal disease (see Chapter 13) (27). Lastly, rheumatologic and kidney disease may co-occur independently.

In this section, we describe three patterns of undifferentiated kidney injury (glomerular, tubulointerstitial, and vascular) and briefly review rheumatologic etiologies of each. While a brief overview of kidney involvement including urinary, histopathologic, and renal-related clinical features for each disease is provided here, later chapters provide a more complete description.

1.3.1 Glomerular Disease

Causes of glomerular disease encompass a wide array of conditions (e.g., autoimmune disease, malignancy, sequelae of infection, genetic mutations, medication toxicity) that lead to injury of the glomerular filtration barrier, enabling the passage of protein and/or blood into the urine (28). Most rheumatologic etiologies of glomerular disease cause immune-mediated damage to the basement membrane, mesangium, podocytes, or capillary endothelium, usually via immune complex or complement fragment deposition (29).

Findings that suggest glomerular injury include:

(1) Glomerular hematuria, as evidenced by the presence of red blood cells (of which a substantial portion are dysmorphic) and/or red blood cell casts

(2) Proteinuria, which can be in a nephrotic or non-nephrotic range (see herein)

(3) Reduction in GFR

Glomerular injury may be further differentiated as a nephritic or nephrotic syndrome, each of which is associated with distinct though overlapping pathophysiology and underlying primary etiology.

Nephritic Syndrome

Nephritic syndrome is characterized by glomerular inflammation (i.e., glomerulonephritis) leading to hematuria, variable degrees of proteinuria (though mainly in a non-nephrotic range), hypertension, and rarely significant edema, except the kidney function is significantly impaired. Suspected glomerulonephritis usually demands a diagnostic kidney biopsy. IF performed on unfixed frozen tissue may determine the nature and location of immune complex deposits, further refining the categorization of the glomerulonephritis for the rheumatologist (30).

Lupus Nephritis and Related Overlap Connective Tissue Disease Syndromes

LN is a leading cause of morbidity and mortality in patients with systemic lupus erythematosus (SLE) (31). It occurs in up to 38% of SLE patients, usually within 5 years of disease onset and frequently at the time of initial presentation (32). It most frequently affects individuals of African American, Hispanic, and Asian ethnicities (33).

Antibodies arising as a result of failures in self-tolerance precipitate LN by binding to multiple intrarenal nuclear autoantigens, leading to associated tertiary lymphoid tissue formation with subsequent local antibody production and immune complex formation (34). Immune deposits, primarily complexes of anti-double stranded DNA antibody—nucleosomal antigens—subsequently trigger the activation of the classical complement pathway.

Patterns of this deposition are the basis for the International Society of Nephrology and Renal Pathology Society's classification of LN and account for the various clinical presentations and degree of proteinuria and/or hematuria (29, 33, 35). The definitive diagnosis of LN requires kidney biopsy. On IF, the pathognomonic glomerular deposits stain for IgG with co-deposits of IgA, IgM, C3, and C1q in a "full house" pattern (29).

Nephrotic syndrome in SLE is classically associated with WHO class V (membranous nephropathy) LN on histopathology. However, nephrotic syndrome in SLE may coincide as lupus podocytopathy with class I or II LN (mesangial pattern), which should be managed as minimal change disease (33). Biopsy is thus instrumental in differentiating histopathological changes and guiding treatment.

Immunosuppression is guided by histologic findings and the degree of activity versus chronicity. Depending on the class of LN, up to 30% of patients will progress to ESKD (33).

Cryoglobulinemic Glomerulonephritis

Cryoglobulinemia is defined by the presence of one (monoclonal) or more (mixed) immunoglobulins that precipitate *in vitro* at cold temperatures (i.e., < 37 °C) and redissolve on warming for poorly understood and likely variable reasons (36). Three subgroups are distinguished based on the clonality and class of involved immunoglobulin. Kidney involvement occurs more frequently in types 2 and 3, representing mixed cryoglobulinemia characterized by a monoclonal component (IgM, IgG, or IgA) with polyclonal IgG and polyclonal Ig (any isotype), respectively (36). Hepatitis C is the leading cause of mixed cryoglobulinemia, but additional etiologies include essential cryoglobulinemia (approximately 45% of cases), rheumatologic conditions (i.e., Sjögren's disease and SLE), other infections, and lymphoproliferative disorders.

Kidney involvement occurs in 20–60% of patients with cryoglobulinemia and is caused by the deposition of immune complexes in small glomerular vessels. Biopsy shows a membranoproliferative pattern with the deposition of immunoglobulins, C3, and C1q on IF (33). Differentiation from LN class IV requires EM, demonstrating cryoglobulins identified by their microtubular substructure (29).

The treatment of cryoglobulinemia is dictated by the extent of organ involvement and the speed of organ damage. In patients with life-threatening organ involvement, exemplified by kidney failure, urgent treatment initiation should include a combination of plasma exchange, rituximab or other potent immunosuppressants, and high doses of glucocorticoids. After stabilization, treatment is directed at the underlying condition. A careful review of systems, physical exam, and r workup are necessary to rule out underlying systemic autoimmune diseases.

IgA Vasculitis

IgA vasculitis is the most common systemic vasculitis affecting children, but kidney involvement is more likely to occur in older children and adults (29). IgA vasculitis classically presents with the tetrad of palpable purpura, arthralgia ± arthritis, abdominal pain, and kidney disease. Histologically, the pattern of renal injury is similar to that of IgA nephropathy, with kidney biopsy showing the mesangial deposition of IgA with C3 predominantly and occasional IgG or IgM (29). The renal prognosis is usually favorable in children but varies in adults, with 10–15% of patients developing severe renal involvement with possible progression to ESRD (27).

Antineutrophilic Cytoplasmic Antibody (ANCA)-Associated Glomerulonephritis

Renal involvement among those with ANCA-associated vasculitis, including microscopic polyangiitis (MPA), granulomatosis with polyangiitis (GPA), and eosinophilic granulomatosis with polyangiitis (EGPA), may cause kidney failure, particularly in those older than 60 years (33).

Kidney involvement is a key feature of both MPA (affecting 80–100% of patients) and GPA, though occurring less frequently in the latter (60%) (37). Fewer EGPA patients are affected by renal pathology (25%). Interestingly, the presence of ANCA in EGPA predicts renal involvement, with approximately 75% of all patients with renal involvement demonstrating ANCA positivity versus just 25% of those without renal involvement (38). Severity ranges from asymptomatic active urine sediment to rapid progression to kidney failure (37).

Kidney biopsy demonstrates focal segmental necrotizing vasculitis with few or no immune deposits predominantly affecting the small vessels, classically referred to as a "pauci-immune" phenomenon (39). Non-glomerular regions may be affected as well, as evidenced by interstitial inflammation, eventually leading to interstitial fibrosis and tubular atrophy in up to 50% of patients (40).

Renal involvement is relevant for the choice of treatment, which involves induction and maintenance phases. First-line induction agents are cyclophosphamide or rituximab alongside glucocorticoids, though avacopan is an emerging alternative to glucocorticoids (41). Rituximab is the recommended first-line maintenance agent, though azathioprine and methotrexate may be appropriate alternatives if rituximab is contraindicated. Longer maintenance treatment duration reduces relapse rates (41).

Anti-GBM Disease

Anti-GBM disease most often presents with severe kidney disease, with concurrent lung hemorrhage observed in 50% of affected patients. It follows a bimodal age and gender distribution in those in third, sixth, and seventh decades of life (33). Serologic testing for anti-GBM antibodies has a variable sensitivity of 60–100%, necessitating kidney biopsy, which demonstrates a crescentic glomerulonephritis and pathognomonic IgG linear staining along glomerular capillaries (33). A variant of anti-GBM disease seen in 10–50% of patients is distinguished by the concomitant presence of ANCA (usually p-ANCA/myeloperoxidase) (29). Treatment consists of rapid removal of the pathologic antibody with plasma exchange, high doses of steroids, and cyclophosphamide (33).

Nephrotic Syndrome

Diverse primary (idiopathic) and secondary glomerular perturbations causing increased permeability to large molecules (mainly albumin) may result in massive urinary protein loss. Nephrotic syndrome is defined as a urine protein excretion of >3500 mg in 24 hours or uPCR of >3000 mg/g and hypoalbuminemia, hypercholesterolemia, and peripheral edema (42).

Rheumatologic conditions that often present with nephrotic syndrome include lupus nephritis (class V membranous pattern) and related overlap connective tissue diseases, secondary amyloidosis from rheumatologic conditions driving chronic inflammation, and drug-induced injury (i.e., gold, NSAIDs, etc.)

Secondary Amyloidosis

Serum amyloid A protein (AA) amyloidosis results from chronic inflammation and is characterized by the multi-organ deposition of AA protein, leading to organ dysfunction. The kidney is the most commonly involved organ in AA amyloidosis, typically leading to nephrotic syndrome (43). Periodic fever syndromes and inflammatory arthropathies, such as rheumatoid arthritis (RA) and spondyloarthropathies (SpA), are associated with systemic AA amyloidosis. Kidney biopsy is the gold standard for diagnosis, demonstrating amorphous, extracellular, lightly eosinophilic amyloid material staining positively for Congo red (43).

1.3.2 Tubulointerstitial Nephritis

The presentation of tubulointerstitial nephritis is non-specific and highly variable given a broad range of potential pathologies. Possible laboratory manifestations include a decline in GFR, Fanconi syndrome (kidney wasting of glucose, phosphate, uric acid, bicarbonate, and amino acids), normal anion gap acidosis (from either proximal or distal renal tubular acidosis [RTA] and decreased ammonia production), polyuria and isosthenuria (decreased concentrating and diluting ability), non-nephrotic range proteinuria (from the decreased tubular reabsorption of low-molecular weight proteins causing a typical gap between uPCR and uACR), hyper-/hypokalemia depending on the type of RTA, leukocyturia, eosinophiluria, and anemia (44). The classical hypersensitivity triad (skin rash, peripheral blood eosinophilia, and fever) is seen only in a small portion of patients (12). Diagnosis is largely driven by clinical suspicion for underlying etiology.

Non-rheumatologic entities represent most cases, including drug-induced, idiopathic, genetic, and infectious (viral, bacterial, parasitic, or fungal) etiologies (45). Rheumatologic-mediated causes represent 10–20% of cases, including Sjögren's disease, sarcoidosis, and IgG4-related disease (44).

Sjögren's Disease

Acute or chronic tubulointerstitial nephritis is the predominant kidney lesion in Sjögren's disease. Distal (type 1) RTA manifesting as non-anion gap metabolic acidosis and hypokalemia secondary to defects in distal acidification is the most common clinical finding, with severity ranging from mild symptoms to life-threatening hypokalemic paralysis. Glomerular disease is less common, but cryoglobulinemic glomerulonephritis and membranous nephropathy have been reported (31, 35). Treatment depends on the type and degree of renal involvement, with supportive therapy via bicarbonate and electrolyte supplementation being the predominant treatment strategy in RTA and immunosuppressive medications in glomerular disease (31).

Sarcoidosis

The involvement of the kidneys and the urinary tract in sarcoidosis is highly variable, including (but not limited to) nephrocalcinosis secondary to hypercalciuria with or without hypercalcemia, obstructive uropathy due to enlarged lymph nodes or nephrolithiasis, and granulomatous interstitial nephritis (about 7–23%) (46). Glomerulonephritis secondary to amyloidosis is rare.

IgG4-Related Disease

IgG4-related kidney disease most frequently presents as tubulointerstitial nephritis with laboratory findings of low complement and peripheral blood eosinophilia alongside elevated serum IgG4 levels. Histologic findings include the lymphoplasmacytic infiltration of the kidney interstitium, increased numbers of IgG4-positive plasma cells, and (rarely) the presence of storiform fibrosis (47). Glomerular manifestations of IgG4-related kidney disease are rare but usually present as membranous nephropathy, with a predominance of IgG4 deposition (48).

Drug Induced

The most common cause of tubulointerstitial nephritis is secondary to a medication (45). About half of all patients with biopsy-proven drug-induced tubulointerstitial nephritis present with AKI, while others demonstrate a slow, progressive loss of kidney function (49, 50). Though classically ascribed, urinary markers, including eosinophiluria, pyuria, and white blood cell casts, are unreliable (50, 51). A careful history with review of medications should be performed. Implicated medications commonly used by rheumatologists include NSAIDs, antibiotics (e.g., beta-lactams, fluoroquinolones), allopurinol, alendronate, and sulfasalazine (12, 45).

Vascular Renal Injury

The presentation of vascular injury to the kidneys can be classified as renal vascular disease or thrombotic microangiopathy. Renal vascular disease refers to conditions that affect blood flow to and from the kidneys, including renal artery stenosis, microaneurysms, and renal artery/vein thromboses, leading to infarcts and/or parenchymal bleeds. Thrombotic microangiopathy is defined as endothelial damage leading to microvascular thrombosis. Both can present with dramatic organ dysfunction and require immediate attention.

Medium-Vessel Vasculitis

Renal vascular disease can be seen in any vessel size vasculitis but is mostly seen in large- and medium-vessel vasculitides that cause eccentric inflammation of the vessel wall with subsequent aneurysm, predisposing the patient to thrombosis.

Polyarteritis Nodosa (PAN)

The classic medium-vessel vasculitis involving the kidneys is polyarteritis nodosa, defined by the segmental eccentric inflammation of medium vessels leading to aneurysm, hematoma, and thrombotic occlusion resulting in renal infarct (27). While most cases are idiopathic, roughly 33% are associated with chronic hepatitis B infection. Acute-onset hematuria, proteinuria, and hypertension in the setting of suspected PAN should prompt the consideration of renal involvement (52). Renal biopsy may show inflammatory fibrinoid necrosis of medium-sized arteritis, though the absence of such changes does not exclude the diagnosis (52). Renal arteriography is a valuable alternative diagnostic tool (31).

Thrombotic Microangiopathy

Thrombotic microangiopathy is the underlying pathologic process causing kidney injury in both scleroderma renal crisis and antiphospholipid syndrome.

Scleroderma Renal Crisis (SRC)

SRC is a rare (2–5%) but life-threatening complication of systemic sclerosis. Predictive factors include diffuse skin involvement, the rapid progression of skin involvement, a duration of onset less than 4 years, the presence of anti-RNA polymerase III antibody, and preceding high steroid use greater than 15 mg per day (27, 35, 53). Clinical presentation is usually characterized by sudden-onset severe arterial hypertension and acute kidney injury without abnormal urinary sediment. Laboratory markers of thrombotic microangiopathy may also be present such as thrombocytopenia, anemia, elevated lactate dehydrogenase, low haptoglobin, and schistocytes on a peripheral blood smear. Glomerulonephritis is not a feature of SRC; the primary histopathologic changes are intimal proliferation and thickening, leading to vascular luminal narrowing of the small arcuate and interlobular arteries (27). In cases of glomerulonephritis, the presence of ANCA, especially MPO-ANCA, needs to be tested, as there is an association between scleroderma and AAV (54).

Antiphospholipid Syndrome (APS)

APS can be primary or secondary to numerous rheumatologic conditions (27). Thrombosis may occur in arteries and veins of any size, commonly involving the renal vasculature.

The involvement of the renal vein may result in nephrotic range proteinuria (35). In addition to thrombosis, APS-associated chronic arteriosclerosis and intimal hypertrophy may result in intrarenal vascular damage. Most cases are managed with blood pressure control and anticoagulation, as well as treatment of the underlying etiology as indicated (if present). Immunosuppression is warranted, however, for those with catastrophic APS, characterized by multi-organ dysfunction (35).

1.4 CLINICAL APPROACH TO RENAL INVOLVEMENT IN RHEUMATOLOGIC DISEASE

In this section, we suggest an approach to ruling out rheumatologic etiologies of kidney disease. While this framework can guide the clinician's initial historical, physical, and associated diagnostic workup, it is important to note that many rheumatologic conditions have overlapping features of renal pathology and often do not exclusively fit one pattern of kidney injury.

1.4.1 Clinical Features of Rheumatologic Diseases with Kidney Involvement

Many rheumatologic diseases may present with shared features of kidney disease. In such cases, a targeted clinical history and examination are indispensable, as non-renal signs and symptoms may narrow the differential diagnosis or even highlight the underlying etiology. Table 1.3 non-exhaustively describes such features that can help guide a systematic approach to evaluate for underlying rheumatologic conditions driving renal disease. For a more complete list of extra-renal symptoms, we refer to the respective chapters in this book.

Table 1.3: Non-Renal Historical and Physical Examination Features of Rheumatologic Diseases Associated with Kidney Disease

Pattern of Renal Injury	Rheumatologic Disease	Non-Renal Manifestations
Glomerulonephritis (immune complex deposition)	Systemic lupus erythematous*	Fatigue, fever, and weight loss; asymmetric, migratory small-joint arthralgia/arthritis; neurologic (psychosis, seizure), serositis (pleural/pericardial effusion), cutaneous (malar rash, photosensitivity, discoid lesion, alopecia, Raynaud phenomenon), hematologic (cytopenia), thrombotic history (60)
	Mixed connective tissue disease	Overlapping features of SLE, SSc, inflammatory myositis (anti-synthetase syndrome, dermatomyositis, necrotizing myositis, inclusion body myositis, polymyositis), and/or RA (61)
	Cryoglobulinemia	Cutaneous (palpable purpura, Raynaud phenomenon, livedo lesions, ulcers, acrocyanosis); arthralgias; peripheral neuropathy and/or mononeuritis multiplex (62)
	IgA vasculitis	Recent upper respiratory or gastrointestinal illness; palpable purpura; abdominal pain; arthralgias (39)

(Continued)

Table 1.3: (Continued)

Pattern of Renal Injury	Rheumatologic Disease	Non-Renal Manifestations
Glomerulonephritis (pauci-immune)	ANCA-associated vasculitis	Fatigue, fever, and weight loss
	Granulomatosis polyangiitis	Ear, nose, and throat (crusting, rhinorrhea, recurrent sinusitis, chronic otitis media, facial cartilage damage); lung nodules, orbital disease, lower respiratory tract (alveolar hemorrhage, tracheal and subglottic stenosis); cutaneous (63)
	Eosinophilic granulomatous polyangiitis	Ear, nose, and throat (otitis media, allergic rhinitis, nasal polyps); asthma and atopy; eosinophilia; cardiac (heart failure, pericarditis, arrhythmias); mononeuritis multiplex, cutaneous (39)
	Microscopic polyangiitis	Pulmonary (alveolar hemorrhage, interstitial fibrosis); skin (palpable purpura, livedo lesions, urticaria, ulcers); neurologic (peripheral neuropathy) (37)
Nephrotic (secondary to AA amyloidosis)	Rheumatoid arthritis	Symmetric, destructive arthritis of small joints with morning stiffness; anemia; systemic vasculitis causing cutaneous (rheumatoid nodules, ulcers), gastrointestinal, cardiac (pericarditis, atherosclerosis, valvular), and pulmonary (pleuritis, pulmonary fibrosis) manifestations (64)
	Spondyloarthritis Ankylosing spondylitis	Insidious-onset axial and peripheral joint pain with morning stiffness
	Inflammatory bowel disease-related arthritis	Sacroiliitis and stiffness not improving with rest, typically age < 40 years; symmetric and continuous peripheral arthritis; enthesitis; history of uveitis; +family history (65)
	Reactive arthritis	Similar to AS (symmetric, continuous, non-erosive sacroiliitis and/or peripheral oligo- or polyarthritis) with concomitant inflammatory bowel disease (66)
	Psoriatic arthritis	Asymmetric, non-continuous peripheral oligoarthritis with preceding symptoms of enteritis or urethritis; sacroiliitis; extra-articular (urethritis or cervicitis, conjunctivitis or uveitis, skin changes including keratoderma blennorrhagicum) (67)
		Asymmetric, non-continuous peripheral oligo- or polyarthritis with cutaneous psoriasis; sacroiliitis; dactylitis (65)
	Autoinflammatory syndromes	Recurrent fever with associated inflammatory cutaneous, mucosal, serosal, and musculoskeletal changes
	Familial Mediterranean fever	Recurrent episodes of fever, serositis (abdominal and/or pleuritic chest pain), and non-erosive arthritis lasting 12–72 hours, typically age < 20 years
Tubulointerstitial nephritis	Sjögren's syndrome	Oral and ocular dryness; dyspareunia; upper respiratory tract dryness; extraglandular (fatigue, Raynaud's phenomenon, other autoimmune end-organ disease, lymphoma)
	Sarcoidosis	Fatigue, fever, weight loss, lymphadenopathy; respiratory (chronic cough, dyspnea, chest pain); cutaneous (lupus pernio), other end-organ involvement (cardiac, liver, central nervous system, etc.) (68)

Table 1.3: (Continued)

Pattern of Renal Injury	Rheumatologic Disease	Non-Renal Manifestations
	IgG4-related disease	Multi-organ inflammation and fibrosis causing end-organ dysfunction (i.e., lacrimal and salivary gland enlargement, autoimmune pancreatitis, hypophysitis, Riedel thyroiditis, interstitial pneumonitis, retroperitoneal fibrosis, etc.) (69)
	Drug-induced	Recent initiation (i.e., 2–3 days, though may be delayed for weeks to months) of antibiotic, non-steroidal anti-inflammatory drug, or proton pump inhibitor with concomitant development of rash, fever, and eosinophilia (classic triad only present in ~10%) (51, 70)
Vascular	Medium- or large-vessel vasculitis	Fever, weight loss, malaise, fatigue, arthralgia, rash
	Polyarteritis nodosa	End-organ ischemia (abdominal pain, chest pain, headache, neurologic deficit)
	Scleroderma renal crisis	Acute-onset anemia, thrombocytopenia, congestive heart failure, arrhythmia, pericardial effusion
	Limited systemic sclerosis	Acral skin fibrosis, sclerodactyly, Raynaud phenomenon, acro-osteolysis, calcinosis cutis; late and slow gastrointestinal and pulmonary involvement (71)
	Diffuse systemic sclerosis	Axial and proximal cutaneous changes as above; early and fast cardiac, lung, gastrointestinal, and nervous system involvement (71)
	Antiphospholipid antibody syndrome	Venous, arterial, or small-vessel thrombosis; pregnancy morbidity**

* SLE may also present as nephrotic syndrome as reviewed in Section II.
** Pregnant morbidity is defined as 1+ of the following: (a) unexplained death of one or more morphologically normal fetuses at or beyond the 10th week of gestation; (b) premature birth of one or more morphologically normal neonates before the 34th week of gestation due to placental insufficiency; (c) three or more unexplained, consecutive spontaneous abortions before the 10th week of gestation.

1.4.2 Non-Rheumatologic Diagnostic Workup of Kidney Disease

The approach to kidney disease diagnosis presented herein assumes a complete workup of non-rheumatologic disease. Ruling out infectious (HIV, hepatitis B, hepatitis C), clonal hematologic (myeloma, Waldenström macroglobulinemia), and kidney-limited etiologies is essential. Age-appropriate malignancy screening is advised. Additional serological workup for membranous nephropathy may facilitate a non-invasive diagnosis, particularly among patients with nephrotic syndrome. This includes testing for antibodies targeting M-type phospholipase A2 receptor (PLA2R) and eventually neural epidermal growth factor-like protein 1 (NELL1), the two most common antigens/antibodies in membranous nephropathy. Although membranous nephropathy secondary to underlying systemic autoimmune disease has been associated with additional target antigens, including exostosin (EXT) 1 and 2, transforming growth factor ß receptor 3 (TGFBR3), and neural cell adhesion molecule 1 (NCAM1), testing is not widely available (55).

1.4.3 Rheumatologic Diagnostic Workup of Kidney Disease

The initial workup to consider a rheumatologic etiology of kidney disease varies by the pattern of injury. Further diagnostic testing should be guided by the presence (or absence) of clinical features associated with rheumatologic diseases associated with the pattern of injury. Figure 1.2 demonstrates our suggested clinical approach.

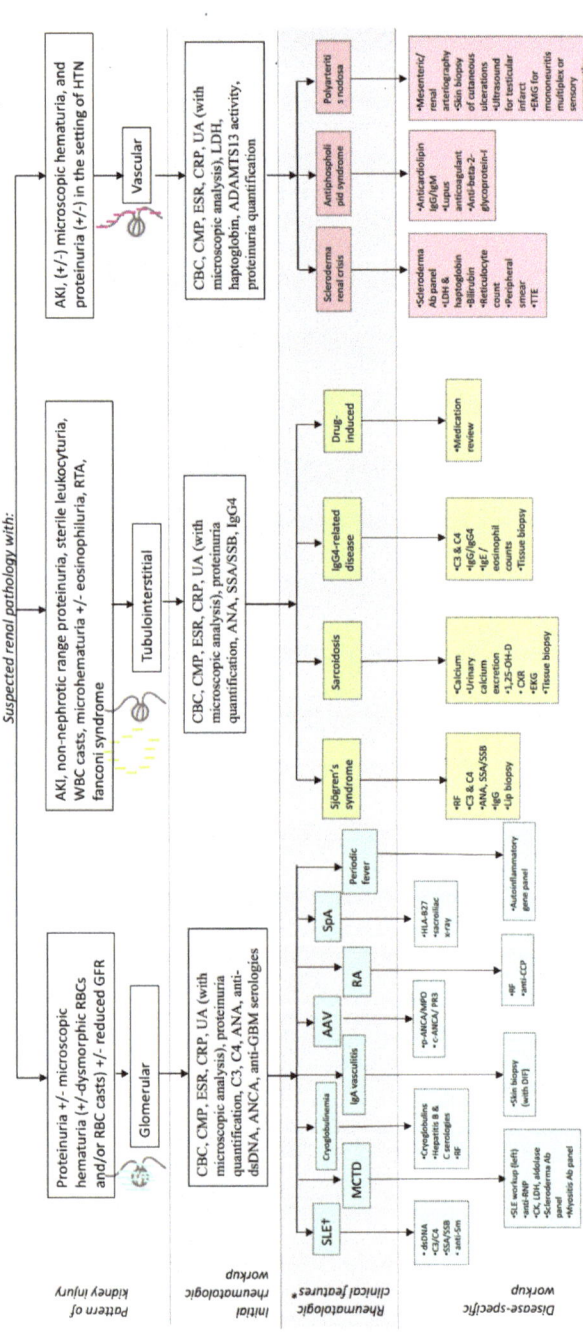

Figure 1.2 Suggested clinical approach to evaluate for rheumatologic etiologies of kidney injury, including initial rheumatologic workup and advanced workup based on disease-specific features.

*See Table 1.3 for clinical features suggestive of each individual rheumatologic diagnosis.

†Renal involvement in SLE may manifest as glomerulonephritis and/or nephrotic syndrome

CTD = connective tissue disease; RBC = red blood cell; GFR = glomerular filtration rate; AKI = acute kidney injury; WBC = white blood cell; HTN = hypertension; CBC = cell blood count; CMP = complete metabolic panel; ESR = erythrocyte sedimentation rate; CRP = c-reactive protein; UA = urinalysis; ANA = antinuclear antigen; ANCA = antineutrophilic cytoplasmic antibody; anti-GBM = anti-glomerular basement membrane; LDH = lactate dehydrogenase; SLE = systemic lupus erythematosus; MCTD = mixed connective tissue disease; AAV = ANCA-associated vasculitis; RA = rheumatoid arthritis; SSA/SSB = anti-Ro and anti-La antibodies; anti-Sm = anti-Smith antibody; anti-RNP = anti-ribonucleoprotein antibody; CK = creatine kinase; Ab = antibody; RF = rheumatoid factor; p-ANCA= perinuclear ANCA; MPO = myeloperoxidase antibody; c-ANCA = cytoplasmic ANCA; PR3 = anti-proteinase-3 antibody; HLA-B27 = human leukocyte antigen B27; EMG = electromyogram; DIF = direct immunofluorescence.

REFERENCES

1. Group KDIGOKBPW. KDIGO 2021 clinical practice guideline for the management of blood pressure in chronic kidney disease. Kidney Int. 2021;99(3S):S1–S87.
2. Shannon JA, et al. The excretion of inulin, xylose and urea by normal and phlorizinized man. J Clin Invest. 1935;14(4):393–401.
3. Levey AS, et al. A new equation to estimate glomerular filtration rate. Ann Intern Med. 2009;150(9):604–12.
4. Inker LA, et al. Estimating glomerular filtration rate from serum creatinine and cystatin C. N Engl J Med. 2012;367(1):20–9.
5. Inker LA, et al. New creatinine- and cystatin C-based equations to estimate GFR without race. N Engl J Med. 2021;385(19):1737–49.
6. Inker LA, et al. Measurement and estimation of GFR for use in clinical practice: Core curriculum 2021. Am J Kidney Dis. 2021;78(5):736–49.
7. Tsai JJ, et al. Comparison and interpretation of urinalysis performed by a nephrologist versus a hospital-based clinical laboratory. Am J Kidney Dis. 2005;46(5):820–9.
8. Cavanaugh C, et al. Urine sediment examination in the diagnosis and management of kidney disease: Core curriculum 2019. Am J Kidney Dis. 2019;73(2):258–72.
9. Ingelfinger JR. Hematuria in adults. N Engl J Med. 2021;385(2):153–63.
10. Barocas DA, et al. Microhematuria: AUA/SUFU guideline. J Urol. 2020;204(4):778–86.
11. Köhler H, et al. Acanthocyturia—a characteristic marker for glomerular bleeding. Kidney Int. 1991;40(1):115–20.
12. Muriithi AK, Let al. Biopsy-proven acute interstitial nephritis, 1993–2011: A case series. Am J Kidney Dis. 2014;64(4):558–66.
13. Kdigokbpw G. Kidney disease: Improving global outcomes (KDIGO) CKD work group. KDIGO 2024 clinical practice guideline for the evaluation and management of chronic kidney disease. Kidney Int. 2024 Apr;105(4S):S117–S314.
14. Bajema IM, et al. Revision of the international society of nephrology/renal pathology society classification for lupus nephritis: Clarification of definitions, and modified national institutes of health activity and chronicity indices. Kidney Int. 2018;93(4):789–96.
15. Zhang WR, et al. Biomarkers of acute and chronic kidney disease. Annu Rev Physiol. 2019;81:309–33.
16. Jayne DRW, et al. Randomized trial of C5a receptor inhibitor avacopan in ANCA-associated vasculitis. J Am Soc Nephrol. 2017;28(9):2756–67.
17. Jayne DRW, et al. Avacopan for the treatment of ANCA-associated vasculitis. N Engl J Med. 2021;384(7):599–609.
18. Mejia-Vilet JM, et al. Urinary soluble CD163: A novel noninvasive biomarker of activity for lupus nephritis. J Am Soc Nephrol. 2020;31(6):1335–47.
19. Moran SM, et al. The clinical application of urine soluble CD163 in ANCA-associated vasculitis. J Am Soc Nephrol. 2021;32(11):2920–32.
20. Wong-You-Cheong JJ, et al. ACR appropriateness criteria® renal failure. J Am Coll Radiol. 2021;18(5S):S174–88.
21. Koratala A, et al. Venous excess doppler ultrasound for the nephrologist: Pearls and pitfalls. Kidney Med. 2022;4(7):100482.
22. Takata T, et al. Left renal cortical thickness measured by ultrasound can predict early progression of chronic kidney disease. Nephron. 2016;132(1):25–32.
23. Najafian B, et al. Approach to kidney biopsy: Core curriculum 2022. Am J Kidney Dis. 2022;80(1):119–31.
24. Luciano RL, et al. Update on the native kidney biopsy: Core curriculum 2019. Am J Kidney Dis. 2019;73(3):404–15.
25. Poggio ED, et al. Systematic review and meta-analysis of native kidney biopsy complications. Clin J Am Soc Nephrol. 2020;15(11):1595–602.
26. Group KDIGOKGDW. KDIGO 2021 clinical practice guideline for the management of glomerular diseases. Kidney Int. 2021;100(4S):S1–S276.
27. Mittal T, et al. Rheumatological diseases and kidneys: A nephrologist's perspective. Int J Rheum Dis. 2014;17(8):834–44.
28. Hebert LA, et al. Differential diagnosis of glomerular disease: A systematic and inclusive approach. Am J Nephrol. 2013;38(3):253–66.

29. Kronbichler A, et al. Novel aspects in the pathophysiology and diagnosis of glomerular diseases. Ann Rheum Dis. 2023;82(5):585–93.
30. Amann K, et al. What you should know about the work-up of a renal biopsy. Nephrol Dial Transplant. 2006;21(5):1157–61.
31. Alobaidi S, et al. Renal system and rheumatology. In: Almoallim H, Cheikh M, editors. *Skills in Rheumatology*. Singapore: Springer; 2021.
32. Hanly JG, et al. The frequency and outcome of lupus nephritis: Results from an international inception cohort study. Rheumatology (Oxford). 2016;55(2):252–62.
33. Sethi S, et al. Acute glomerulonephritis. Lancet. 2022;399(10335):1646–63.
34. Lech M, et al. The pathogenesis of lupus nephritis. J Am Soc Nephrol. 2013;24(9):1357–66.
35. Kronbichler A, et al. Renal involvement in autoimmune connective tissue diseases. BMC Med. 2013;11:95.
36. Ferri C, et al. Cryoglobulins. J Clin Pathol. 2002;55(1):4–13.
37. Chung SA, et al. Microscopic polyangiitis. Rheum Dis Clin North Am. 2010;36(3):545–58.
38. Sinico RA, et al. Renal involvement in Churg-Strauss syndrome. Am J Kidney Dis. 2006;47(5):770–9.
39. Jennette JC, et al. 2012 revised international Chapel Hill consensus conference nomenclature of vasculitides. Arthritis Rheum. 2013;65(1):1–11.
40. Savage CO, et al. Microscopic polyarteritis: Presentation, pathology and prognosis. Q J Med. 1985;56(220):467–83.
41. Samman KN, et al. Update in the management of ANCA-associated vasculitis: Recent developments and future perspectives. Int J Rheumatol. 2021;2021:5534851.
42. Hull RP, et al. Nephrotic syndrome in adults. BMJ. 2008;336(7654):1185–9.
43. Thorne J, et al. Serum Amyloid a protein-associated kidney disease: Presentation, diagnosis, and management. Kidney Med. 2022;4(8):100504.
44. Oliva-Damaso N, et al. Acute and chronic tubulointerstitial nephritis of rheumatic causes. Rheum Dis Clin North Am. 2018;44(4):619–33.
45. Joyce E, et al. Tubulointerstitial nephritis: Diagnosis, treatment, and monitoring. Pediatr Nephrol. 2017;32(4):577–87.
46. Bergner R, et al. Renal sarcoidosis: Approach to diagnosis and management. Curr Opin Pulm Med. 2018;24(5):513–20.
47. Salvadori M, et al. Immunoglobulin G4-related kidney diseases: An updated review. World J Nephrol. 2018;7(1):29–40.
48. Cortazar FB, et al. IgG4-related disease and the kidney. Nat Rev Nephrol. 2015;11(10):599–609.
49. Chu R, et al. Assessment of KDIGO definitions in patients with histopathologic evidence of acute renal disease. Clin J Am Soc Nephrol. 2014;9(7):1175–82.
50. Moledina DG, et al. Drug-induced acute interstitial nephritis. Clin J Am Soc Nephrol. 2017;12(12):2046–9.
51. Perazella MA. Clinical approach to diagnosing acute and chronic tubulointerstitial disease. Adv Chronic Kidney Dis. 2017;24(2):57–63.
52. Dillon MJ, et al. Medium-size-vessel vasculitis. Pediatr Nephrol. 2010;25(9):1641–52.
53. Steen VD, et al. Case-control study of corticosteroids and other drugs that either precipitate or protect from the development of scleroderma renal crisis. Arthritis Rheum. 1998;41(9):1613–19.
54. Kant S, et al. ANCA-associated vasculitis in scleroderma: A renal perspective. Clin Nephrol. 2018;90(6):413–18.
55. Sethi S, et al. Mayo Clinic consensus report on membranous nephropathy: Proposal for a novel classification. Kidney Int. 2023 Dec;104(6):1092–102.
56. Perazella MA, et al. Etiology and evaluation of hematuria in adults. In: TW P, editor. *UpToDate*. Wolters Kluwer [cited 2023 Nov 29]. Available from: www.uptodate.com.
57. Liu JJ, et al. Urinalysis in the evaluation of hematuria. JAMA. 2016;315(24):2726–7.
58. Schröder FH. Microscopic haematuria. BMJ. 1994;309(6947):70–2.
59. Fogazzi GB, et al. Urinalysis: Core curriculum 2008. Am J Kidney Dis. 2008;51(6):1052–67.
60. Cojocaru M, et al. Manifestations of systemic lupus erythematosus. Maedica (Bucur). 2011;6(4):330–6.
61. Ortega-Hernandez OD, et al. Mixed connective tissue disease: An overview of clinical manifestations, diagnosis and treatment. Best Pract Res Clin Rheumatol. 2012;26(1):61–72.

62. Braun GS, et al. Cryoglobulinaemic vasculitis: Classification and clinical and therapeutic aspects. Postgrad Med J. 2007;83(976):87–94.
63. Comarmond C, et al. Granulomatosis with polyangiitis (Wegener): Clinical aspects and treatment. Autoimmun Rev. 2014;13(11):1121–5.
64. Radu AF, et al. Management of rheumatoid arthritis: An overview. Cells. 2021;10(11).
65. Akgul O, et al. Classification criteria for spondyloarthropathies. World J Orthop. 2011;2(12):107–15.
66. Arvikar SL, et al. Inflammatory bowel disease associated arthropathy. Curr Rev Musculoskelet Med. 2011;4(3):123–31.
67. Bentaleb I, et al. Reactive arthritis: Update. Curr Clin Microbiol Rep. 2020;7(4):124–32.
68. Sève P, et al. Sarcoidosis: A clinical overview from symptoms to diagnosis. Cells. 2021;10(4).
69. Kubo K, et al. IgG4-related disease. Int J Rheum Dis. 2016;19(8):747–62.
70. Perazella MA, et al. Drug-induced acute interstitial nephritis. Nat Rev Nephrol. 2010;6(8):461–70.
71. Sobolewski P, et al. Systemic sclerosis—multidisciplinary disease: Clinical features and treatment. Reumatologia. 2019;57(4):221–33.

2 Dosing and Monitoring of Rheumatologic Medications in Patients with Renal Disease

Jennifer Strouse, M. Lee Sanders, Chelsea McIntire, and Priyanka Iyer

2.1 INTRODUCTION

A myriad of medications are prescribed in the treatment of patients with rheumatic disease. Given the increased risk of renal disorders associated with some rheumatologic diseases, these drugs may require dosing modifications, additional monitoring, or avoidance altogether. In addition, some rheumatologic medications may directly lead to nephrotoxicity. Therefore, both renal function and toxicity are important to consider when prescribing medications to all patients.

Rheumatologic drug classes include non-steroidal anti-inflammatory drugs (NSAIDs), conventional synthetic disease-modifying antirheumatic drugs (csDMARDs), biologic DMARDs, targeted synthetic DMARDs, and uricosurics. In this chapter, clinical guidance for the dosing and monitoring of commonly used rheumatologic medications is provided, along with nephrotoxicity considerations.

2.2 NON-STEROIDAL ANTI-INFLAMMATORY DRUGS (NSAIDS)

NSAIDs are frequently used analgesics and anti-inflammatory agents in rheumatology. The frequency of use is likely underrepresented given their availability over-the-counter. Oral NSAIDs may contribute to acute kidney injury by several different mechanisms: vasoconstrictive effects on the afferent arteriole (1), the development or worsening of systemic hypertension, the promotion of sodium and water retention contributing to clinically apparent edema, and acute interstitial nephritis (1, 2).

In healthy individuals, with prolonged use of oral NSAIDs, close monitoring of renal function is advised. Stringent monitoring in patients with pre-existing comorbidities such as concomitant diuretic use or anti-hypertensive use (particularly those that inhibit the renin–angiotensin system) and those with cirrhosis and heart failure is recommended.

Clinical guidance regarding dose adjustments in patients with moderate to severe renal impairment differs between individual NSAIDs. Avoiding prolonged use in patients with an estimated glomerular filtration rate (eGFR) 30–45 mL/minute/1.73 m^2 is recommended. Absolute oral NSAID avoidance is recommended in those with an eGFR of < 30 mL/minute/1.73 m^2, in dialysis patients who continue to possess residual renal function, and in those who are at high risk for kidney injury (2). If NSAIDs must be used, it is recommended to use them for a brief period of time while closely monitoring renal function, electrolytes, and volume status (2). In patients on hemodialysis (HD), NSAIDs may be used if a patient is anuric. In patients post renal transplant, avoidance of NSAID use is recommended. NSAIDs should be avoided in patients with nephrotic syndrome with decreased effective arterial volume due to the increased risk of AKI in this setting. NSAIDs may be causally related to some cases of membranous nephropathy and minimal change disease.

The systemic absorption of topical NSAIDs is negligible. However, the effects of topical NSAIDs have been inadequately studied in patients with advanced CKD.

2.3 CONVENTIONAL SYNTHETIC DISEASE-MODIFYING ANTIRHEUMATIC DRUGS (CSDMARDS)

A summary of dosing recommendations for the conventional disease-modifying antirheumatic drugs intravenous immunoglobulin (IVIG) and calcineurin inhibitors is provided in Table 2.1.

2.3.1 Methotrexate

Methotrexate (MTX) is commonly used for several rheumatologic conditions, including rheumatoid arthritis. Renal toxicity at doses used in rheumatology is uncommon; however, patients with pre-existing renal impairment and decreased renal clearance are at higher risk, as renal excretion accounts for approximately 90% of MTX clearance (1). It is contraindicated in patients with CKD stage 4 and 5 (1). In patients with concomitant NSAID use, there is a theoretical possibility of a decline in eGFR. High-dose MTX used for oncologic indications may cause the precipitation of MTX or its metabolites in renal tubules, where it is thought to be directly toxic as a result of oxidative stress (2).

DOI: 10.1201/9781003438373-3

Table 2.1: Considerations for the Dosing of Commonly Used in Rheumatology

Drug	Dosing			Comments
	CKD3*	CKD4*	CKD5*	
Methotrexate (1)	Dose reduction is recommended. No clear guidelines—consider 50–100% dose (max dose 15 mg weekly).	Contraindicated	Contraindicated	Can be used in patients on hemodialysis, but not recommended for use in peritoneal dialysis
Hydroxychloroquine (1)	No dose adjustments recommended	Recommend 25–50% dose (equivalent of 150 mg/day).	Recommend 25–50% dose. Use with caution.	
Sulfasalazine (1)	No dose adjustments recommended	Start lower dose with caution.	Start lower dose with caution.	
Leflunomide (1)	No dose adjustments recommended	Use full dose with caution.	Not recommended	No dose adjustments recommended in HD.
Azathioprine (1)	No dose adjustments recommended	Administer 75% of dose.	Administer 50% of dose.	
Mycophenolate mofetil (1)	No dose adjustments recommended	Consider 1 g twice a day.	Consider 1 g twice a day.	
Cyclophosphamide (1)	No dose adjustments recommended	Administer 75% of dose.	Administer 50% dose.	Moderately dialyzable with HD—dose reduction to 50 or 75% is recommended (7). On dialysis days, administer after HD, allowing at least 12 hours before the next HD session.
Tacrolimus	No dose adjustments recommended	Contraindicated	Contraindicated	
Voclosporin		Not clearly defined. The package insert does not recommend use in patients with eGFR < 45 unless benefit outweighs risk. Recommended starting dose is 15.8 mg twice a day.	Not defined, relatively contraindicated	If eGFR < 60 mL/minute/1.73 m2 and reduced from baseline by > 20% and < 30%, reduce the dose by 7.9mg twice a day. Re-assess eGFR within 2 weeks. If eGFR is still reduced from baseline by > 20%, reduce the dose again by 7.9 mg twice a day. If eGFR < 60 mL/minute/1.73 m2 and reduced from baseline by > 30%, discontinue medication. Re- assess eGFR within 2 weeks; consider re-initiating at a lower dose (7.9mg twice a day) only if eGFR has returned to > 80% of baseline. For patients that had a decrease in dose due to eGFR, consider increasing the dose by 7.9 mg twice a day for each eGFR measurement that is > 80% of baseline; do not exceed the starting dose.
IVIG	Start at a lower infusion rate	Start at a lower infusion rate	Start at a lower infusion rate	Start at a lower infusion rate in patients with CKD 3-5.

*CKD3, eGFR > 30 mL/minute/1.73m2; CKD 4, eGFR 15–29 mL/minute/1.73 m2; CKD 5, eGFR <15 mL/minute/1.73 m2

In healthy individuals, the American College of Rheumatology (ACR) recommends obtaining routine monitoring labs every 2–4 weeks during the first few weeks of therapy and at least every 12 weeks thereafter (3). Dose adjustment in renal impairment is recommended, although exact modified dosing guidelines are not available. In patients on HD, caution is recommended, while use is contraindicated in patients on peritoneal dialysis (PD).

2.3.2 Hydroxychloroquine

Hydroxychloroquine has several indications in rheumatology, including systemic lupus erythematosus (SLE). Nephrotoxicity is extremely rare, and it may even have a reno-protective benefit. Dose modification in renal impairment is recommended by some as follows: for eGFR ranging between 10 and 50 mL/minute/1.73 m^2, a 25–50% reduction in the normal dose (4), although specific dose adjustment is not addressed in the package insert. Ophthalmic monitoring is advised in patients with CKD due to the potential risk of retinopathy (5). Formal dose modifications in CKD are not available (5). Rare cases of nephropathy have been reported with proteinuria and biopsy-confirmed renal phospholipidosis (1).

2.3.3 Sulfasalazine

Sulfasalazine may be used as a part of a triple drug therapy regimen for the treatment of rheumatoid arthritis. Rare reports of interstitial nephritis, crystalluria, and minimal change disease have been reported (2). No specific dose adjustment for renal function is recommended.

2.3.4 Leflunomide

Leflunomide is used in the treatment of rheumatoid arthritis. It converts to an active metabolite, teriflunomide, which may contribute to acute kidney injury and hyperkalemia (2). It may contribute to incident or worsening pre-existing hypertension (1). The Federal Drug Administration (FDA) urges caution while prescribing leflunomide in the context of kidney disease (Table 2.1).

2.3.5 Azathioprine

Azathioprine (AZA) is often used in the treatment of SLE and vasculitis and has no direct nephrotoxic effects (1). Acute interstitial nephritis has been reported in some cases of hypersensitivity reactions (1). The amount of 6-mercaptopurine, the active metabolite, excreted through the kidneys varies greatly among individuals. The accumulation of 6-mercaptopurine can result in hepatotoxicity and bone marrow toxicity, and renal dose adjustment is suggested (Table 2.1).

2.3.6 Mycophenolate Mofetil

Mycophenolate mofetil is commonly used in the treatment of SLE and lupus nephritis (LN) but also has several other indications. It has no known nephrotoxic effects (1). Its use has not been associated with nephrotoxicity, and individuals with CKD 4–5, including those receiving dialysis and post-transplant, require only minor dose adjustment (See Table 2.1).

2.3.7 Cyclophosphamide

Intravenous pulse therapy with cyclophosphamide (CYC) is typically used as a treatment for severe SLE, systemic sclerosis, refractory myositis and vasculitis (2). It is widely believed that continuous oral CYC administration has a higher propensity for toxicity and is now rarely utilized in rheumatology (6). Since the kidney excretes CYC and its metabolites, dose lowering is recommended in the presence of renal impairment (1, 7) (Table 2.1).

Another side effect attributed to CYC is hyponatremia (1). CYC has also been reported to cause hematuria, pyelitis, ureteritis, and hemorrhagic cystitis due to its metabolite acrolein, which is excreted in the urine (6, 8). It is important to routinely examine urine sediment for the presence of erythrocytes and other indicators of nephrotoxicity or urotoxicity. Exercise caution when considering the administration of CYC in the presence of a urinary tract infection. CYC is a pro-drug that is activated by cytochrome P450—hence, there is a potential of drug interactions and thus increased nephrotoxicity (8).

2.3.8 Intravenous Immunoglobulin

IVIG is used in several rheumatic conditions, including lupus and myositis. Nephrotoxicity is attributed to two main mechanisms: direct toxicity because of lysosomal damage and pigment nephropathy. Sucrose macromolecules, historically used as an additive in IVIG solutions to prevent immunoglobulin dimerization and subsequent infusion reactions, may accumulate in the lysosomes of the proximal tubules, resulting in cell swelling progressing to tubular obstruction in severe cases (2). Coomb's positive hemolysis triggered by IVIG may contribute to pigment nephropathy.

Nephrotoxicity manifests as oliguria and occurs a few days after IVIG therapy. Cytoplasmic vacuolization, proximal tubular cell degeneration, and tubular lumina narrowing or obstruction are the hallmarks on biopsy (2). Up to 40% of patients require short-term dialysis, and recovery usually happens within weeks of ceasing therapy.

Experts advise avoiding sucrose-stabilized solutions and considering slower infusion rates for those with CKD (2, 8). IVIG is thought to be safe for patients on HD (2).

2.3.9 Calcineurin Inhibitors

Cyclosporine and tacrolimus are calcineurin inhibitors (CNIs) that have been used for several years as adjuncts in the management of active LN and other refractory rheumatic diseases (2). A third CNI, voclosporin, was FDA approved for use in LN in 2021 (9).

Nephrotoxicity and angioedema were first reported in a case of SLE where cyclosporine was used at a high dose of 10 mg/kg (10). Since then, CNIs have been safely used at much lower doses with close monitoring of renal function and trough levels. CNIs may contribute to renal afferent arteriolar vasoconstriction (6), tubular atrophy (6), interstitial fibrosis (2), thrombotic microangiopathy, and glomerular sclerosis (2, 6). Hyperkalemia, hypomagnesemia, hyperuricemia, metabolic acidosis, and hypertension have been reported (2). Hypertension is usually dose dependent (6).

The use of CNIs in older patients, particularly with concomitant NSAID use, pre-existing renal dysfunction, and volume depletion, may contribute to nephrotoxicity (2, 6). The simultaneous use of cytochrome P450 isoenzyme CYP3A4 inhibitors may increase serum CNI levels (6).

CNIs should be avoided in those with CKD 3–5 (2). They are safely used in the transplant population for anti-rejection when the lowest acceptable trough level is targeted (2). CNIs are not dialyzable because they are highly protein bound (2).

The starting dose of the voclosporin is 23.7 mg twice a day. Assessing eGFR every 2 weeks for the first month and every 4 weeks thereafter is recommended. Depending on eGFR values, modifying the dose (Table 2.1) or discontinuing treatment is recommended. Close attention should be paid to blood pressure after initiation, with initial checks at least every 2 weeks. If BP > 165/105 mmHg or with hypertensive emergency, discontinue its use. Safety and efficacy have not been established beyond 1 year of use or in patients with eGFR < 45 (8).

2.4 BIOLOGIC DISEASE-MODIFYING ANTIRHEUMATIC DRUGS (DMARDS)

Biologic DMARDs are increasingly used to treat a multitude of rheumatic diseases. They are not well studied in individuals with kidney disease. The high molecular weight of most biologic DMARDs limits renal clearance, as the cutoff for renal clearance is about 60 kDa (11). There is a theoretical risk that in patients with proteinuria there could be increased clearance with decreased efficacy. Rare reports of nephrotoxicity exist, with possible etiologies of infection, induced autoimmune disease, and immune-complex deposition proposed (1, 2, 8).

Anakinra is the only exception in this group (see Table 2.2 for summary). It is predominantly renally cleared, with a smaller molecular size. Every-other-day dosing in individuals with a creatinine clearance (CrCl) of < 30 mL/minute is recommended (8).

2.5 TARGETED SYNTHETIC DISEASE-MODIFYING ANTIRHEUMATIC DRUGS (TSDMARDS)

2.5.1 Janus Kinase (JAK) Inhibitors

JAK inhibitors have been approved for a variety of diseases in rheumatology. There are three JAK inhibitors that are currently FDA approved for rheumatic indications—tofacitinib, baricitinib, and upadicitinib. The data regarding dose modifications and renal monitoring is varied (Table 2.3), and nephrotoxicity has been limited to a small increase in serum creatinine observed in patients on baricitinib and tofacitinib (1). While the exact mechanism is unclear, this might be related to the inhibition of the tubular secretion of creatinine or an increase in creatine kinase levels (1). However, the significance of this mild increase is unknown. In trials with tofacitinib, an increase in serum creatinine of greater than 50% from the baseline value led to drug discontinuation in up to 2% of participants (8). With upadicitinib, there are no dose adjustments recommended for patients with impaired renal function. With baricitinib, the manufacturers recommend a 50% dose reduction for patients with an eGFR of 30–59 mL/minute/1.73 m^2 and do not recommend use with eGFR < 30 mL/minute/1.73 m^2 (1). In patients on tofacitinib with moderate to severe renal

Table 2.2: Considerations for the Dosing of Biologic Commonly Used in Rheumatology

Drug	Nephrotoxicity/ Pharmacokinetic Summary	Dosing eGFR > 30 mL/ minute/1.73 m²	Dosing CKD 4 eGFR 15–29 mL/minute/1.73 m²	Dosing CKD 5 eGFR < 15 mL/ minute/1.73 m²	Comments
Anakinra		No dose adjustments recommended	Consider every-other-day dosing if CrCl < 30.	Consider every-other-day dosing if CrCl < 30.	
Other biologic DMARDs	Rare reports of nephrotoxicity	No dose adjustments recommended			

Table 2.3: Considerations for the Dosing of Targeted Synthetic Commonly Used in Rheumatology

Drug	Nephrotoxicity/ Pharmacokinetic Summary	Dosing eGFR > 30 mL/ minute/1.73 m²	Dosing CKD 4 eGFR 15–29 mL/ minute/1.73 m²	Dosing CKD 5 eGFR < 15 mL/ minute/1.73 m²	Comments
Tofacitinib	Small increase in creatinine observed	No dose adjustment recommended	Switching from the extended-release formulation to the immediate-release formulation and decreasing the dose by 50%	Switching from the extended-release formulation to the immediate-release formulation and decreasing the dose by 50%	
Baricitinib	Small increase in creatinine observed	50% dose reduction	Contraindicated	Contraindicated	
Upadacitinib		No dose adjustments recommended	Dose adjustment recommended in non-rheumatologic disease, but has not been recommended in rheumatologic disease		

impairment, the manufacturer recommends switching from the extended-release formulation to the immediate-release formulation and decreasing the dose by 50% (1, 2, 8).

2.6 PHARMACOLOGIC TREATMENT OF GOUT

Gout and CKD commonly co-occur. CKD stage 3–5 is a comorbid condition listed in the ACR guidelines to suggest the initiation of allopurinol after a first attack of gout (12).

2.6.1 Colchicine

Colchicine has various mechanisms of action, including neutrophil cell division interruption and inflammasome inhibition. It is most frequently used in the treatment and prevention of gout flares. While there is no significant data suggesting direct nephrotoxicity, renal failure following overdose has been reported (13). Systemic toxicity can cause diarrhea, leading to volume depletion and acute tubular necrosis (ATN). A second phase of the toxicity can result in multiorgan failure, which can lead to shock and ATN (13). Neuromyopathy can lead to elevated creatine kinase, with rhabdomyolysis leading to acute kidney injury (8). Rarely, death has been reported (14).

Table 2.4: Considerations for the Dosing of Gout Therapies

Drug	Nephrotoxicity/ Pharmacokinetic Summary	Dosing eGFR > 30 mL/ minute/1.73 m²	Dosing CKD 4 eGFR 15–29 mL/ minute/1.73 m²	Dosing CKD 5 eGFR < 15 mL/ minute/1.73 m²	Comments
Colchicine	Case report of renal failure with overdose	No dose adjustment recommended	50% dose reduction	Complete avoidance	Case reports of death due to toxicity
Allopurinol	Rare AIN Reports of renal failure in neoplastic disease and gouty nephropathy	Start at 50 mg with slow titration	Start at 50 mg with slow titration	Do not exceed 100 mg if CrCl < 10 mL/minute	
Febuxostat	Multiple uncommon effects	No dose adjustment recommended	Do not exceed 40 mg	Not defined	Post-marketing suggestion to use in dialysis is reasonable and to consider a dose of 20 mg/day in PD
Probenecid	Hematuria, renal colic, uric acid stone formation, nephrotic syndrome	May be less effective in CKD with a higher dose required, up to 2000 mg per day	Likely ineffective	Likely ineffective	

The FDA recommends a dose reduction for eGFR < 30 mL/minute/1.73 m^2 (Table 2.4) (8). However, these recommendations are largely empirical (15). Drug interactions with strong CYP3A4 inhibitors or with P-glycoprotein inhibitors can occur (8).

2.6.2 Xanthine Oxidase Inhibitors

2.6.2.1 Allopurinol

Allopurinol lowers uric acid through xanthine oxidase inhibition and is used to prevent gout attacks. Nephrotoxicity has been rarely reported and is usually associated with acute interstitial nephritis (AIN). Proteinuria and hematuria can also occur. The treatment of AIN is the discontinuation of allopurinol and consideration of corticosteroids (16). Case reports of renal failure have been described with use for neoplastic disease and in gouty nephropathy (8).

Allopurinol is renally excreted, necessitating lower starting doses in individuals with CKD (Table 2.4). The starting dose is a risk factor for allopurinol hypersensitivity syndrome. Guidelines recommend starting at a lower dose (50 mg daily) in individuals with CKD 3–5 or ESRD (12), followed by slow titration with increases of 50 to 100 mg daily every 2 to 4 weeks until uric acid is at goal. Doses above 300 mg/day may be needed. Doses should not be > 100 mg/day if the CrCl is < 10 mL/minute; when CrCl is < 3 mL/minute a longer dosing interval may be needed (8).

2.6.2.2 Febuxostat

Febuxostat is lowers urate through xanthine oxidase inhibition with primary hepatic metabolism. Less common renal adverse effects include hematuria, nephrolithiasis, proteinuria, tubulointerstitial nephritis, renal insufficiency, and elevated BUN/creatinine ratio (8). In individuals with a CrCl of 15 to 29 mL/minute, it is recommended to limit the dose to 40 mg/day (Table 2.4). Postmarketing information suggests it is tolerated and effective for patients on dialysis (17). For those on PD, a dose of 20 mg/day may be better tolerated (18).

2.6.3 Probenecid

Probenecid blocks the renal tubular transport of uric acid, thereby increasing secretion by the kidneys. Hematuria, renal colic, and uric acid stone formation have been reported with use. Alkalization of the urine and increased fluid intake can help prevent these complications. Probenecid is not recommended in patients with urate urolithiasis and should not be commenced during a gout attack.

Dosage requirements are increased in individuals with renal impairment. Dosing should not be increased above 2000 mg/day. When eGFR is ≤ 30 mL/minute/1.73 m^2, it may be ineffective, and other treatments are recommended. There are also multiple drug interactions frequently resulting in increased levels of other medications such as penicillin, methotrexate, and sulfonylureas (8).

2.6.4 Pegloticase

Pegloticase is a uric acid-specific enzyme used to treat refractory gout that is primarily excreted by the kidneys. No dose adjustment is recommended for individuals with renal impairment (8). More recently, the addition of methotrexate has been recommended to prevent anti-drug antibody formation. However, individuals with eGFR < 40 mL/minute/1.73 m^2 were excluded from the clinical trials with methotrexate (19). CKD will need to be considered in patients related to use of methotrexate in this population.

Pegloticase is contraindicated in glucose-6-phosphate dehydrogenase deficiency. Anaphylaxis has been reported in 6.5% of patients. Infusion reactions and gout flares are common. It is important to stop oral antihyperuricemic drugs prior to initiation (8).

2.6.5 Other Agents Used to Treat Gout

Anakinra is also used in the treatment of gout, and canakinumab was recently FDA approved for the treatment of gout. NSAIDs are also commonly used in the treatment of gout. See other sections related to these medications.

2.7 OTHER RHEUMATOLOGIC MEDICATIONS

2.7.1 Apremilast

Apremilast can be used in the treatment of psoriatic arthritis and Behcet's disease. It is a phosphodiesterase-4-inhibitor. Slow titration to 30 mg twice daily is recommended to reduce gastrointestinal side effects. For initial titration in individuals with a CrCl of < 30 mL/minute, the morning dose of the titration regimen should be used with a final dose of 30 mg once daily (8).

2.8 CONCLUSION

Many individuals with rheumatologic disease have co-existing renal disease. Patients with severe CKD are already in an immunocompromised state. Given the increased risk of infections, caution is recommended with the concomitant use of biologics, targeted synthetic DMARDs, and csDMARDs. Several rheumatologic medications have recommendations regarding avoidance or modified dosing in individuals with renal dysfunction. Some may directly lead to renal toxicity. A multidisciplinary approach involving rheumatologists, nephrologists, and pharmacists may contribute to optimal care.

REFERENCES

1. Harty T, et al. Therapeutics in rheumatology and the kidney. Rheumatology. 2023;62(3):1009–20.
2. Woodell T, et al. Nephrotoxicity of select rheumatologic drugs. Rheum Dis Clin North Am. 2018;44(4):605–17.
3. Saag KG, et al. American college of rheumatology 2008 recommendations for the use of nonbiologic and biologic disease-modifying antirheumatic drugs in rheumatoid arthritis. Arthritis Rheum. 2008;59(6):762–84.
4. Ashley C, et al. *The Renal Drug Handbook* [Internet]. CRC Press; 2017 [cited 2023 Aug 21]. Available from: www.taylorfrancis.com/books/9781498794619.
5. Rosenbaum JT, et al. American college of rheumatology, American academy of dermatology, rheumatologic dermatology society, and American academy of ophthalmology 2020 joint statement on hydroxychloroquine use with respect to retinal toxicity. Arthritis Rheumatol. 2021;73(6):908–11.
6. Bingham S, et al. Renal toxicity of anti-rheumatic drugs. In: Adu D, Emery P, Madaio M, editors. *Rheumatology and the Kidney* [Internet]. Oxford University Press; 2012, pp. 385–98 [cited 2023 Jul 17]. Available from: https://academic.oup.com/book/25010/chapter/189028156.
7. Krens SD, et al. Dose recommendations for anticancer drugs in patients with renal or hepatic impairment. Lancet Oncol. 2019;20(4):e200–7.
8. FDA Label Search [Internet]. 2023 [cited 2023 Oct 11]. FDA Label Search. Available from: https://labels.fda.gov/proprietaryname.cfm.
9. Rovin BH, et al. Efficacy and safety of voclosporin versus placebo for lupus nephritis (AURORA 1): A double-blind, randomised, multicentre, placebo-controlled, phase 3 trial. Lancet. 2021;397(10289):2070–80.
10. Isenberg DA, et al. Cyclosporin A for the treatment of systemic lupus erythematosus. Int J Immunopharmacol. 1981;3(2):163–9.
11. Meibohm B, Zhou H. Characterizing the impact of renal impairment on the clinical pharmacology of biologics. J Clin Pharmacol. 2012;52(1 Suppl):54S–62S.
12. FitzGerald JD, et al. 2020 American college of rheumatology guideline for the management of gout. Arthritis Care Res (Hoboken). 2020;72(6):744–60.
13. Huang WH, et al. Colchicine overdose-induced acute renal failure and electrolyte imbalance. Ren Fail. 2007;29(3):367–70.
14. Maxwell MJ, et al. Accidental colchicine overdose. A case report and literature review. Emerg Med J. 2002;19(3):265–7.
15. Marinaki S, et al. Colchicine in renal diseases: Present and future. Curr Pharm Des. 2018;24(6):675–83.
16. Gelbart DR, et al. Allopurinol-induced interstitial nephritis. Ann Intern Med. 1977;86(2):196–8.
17. Choi SY, et al. Efficacy and tolerability of febuxostat in gout patients on dialysis. Intern Med J. 2021;51(3):348–54.
18. Ma J, et al. The safety and urate-lowering efficacy of febuxostat in patients undergoing peritoneal dialysis: A retrospective single-arm cohort study of 84 patients. Ann Palliat Med. 2022;11(7):2443–50.
19. Botson JK, et al. A randomized, placebo-controlled study of methotrexate to increase response rates in patients with uncontrolled gout receiving pegloticase: Primary efficacy and safety findings. Arthritis Rheumatol. 2023;75(2):293–304.

3 Renal Disease in the Pregnant Patient with Rheumatic Disease

Lauren He, Namrata Parikh, Silvi Shah, and Cuoghi Edens

3.1 INTRODUCTION

Pregnancy is often a joyous time; however, for those with a known or soon-to-be-unmasked rheumatic disease (RD) with renal involvement, pregnancy or trying to conceive may become more fearful than joyful. Advances in the fields of both rheumatology and nephrology, including pregnancy-compatible medications, hemodialysis, and kidney transplantation, have made it safer for women with significant renal disease to conceive and have markedly improved pregnancy outcomes. Worry, guilt, and anxiety, however, may persist in these high-risk pregnancies for patients, families, and medical professionals. Chronic kidney disease (CKD) has emerged as one of the leading causes of morbidity and mortality worldwide, with 12% of women afflicted with CKD, existing in at least 3% of pregnancies (1). The leading rheumatic causes of CKD in women of childbearing age are systemic lupus erythematosus (SLE) with lupus nephritis (LN) and antiphospholipid antibody syndrome (APS) (2). This chapter will touch on specific considerations for the pregnant/contemplating patient with an RD with renal involvement or impact as well as medication and contraception safety.

When counseling a nephrology patient regarding childbearing, it is essential to review the entirety of their medical diagnoses to assess for relative contraindications to pregnancy that may prove detrimental to their health and/or their baby. This also helps with appropriate contraceptive counseling and the investigation of alternate paths to parenthood. Congestive heart failure, severe valvular heart disease, liver disease, significant restrictive lung disease, pulmonary hypertension, recent cerebrovascular event, HELLP or eclampsia while on treatment, and, notable for this review, teratogenic medications and significant CKD, are conditions that respective medical societies have put forth as relative or absolute pregnancy contraindications. A low glomerular filtration rate (GFR) from any cause is associated with fetal loss, preterm delivery, Cesarean section, low birth weight, intrauterine growth restriction (IUGR), preeclampsia, and anemia. These may be amplified by an underlying diagnosis like SLE or vasculitis. CKD stage 3 and higher is more likely to have poor outcomes versus lower stages, although CKD should be thought of as a continuum and less as a dichotomy (3). The progression of CKD is a feared complication that can occur both during pregnancy and postpartum. This likelihood increases in those with concomitant hypertension and pre-pregnancy CKD stage ≥3 (4); preconception dialysis counseling is recommended in this instance. Dialysis-dependent women have more difficulty conceiving and, once pregnant, not unexpectedly, have increased negative outcomes.

Being familiar with expected renovascular changes seen in pregnancy is essential to understanding contraindications and detecting new or monitoring known diagnoses. Early in pregnancy, maternal cardiac output increases, and at the same time, there is a reduction in vascular resistance in renal circulation (5). As a result, there is increased intravascular volume, and this can aggravate underlying, often undiagnosed, congestive heart failure or pulmonary artery hypertension from RDs. Moreover, GFR increases, and renal plasma flow contributes to glomerular hyperfiltration. Creatinine decreases in the first trimester, plateaus in second trimester, and slowly increases to pre-pregnancy levels in the third trimester (4). A failure of serum creatinine to decrease during early pregnancy warrants attention, as this is also a risk factor for adverse pregnancy outcomes.

Studies have shown that protein excretion can increase during pregnancy, typically after the 20th week of gestation, and the upper limit of proteinuria in pregnancy, coined "gestational proteinuria", is defined as 300 mg/day (6). The urine protein-to-creatinine ratio increases more than the albumin-to-creatinine ratio, so it appears that hyperfiltration is not responsible for the increase (7). Importantly, the appearance of new proteinuria or worsening of proteinuria during pregnancy, especially before 20 weeks, requires more detailed evaluation for causation and should not be presumed secondary to one's pregnant state (Table 3.1).

Since it is not unusual for glomerular diseases to manifest for the first time during pregnancy or for known diagnoses to flare, a renal biopsy is often warranted to solidify an accurate diagnosis and guide appropriate treatment if non-invasive evaluations have been unrevealing. Distinguishing preeclampsia from LN, for example, would dramatically change management and outcomes for the mom and baby. Renal biopsies should be performed as early in pregnancy

DOI: 10.1201/9781003438373-4

Table 3.1: Causes of Proteinuria in Pregnancy

Renal Limited	Systemic
Chronic vesicoureteral reflux	Amyloidosis
Focal segmental glomerulosclerosis	ANCA-associated vasculitis
IgA nephropathy	Antiphospholipid antibody syndrome
Interstitial nephritis	Chronic hypertension
Membranous nephropathy	Diabetic nephropathy
Minimal change disease	Hemolytic-uremic syndrome
Primary glomerulonephritis	Infection-related glomerulonephritis
Polycystic kidney disease	Multiple myeloma
Urinary obstruction	Preeclampsia
	Polyarteritis nodosa
	Scleroderma renal crisis
	Systemic lupus, rarely can present only as lupus nephritis
	Thrombotic thrombocytopenic purpura

as possible and avoided after 23–26 weeks due to the increased risk of procedure-related bleeding secondary to pregnancy hemodynamics and procedural difficulties (8). There have been case reports of fetal complications, including placental abruption and preterm delivery; however, it was impossible to determine if this outcome was due to the renal biopsy itself or the reason for said biopsy (9).

Needless to say, pregnancies in patients with RD with renal involvement are high risk and require extensive counseling and closely coordinated care by a cohesive team involving nephrology, rheumatology, pharmacology, obstetrics, maternal fetal medicine, pharmacy, and others. These pregnancies can be associated with complications like a deterioration in kidney function, flare of underlying autoimmune conditions, and hypertensive disorders of pregnancy, in addition to the repercussions of such to the offspring. Informed, shared decision making is key in these pregnancies where medications and procedures are often essential to success and can lower risk.

3.2 SYSTEMIC LUPUS ERYTHEMATOSUS

Females with systemic lupus erythematosus (SLE) have a higher risk of developing gestational diabetes, preeclampsia, and lupus nephritis (LN) during pregnancy. While most disease manifestations do not flare during pregnancy, LN does. In fact, some patients' initial presentation of SLE is LN during pregnancy. Differentiating active LN from other hypertensive disorders of pregnancy can be challenging; however, clinical features can help to distinguish between these conditions (Table 3.2). Risk factors for pregnant women with SLE developing adverse outcomes include a history of LN, the presence of antiphospholipid antibodies (aPLs), being on anti-hypertensive agents, and being non-white or Hispanic (10–11).

For females who have pre-existing LN, higher disease activity at conception reflected by low complement and high anti-dsDNA levels is a predictor of renal flare. Severe flares occur in 3–5% of pregnancies. In a meta-analysis involving 2751 pregnancies, the most common adverse events in pregnancies with pre-existing LN were lupus flare (25.6%), hypertension (16.3%), nephritis (16.1%), preeclampsia (7.6%), and eclampsia (0.8%) (10). Fetal complications included spontaneous abortion (16%), IUGR (12.7%), stillbirth (3.6%), and neonatal death (2.5%). Active nephritis was associated with hypertension and premature birth, while a history of LN (without increased activity during pregnancy) was associated with hypertension and preeclampsia. In females who had a history of LN but quiescent disease from conception through pregnancy, over 80% of pregnancies were uncomplicated (10). Notably, an LN flare is not an absolute contraindication to an ongoing pregnancy. A patient-centered approach involving a discussion of the risks and benefits of continuing the pregnancy is warranted, particularly since teratogens may be needed and pregnancy loss may be high (Table 3.3).

Ideally, SLE patients should have a preconception visit where complete blood count, comprehensive metabolic panel, urine protein measurement, and aPLs are collected. Those with a history of LN should have quiescent disease for at least 6 months prior to conception. During pregnancy and through the fourth trimester, patients should get periodic assessments including blood work

Table 3.2: Distinguishing a Rheumatic Disease Flare from Hypertensive Disorders of Pregnancy

	Normal Pregnancy	Lupus Nephritis	Preeclampsia	HELLP	ANCA-Associated Vasculitis	Scleroderma Renal Crisis (SRC)
Typical timing		<20 weeks gestation	>20 weeks gestation	>20 weeks gestation	Any time	Between 16 and 28 weeks gestation
Common clinical features	—Decrease in BP until 20 weeks gestation, then gradually increases back to baseline —Can see dilutional anemia due to increased circulating blood volume	—HTN —Renal dysfunction (40–80%)	—HTN: Systolic ≥140 or diastolic ≥90 on two occasions at least 4 hours apart OR Systolic ≥160 or diastolic ≥110 once —Renal dysfunction —Pulmonary edema —Headache and visual problems —Elevated uric acid	—HTN (absent in 10–12%) —Hemolysis (schistocytes on peripheral smear)	—HTN —Pulmonary involvement (hemoptysis, infiltrates, diffuse alveolar hemorrhage) —Renal dysfunction —Sinus involvement (for GPA)	—Abrupt-onset HTN —Headache —Fever —Hypertensive retinopathy —Encephalopathy —Pulmonary edema
Transaminitis	—	+ More common if aPL+	+	+ >2. upper limit of normal	—	+/–
Thrombocytopenia	+ Mild	+	+	+ (<150,000)	—	+
Urinalysis	—Proteinuria <300 mg/24 hour collection	—Increased proteinuria (varying levels) — Dysmorphic RBCs, RBC casts	—Proteinuria: ≥300 mg/24 hour collection OR Protein/Cr ≥0.3 mg/dL OR Dipstick 2+ *Not required for diagnosis	—Proteinuria (absent in 10–15%)	—Hematuria —Dysmorphic RBCs, RBC casts Proteinuria: ≥300 mg/24 hour collection —Pyuria	—Hematuria, proteinuria, granular casts
Labs and serology	—Increased complement —Decreased creatinine	—Normal angiogenic markers (sFLT-1/sENG, P1GF/VEGF) —Decreased complement —Increased dsDNA	—Abnormal angiogenic markers (sFLT-1/sENG, P1GF/VEGF) —Normal dsDNA —Serum renin low–normal	—Abnormal angiogenic markers (sFLT-1/sENG, P1GF/VEGF) —Normal dsDNA	—c-ANCA or p-ANCA —High-titer MPO or PR3 —Anemia	—Serum renin elevated (secondary to renocortical ischemia) —Elevated pro-BNP
Other considerations		Typically have extra-renal evidence of lupus flare				Risk factors for SRC include diffuse skin involvement, use of steroids, and +RNA polymerase III antibodies

28

Table 3.3: Safety Profiles of Commonly Used Medications in Rheumatic Diseases

Medication	Diagnoses Commonly Prescribed for	Preconception	Pregnancy	Lactation
General				
NSAIDs	Inflammatory arthritis	Discontinue if difficulty conceiving	Discontinue by 20 weeks	Restart, ibuprofen preferred
Colchicine	Gout, pseudogout, FMF, other periodic fever syndromes	Continue	Continue	Continue
Prednisone+	Majority of diseases	*Continue:* Taper <20 mg/day, may need to replace with steroid-sparing agents	*Continue:* Taper <20 mg/day, may need to replace with steroid-sparing agents	*Continue:* After a dose >20 mg, delay breastfeeding for 4 hours
Conventional DMARDs				
Hydroxychloroquine	SLE, RA, Sjögren's, skin-limited lupus	Continue Start in SLE and +SSA patients	Continue Start in SLE and +SSA patients	Continue
Azathioprine+	SLE, inflammatory myositis, vasculitis, RA, IBD, autoimmune hepatitis	Continue	Continue	Continue
Sulfasalazine	RA and other inflammatory arthritides, IBD	Continue	Continue Take extra folic acid	Continue
Cyclosporine+, tacrolimus+	SLE, psoriasis, inflammatory myositis	*Continue:* Monitor blood pressure	*Continue:* Monitor blood pressure monthly serum levels	*Continue:* Monthly serum levels
Methotrexate+	RA, PsA, axial spondyloarthropathy, JIA, SLE, psoriasis, IBD, vasculitis, inflammatory myositis, inflammatory eye disease	Discontinue 1–3 months prior to conception	*Discontinue:* Give folic acid Assess pregnancy intentions Counsel on miscarriage and congenital malformation risk	*Avoid:* Limited data, likely low transfer
Leflunomide+	RA, PsA, JIA	*Discontinue:* Requires cholestyramine washout if detectable levels	*Discontinue:* Give cholestyramine washout	*Avoid:* Limited data, likely low transfer
Mycophenolate mofetil+ / mycophenolic acid+	SLE (especially if renal involvement), vasculitis, systemic sclerosis, inflammatory eye disease	Discontinue >6 weeks prior to conception For lupus nephritis, discontinue 3 months prior to allow disease stabilization or flare	Discontinue	*Avoid:* Limited data, likely low transfer
Biologics				
Rituximab+	RA, vasculitis, Sjögren's, SLE	Consider giving preconception, first trimester	*Second and third trimester use:* Life- or organ-threatening disease	Continue

(*Continued*)

Table 3.3: (Continued)

Medication	Diagnoses Commonly Prescribed for	Preconception	Pregnancy	Lactation
Certolizumab+	RA, PsA, axial spondyloarthropathy, IBD	Continue	Continue	Continue
Other TNF inhibitors+ (infliximab, etanercept, adalimumab, golimumab)	RA, PsA, axial spondyloarthropathy, JIA, psoriasis, inflammatory eye disease, IBD (except etanercept)	Continue	Continue in first and second trimesters; discuss discontinuation in third trimester, if possible	Continue Restart if stopped
JAK inhibitors+ (tofacitinib, upadacitinib, baricitinib)	RA, PsA, axial spondyloarthropathy, JIA, psoriasis, alopecia, eczema, IBD	*Discontinue:* Limited data, small molecule and likely passes to fetus	*Discontinue:* Limited data	No available data
IL-17/23/12+ (secukinumab, ustekinumab, ixekizumab)	PsA, axial spondyloarthropathy, JIA, enthesitis-related arthritis, psoriasis, IBD	Discuss with patient with review of current literature and review of patient history, consider TNFis	Discuss at pregnancy confirmation with review of current literature and review of patient history, consider TNFis	*Limited data:* Likely minimal transfer due to large molecular size
Other biologics+ (anakinra, belimumab, abatacept, tocilizumab)	RA, JIA, adult-onset Still's disease, gout, systemic sclerosis, periodic fever syndromes, SLE	Discuss with patient with review of current literature and review of patient history	Discuss at pregnancy confirmation with review of current literature If stopped and flares, consider restarting	*Limited data:* Likely minimal transfer due to large molecular size
Other Immunosuppressive/Immunomodulatory Medications				
Cyclophosphamide+	Severe complications of SLE, scleroderma, vasculitis, inflammatory myositis	Discontinue 3 months prior to conception	Only in life- or organ-threatening disease in second and third trimesters	Discontinue
IVIg	Inflammatory myositis, SLE, Sjögren's, ITP, hypogammaglobulinemia from rituximab	Continue	Continue	Continue
Recently approved medications (anifrolumab+, voclosporin+, avacopan+)	SLE, vasculitis	Limited data	Limited data	Anifrolumab likely OK due to large molecule size

Antihypertensives

ACEi/ARB		Discontinue, OK to continue up to conception if strong indication (proteinuric kidney disease, HF, MI)	Discontinue by second trimester	Enalapril, captopril, benazepril OK (no data on lisinopril)
Spironolactone		Avoid	Avoid	Safe to use (limited data)
Calcium channel blockers		Extended-release nifedipine preferred	Extended-release nifedipine preferred	Nifedipine and non-dihydropyridine CCB are safe to use
Beta blockers		Labetalol preferred	Labetalol preferred	Safe to use (labetalol may predispose nursing mothers to Raynaud's phenomenon of the nipple)
Diuretics		Continue at minimal dose if strong indication	Continue at minimal dose if strong indication	Continue at minimal dose if strong indication

Other Commonly Used Treatments

Aspirin	Pregnancy with +aPL test, SLE, APS	Continue low dose	Continue low dose / Start if not taking at 12–16 weeks to decrease preeclampsia risks	Low dose (75–325 mg daily) safe / Higher doses are recommended against
Heparin/low-molecular-weight heparin (LMWH)	Pregnancy with history of obstetric APS (prophylactic) or thrombotic APS (therapeutic), proteinuria	Safe	Safe	Safe
Warfarin		Discontinue unless strong indication, change to heparin	Discontinue unless strong indication, avoid during first trimester and 2–4 weeks prior to delivery	Safe (up to 12 mg daily)
Angiogenesis inhibitor (thalidomide, lenalidomide)	SLE, severe skin involvement	Discontinue 3 months prior	Discontinue	No available data
Plasma exchange (TPE or PLEX)	SLE, APS, CAPS, Vasculitis	Safe	Safe (limited data)	Safe

+ = Immunosuppressive

(dsDNA, complement, and renal function studies), urinalysis, and blood pressure. Those with a history of LN require a multidisciplinary approach to ensure the early recognition of preeclampsia given their elevated risk. Ideally, SLE patients should achieve remission, have low levels of proteinuria, and be weaned off teratogenic medications prior to conception, particularly in those with LN on mycophenolate and renin–angiotensin system blockade (Table 3.3). However, this is more of a lofty goal than an achievable actuality for even some of the most medically compliant patients. All patients should be counseled on medication and pregnancy risks, even if LN is not optimally controlled, especially if they share that pregnancy is desired. Depending on timing in pregnancy and other clinical factors, if proteinuria rises to >1 g/day, renal biopsy may be considered to assess for active LN. SLE patients should be on hydroxychloroquine, which has been shown to reduce flares, infections, thrombosis, and even improve renal function (12). Overall, the most important predictor of positive pregnancy outcome in SLE and LN is a planned pregnancy with good disease control prior to and during pregnancy.

3.3 APS/CATASTROPHIC APS

APS is characterized by thrombosis or adverse pregnancy outcome and the presence of aPLs. Patients with aPLs with or without APS have a well-established risk of fetal loss, preeclampsia, and thrombotic events during pregnancy. Given the pro-thrombotic state of pregnancy, having APS or positive aPLs elevates this risk further. Patients with pre-existing glomerular disease may also have worsening proteinuria, increasing the risk of thrombotic events. Other RDs, including SLE, Sjögren's disease, systemic sclerosis, and others, are associated with positive aPLs; these patients also have a higher risk of adverse pregnancy outcomes. Catastrophic APS (CAPS) occurs when severe, life- or organ-threatening thrombotic complications occur in a patient with aPLs. CAPS can present with proteinuria, AKI, or thrombotic microangiopathy and should therefore be considered in pregnant patients presenting with this clinical picture.

The presence of lupus anticoagulant (LAC) is associated with maternal hypertension and premature birth (10–13) and is the most powerful predictor of poor pregnancy outcomes in aPL-positive patients (14). In one prospective cohort study that enrolled 144 patients with at least one positive aPL, 39% of patients with LAC had adverse pregnancy outcomes, including preeclampsia with renal involvement. All patients with positive aPLs and a history of thrombotic events should be treated with therapeutic heparin and low-dose aspirin early in pregnancy (15). The American College of Rheumatology (ACR) guidelines suggest that those with obstetric APS should be treated with prophylactic heparin and low-dose aspirin, while those with positive aPLs without a diagnosis of APS should receive low-dose aspirin only. The UK clinical practice guideline on pregnancy and renal disease published in 2019 recommends that those with nephrotic-range proteinuria (protein:Cr ratio >300 mg/mmol or 3 g/g) use low-molecular-weight heparin in the peripartum period due to an increased risk of thrombosis, even in the absence of previous thrombotic disease or aPLs (16). For patients with renal dysfunction, low-molecular-weight heparin dosing will need adjustment, and levels may be necessary to achieve appropriate dosing.

3.4 VASCULITIS

A broad category of rheumatic diagnoses, vasculitis is rare but important to explore, as it may significantly impact women of childbearing age due the age of onset and sex predominance of each vasculitis subtype. Vasculitis is categorized most often by vessel size involved, which dictates its symptoms and potential complications for pregnancy. Importantly, maternal deaths have been reported in these diseases due to disease flares; in patients with severe renal impairment, cardiac insufficiency, uncontrolled lung or cardiac disease, and uncontrolled hypertension, pregnancy should be entered with caution (17).

Patients with medium- and large-vessel vasculitides, namely polyarteritis nodosa and Takayasu arteritis, can have renal artery and/or abdominal aorta involvement that may be stenotic or aneurysmal. Pregnancy may be associated with worsening hypertension, heart failure, and renal insufficiency in these patients (18). Behcet's disease, a medium-vessel vasculitis, typically does not have renal involvement but has associated arterial and venous thrombotic tendencies and is often associated with spontaneous abortions or preterm deliveries. Patients with a small-vessel vasculitis like granulomatosis with polyangiitis (GPA) or microscopic polyangiitis (MPA), which typically have pulmonary–renal involvement, have the highest incidence of spontaneous abortion, preterm delivery, low birth weight, and high rates of Cesarean delivery across vasculitis subtypes (19). In a systematic review of 84 MPA and GPA pregnancies, one-quarter of these ANCA-associated vasculitis (AAV) patients flared in pregnancy and one-fifth flared post-partum (20). AAV can also present de novo during pregnancy and should be in the differential for renal dysfunction, proteinuria, anemia, and hypertension, especially with respiratory or sinus symptoms (21). Eosinophilic granulomatosis with polyangiitis has similar pregnancy outcomes but does not typically have renal involvement, instead presenting with heart failure and severe asthma. Table 3.2 compares this presentation to other RDs. These pregnancies have significant adverse maternal, pregnancy, and fetal outcomes. Across all subtypes, vasculitis patients should have well-controlled blood pressure and quiescent disease prior to conception, ideally for 6 months on pregnancy-compatible medication(s) (Table 3.3). Due to the high risk of preeclampsia in patients with chronic hypertension and "renal disease", patients with vasculitis should take low-dose aspirin for the duration of pregnancy (22).

3.5 INFLAMMATORY ARTHRITIDES

Rheumatoid arthritis (RA) is one of the most common RDs. It is not uncommon to present in the postpartum period. For those with pre-existing RA, symptoms typically improve during preg-nancy due to changes in the maternal immune system. Disease flares commonly occur after deliv-ery. The biggest determinants of pregnancy outcomes in RA include disease severity, associated comorbidities, and medication management.

The Organization of Teratology Information Specialists Autoimmune Disease in Pregnancy Project was a prospective study including 440 females with RA and found that increasing dis-ease severity at conception or during pregnancy correlated with an increased risk for preterm delivery and small-for-gestational-age (SGA) infants (23). These findings are supported by other large retrospective studies (24). For those with well-controlled RA, pregnancy outcomes are similar to the general population, again emphasizing the importance of RD control prior to conception.

Juvenile idiopathic arthritis (JIA) continues into adulthood in about 50% of patients. It too is female predominant. It is unclear due to small cohorts, global study distribution, alteration of diag-nosis upon transition to adult care, and the availability of superior treatments over time if a true association between JIA and poor pregnancy outcomes exists. There is consistent data to support increased heart disease and hypertension in pregnant patients with a JIA diagnosis (25). While the treatments utilized have changed dramatically in the last 30 years, nonsteroidal antiinflammatory drugs (NSAIDs) have remained a keystone in the treatment of JIA and other arthritides. This treat-ment may explain the increases in cardiovascular disease seen; alternately, chronic inflammation in childhood may play a role in vascular changes leading to hypertension (26).

Renal involvement is generally uncommon in inflammatory arthritides; however, important renal considerations remain. For patients with RA, renal injury is more commonly related to medications such as drug-induced nephropathy secondary to NSAIDs, disease-modifying anti-rheumatic drugs (DMARDs), and some biologics (27–28). Renal disease occurs in less than 2% of patients with SpA (29). Patients with psoriasis do have an increased risk of developing end-stage renal disease (ESRD), including those with psoriatic arthritis and concomitant skin psoriasis (30). NSAIDs are commonly used in autoimmune inflammatory conditions. Non-pregnancy related side effects of these medications can still occur during pregnancy, such as sodium reten-tion, hypertension, and acute interstitial nephritis. If a patient is having difficulty conceiving, it is recommended to stop NSAIDs due to ovulation hindrance. If a pregnant patient is continued on NSAIDs during pregnancy, these should be discontinued ideally by 20 weeks but certainly the third trimester due to the risk of premature closure of the fetal ductus arteriosus, fetal renal impairment, and oligohydramnios (15).

3.6 SJÖGREN'S DISEASE

Sjögren's disease (SD) involves inflammation of the lacrimal and salivary glands, characterized by dry mucosa, glandular enlargement, arthritis, and constitutional symptoms. In a multi-center prospective cohort study involving 106 SD pregnancies, flares occurred in 13% of pregnancies, and adverse out-comes occurred in 9% (31). While not statistically different from controls, there was a higher prevalence of aPLs present. The most common renal involvement in patients with SD is tubulointerstitial nephri-tis (31). Renal tubular acidosis, which can worsen in pregnancy, is seen in 5–10% of SD patients (32). Theoretically, maternal metabolic acidosis can alter fetal growth and development, with resultant loss (33). Glomerulonephritis is rare, although has been reported in the literature in a patient who pre-sented with acute renal failure in the second trimester (34). Renal function should be screened annually in SD patients. Those with SD or any women with a positive SSA should be counseled about the risk of neonatal lupus and offered current screening and prevention interventions (15).

3.7 OTHER CONNECTIVE TISSUE DISEASES

Thankfully rare, systemic sclerosis (SS) has some of the poorest pregnancy outcomes of all RDs due to its cardiopulmonary and renal manifestations (35). Substantially increased rates of miscarriage, IUGR, preterm delivery, and preeclampsia exist, even beyond those of other RDs. Scleroderma renal crisis (SRC), its most feared complication, can present in pregnancy and, like LN, can be difficult to distinguish from preeclampsia (Table 3.2). Renal biopsy is helpful to discern, but patient acuity and hypertension are often barriers to this diagnostic procedure (36). More challenging is that angiotensin-converting enzyme inhibitors (ACEis) are the standard of care for SRC but are teratogenic, particularly later in pregnancy. As SRC carries considerable potential for ESRD, significant morbidity, and death, gold-standard treatment should still be pursued, but not without informed, shared decision making about the continuation of ACEis beyond first trimester, potential risks, and alternatives (15).

Inflammatory myositis can present initially in pregnancy but more often postpartum (37). Those with a known diagnosis can flare during pregnancy and postpartum as well. This group of patients rarely has renal involvement; however, a urinalysis performed in a flare may show hematuria but without red blood cells reported due to myoglobinuria. Although creatinine kinase levels can be significantly elevated in active inflammatory myositis, renal dysfunction does not typically occur (unlike rhabdomyolysis).

Hallmarked with Raynaud's and a solitary RNP antibody, mixed connective tissue disease (MCTD) is an overlap syndrome of SLE, myositis, and SS. SLE and SS, as established, can both have renal involvement; however, MCTD has very low incidence of these associated manifestations (38–39). An increase in gestational hypertension, miscarriage, and stillbirth exists compared to healthy peers. Akin to other diagnoses, positive aPLs increase the risk of poor pregnancy outcomes.

Periodic fevers like familial Mediterranean fever can include amyloidosis as a sequela of chronic inflammation that can lead to renal impairment (40). Blood pressure and renal function are important to watch in pregnancy. Non-NSAID antiinflammatory medications are recommended to be continued in pregnancy, although with limited safety data (Table 3.3).

Rare is the premenopausal woman with gout, as estrogen has a positive uricosuric effect. However, in pregnancy, a patient who has a genetic cause of gout or who may have renal dysfunction, ESRD, or organ transplant may be plagued by this crystal arthropathy (41). Allopurinol can be used with caution in pregnancy for urate lowering with renally dosed colchicine and/or steroids administered in a variety of modalities for acute flares. Anakinra and canakinumab are also options for flare treatment in pregnancy.

3.8 RHEUMATIC MEDICATIONS IN PREGNANCY

Current treatments available for RDs, particularly those that involve the kidneys, have substantially increased over the last quarter of a century. Those with childbearing abilities with diagnoses such as moderate to severe SLE, LN, vasculitis, and SS were historically told that they "can't" or "shouldn't" have children. There may be some small truth in this for the rare patient, but now most can fulfill their childbearing desires, with planning and preparation.

Challenges exist in that the most effective treatments used for renal involvement of RDs are unfortunately teratogenic—mycophenolate mofetil/mycophenolic acid and cyclophosphamide (15). This particularly leaves those with LN in a difficult position, as tapering off these medications can increase disease activity and proteinuria, especially when teratogenic ACEi and angiotensin reception blockers are also stopped. The teratogenicity risk is of such concern that mycophenolate has an optional Risk Evaluation and Mitigation Strategy (REMS) that involves patient education on congenital malformation and miscarriage risk as well as contraception guidance (42). Other teratogens may also be used for non-renal manifestations of RDs, particularly methotrexate and leflunomide. It is essential to review medication safety with patients of childbearing age for their family planning and contraceptive needs but also in the event of an unplanned pregnancy so unsafe medications can be stopped and appropriate ones continued. Table 3.3 reviews common RD medications and their compatibility with conception, pregnancy, and lactation.

The immunosuppressive nature of many RD medications that are compatible with pregnancy is of great concern to the patient's care team members as well as the patient and their family. While there may be hesitancy to continue these medications in the pregnant state, their use greatly improves pregnancy outcomes for both mother and baby due to their ability to maintain RDs with low or no activity. Studies have shown that immunosuppressive medication use in pregnancy does not increase the risk of infections during pregnancy or postpartum for either the mother or infant (43–44). Furthermore, infants born to mothers who had in utero exposure to immunosuppressive medications show appropriate responses to vaccinations and are therefore recommended to receive these with minimal alterations from the standard (45). During pregnancy, those with RDs should receive recommended vaccinations for both their benefit as well as their child's, with guidelines existing on concurrent vaccine administration and immunosuppressive medication usage. As with any condition that has renal involvement, medications used should be renally dosed, especially in pregnancy (43). The close monitoring of renal function and medication side effects should also be carried out with the changing physiology and hemodynamics of pregnancy.

3.9 CONTRACEPTION IN RD PATIENTS WITH KIDNEY DISEASE

Fertility declines as one's GFR worsens, likely due to suppression of the hypothalamic–pituitary–ovarian axis; many patients with ESRD are amenorrheic. Contraception in late-stage CKD is an often-ignored subject due to this. Conception is possible at all stages of renal disease, however, and contraception should be addressed with all patients of childbearing potential. With modalities like daily or nocturnal dialysis and the increasing prevalence of kidney transplantation, pregnancy in patients with CKD is becoming increasingly common. Many patients with SLE, SS, and vasculitis have early-stage CKD or may just have significant proteinuria but normal GFR. These patients have a significant chance of a high-risk unplanned pregnancy, as they are fertile but have proteinuria, hypertension, may have positive aPLs, and are likely on teratogens. In addition to these, there are other reasons to discuss contraception routinely with patients. Most guidelines recommend that pregnancy should be avoided for 1–2 years after kidney transplantation (46). Similarly, pregnancy is not recommended within 6 months of an LN or AAV flare, 3 months after a cyclophosphamide course, or in RDs when disease is active (15). Sexual activity, pregnancy, and contraception use needs should be addressed in all patients of childbearing age, according to guidelines from the American College of Rheumatology. These guidelines also contain evidence-based contraception recommendations for all RDs to support rheumatologists and others in helping their patients understand their contraceptive options.

While combined hormonal contraceptive pills are the most commonly used method by the general public, RD patients often have contraindications to estrogen-containing products, excluding them from not just pills but the patch and ring (47). Estrogen-containing contraceptives increase proteinuria and blood pressure, making them less ideal for renal patients. Overall, progestin-only preparations have a much more favorable safety profile. Progestin-only pills, intrauterine devices, and hormonal arm implants do not appear to be associated with an increased risk of thrombotic events (48–50) when compared to estrogen containing contraceptives. An advantage of progestin-only devices is that they do not require patients to remember to take their contraceptive. Hence, they are becoming increasingly popular as first-line contraception for patients with RDs, with or without kidney disease, including those on immunosuppression. Barrier contraception, such as condoms and diaphragms, are not recommended without another form of contraception due to high failure rates. For women who have completed their families, permanent methods like tubal ligation or partner sterilization may be a medication-free alternative. Emergency contraception has no medical restrictions. Contraception resources for medical professionals and patients include: BEDSIDER Birth Control Support Network, LupusPregnancy.org, and the American College of Rheumatology Guideline for the Management of Reproductive Health in Rheumatic and Musculoskeletal Diseases.

3.10 CONCLUSION

A multitude of RDs have renal involvement or indirectly impact the renovascular system. Childbearing is a desire of most patients with RDs. While these pregnancies may be high risk, patients with RDs with renal involvement can most often have successful pregnancies, with caveats. Due to the high prevalence of teratogen use, propensity for preeclampsia, and other poor outcomes with active disease, it is imperative that those with RDs have pregnancy prevention counseling and frequent pregnancy intention assessment as a part of routine care. In a time where ~50% of pregnancies in the United States are unplanned and restrictions to termination services are increasing, the planning of RD pregnancies allows for cessation of unsafe medications as well as the optimization of medical treatment, underlying diagnosis, and other nonrheumatic social factors, leading to improved outcomes. Presumptively, the best pregnancies can be achieved when those caring for patients with RDs with renal involvement work together and send congruent messages regarding pregnancy risks to the patient and fetus, medication or procedure safety, and possible disease course while engaging the patient in shared decision making.

Funding Disclosure

Silvi Shah is supported by the National Institutes of Health (NIH) K23 career development award under Award Number 1K23HL151816–01A1. The content is solely the responsibility of the authors and does not necessarily represent the official views of the NIH. The funders of the study had no role in study design; collection, analysis, or interpretation of data; writing the report; or the decision to submit the report for publication.

REFERENCES

1. Munkhaugen J, et al. Kidney function and future risk for adverse pregnancy outcomes: A population-based study from HUNT II, Norway. Nephrol Dial Transplant. 2009;24(12):3744–50.
2. Choi HS, et al. The risk of end-stage renal disease in systemic lupus erythematosus: A nationwide population-based study in Korea. Medicine (Baltimore). 2019;98(28):e16420.
3. Wiles K, et al. The impact of chronic kidney disease Stages 3–5 on pregnancy outcomes. Nephrol Dial Transplant. 2021;36(11):2008–17.
4. Webster P, et al. Pregnancy in chronic kidney disease and kidney transplantation. Kidney Int. 2017;91(5):1047–56.
5. Beers K, et al. Kidney physiology in pregnancy. Adv Chronic Kidney Dis. 2020;27(6):449–54.
6. Higby K, et al. Normal values of urinary albumin and total protein excretion during pregnancy. Am J Obstet Gynecol. 1994;171(4):984–9.
7. Hayashi M, et al. Changes in urinary excretion of six biochemical parameters in normotensive pregnancy and preeclampsia. Am J Kidney Dis. 2002;39(2):392–400.
8. Oliverio AL, et al. Kidney biopsy in a pregnant patient with suspected glomerular disease: PRO. Kidney360. 2023;4(10):1353–5.
9. Moss EM, Brewster UC. Kidney biopsy in a pregnant patient with suspected glomerular disease: CON. Kidney360. 2023;4(10):1356–8.
10. Smyth A, et al. A systematic review and meta-analysis of pregnancy outcomes in patients with systemic lupus erythematosus and lupus nephritis. Clin J Am Soc Nephrol. 2010;5(11):2060–8.
11. Yelnik CM, et al. Lupus anticoagulant is the main predictor of adverse pregnancy outcomes in aPL-positive patients: Validation of PROMISSE study results. Lupus Sci Med. 2016;3(1):e000131.
12. Clowse ME, et al. Hydroxychloroquine in lupus pregnancy. Arthritis Rheum. 200;54(11):3640–7.
13. Østensen M, et al. State of the art: Reproduction and pregnancy in rheumatic diseases. Autoimmun Rev. 2015;14(5):376–86.
14. Lockshin MD, et al. Prediction of adverse pregnancy outcome by the presence of lupus anticoagulant, but not anticardiolipin antibody, in patients with antiphospholipid antibodies. Arthritis Rheum. 2012;64(7):2311–18.
15. Sammaritano LR, et al. 2020 American college of rheumatology guideline for the management of reproductive health in rheumatic and musculoskeletal diseases. Arthritis Care Res (Hoboken). 2020;72(4):461–88.
16. Wiles K, et al. Clinical practice guideline on pregnancy and renal disease. BMC Nephrol. 2019;20(1):401.
17. Ross C, et al. Pregnancy outcomes in systemic vasculitides. Curr Rheumatol Rep. 2020;22(10):63.
18. Sims C, et al. A comprehensive guide for managing the reproductive health of patients with vasculitis. Nat Rev Rheumatol. 2022;18(12):711–23.
19. Mettler C, et al. Risk of hypertensive disorders and preterm birth in pregnant women with systemic vasculitides: A nationwide population-based cohort study. Arthritis Rheumatol. 2024 Mar;76(3):429–37.

20. Partalidou S, et al. Pregnancy outcomes in ANCA-associated vasculitis patients: A systematic review and meta-analysis. Joint Bone Spine. 202;90(6):105609.
21. Veltri NL, et al. *De novo* antineutrophil cytoplasmic antibody-associated vasculitis in pregnancy: A systematic review on maternal, pregnancy and fetal outcomes. Clin Kidney J. 2018;11(5):659–66.
22. ACOG committee opinion no. 743: Low-dose aspirin use during pregnancy. Obstet Gynecol. 2018;132(1):e44–e52.
23. Bharti B, et al. Disease severity and pregnancy outcomes in women with rheumatoid arthritis: Results from the organization of teratology information specialists autoimmune diseases in pregnancy project. J Rheumatol. 2015;42(8):1376–82.
24. Wallenius M, et al. Rheumatoid arthritis and outcomes in first and subsequent births based on data from a national birth registry. Acta Obstet Gynecol Scand. 2014;93(3):302–7.
25. Feldman DE, et al. Heart disease, hypertension, gestational diabetes mellitus, and preeclampsia/eclampsia in mothers with juvenile arthritis: A nested case-control study. Arthritis Care Res (Hoboken). 2017;69(2):306–9.
26. Aulie HA, et al. Arterial haemodynamics and coronary artery calcification in adult patients with juvenile idiopathic arthritis. Ann Rheum Dis. 2015;74(8):1515–21.
27. Kronbichler A, et al. Renal involvement in autoimmune connective tissue diseases. BMC Med. 2013;11:95.
28. Kemp E, et al. Newer immunomodulating drugs in rheumatoid arthritis may precipitate glomerulonephritis. Clin Nephrol. 2001;55(1):87–8.
29. Nikiphorou E, et al. Association of comorbidities in spondyloarthritis with poor function, work disability, and quality of life: Results from the assessment of spondyloarthritis international society comorbidities in spondyloarthritis study. Arthritis Care Res (Hoboken). 2018;70(8):1257–62.
30. Lee E, et al. Risk of end-stage renal disease in psoriatic patients: Real-world data from a nationwide population-based cohort study. Sci Rep. 2019;9(1):16581. Erratum in: Sci Rep. 2020;10(1):2284.
31. François H, et al. Renal involvement in primary Sjögren syndrome. Nat Rev Nephrol. 2016;12(2):82–93.
32. Nangaku M, et al. Pregnancy and renal disease. In: Johnson RJ, et al., editors. *Comprehensive Clinical Nephrology*. 6th ed. China: Elsevier; 2018, p. 757.
33. Seong EY, et al. Incomplete distal renal tubular acidosis uncovered during pregnancy: A case report. World J Clin Cases. 2023;11(25):5988–93.
34. Adam FU, et al. Acute renal failure due to mesangial proliferative glomerulonephritis in a pregnant woman with primary Sjögren's syndrome. Clin Rheumatol. 2006;25(1):75–9.
35. Barilaro G, et al. Systemic sclerosis and pregnancy outcomes: A retrospective study from a single center. Arthritis Res Ther. 2022;24(1):91.
36. Sobanski V, et al. Special considerations in pregnant systemic sclerosis patients. Expert Rev Clin Immunol. 2016;12(11):1161 73.
37. Jain N, et al. 2. Pregnancy and myositis. Rheumatol Adv Pract. 2019;3(1):rkz030.001.
38. Radin M, et al. Pregnancy outcomes in mixed connective tissue disease: A multicentre study. Rheumatology (Oxford). 2019;58(11):2000–8.
39. Tardif ML, et al. Mixed connective tissue disease in pregnancy: A case series and systematic literature review. Obstet Med. 2019;12(1):31–7.
40. Turgal M, et al. Pregnancy outcome of five patients with renal amyloidosis regarding familial Mediterranean fever. Ren Fail. 2014;36(2):306–8.
41. Pierre K, et al. Gout in pregnancy: A rare phenomenon. Cureus. 2020;12(11):e11697.
42. Rostas S, et al. Risk evaluation and mitigation strategies: A focus on the mycophenolic acid preparations. Prog Transplant. 2014;24(1):33–6.
43. Matro R, et al. Exposure concentrations of infants breastfed by women receiving biologic therapies for inflammatory bowel diseases and effects of breastfeeding on infections and development. Gastroenterology. 2018;155(3):696–704.
44. Gisbert JP, et al. Vaccines in children exposed to biological agents in utero and/or during breastfeeding: Are they effective and safe? J Crohns Colitis. 2023;17(6):995–1009.
45. Bass AR, et al. 2022 American college of rheumatology guideline for vaccinations in patients with rheumatic and musculoskeletal diseases. Arthritis Care Res (Hoboken). 2023;75(3):449–64.

46. Curtis KM, et al. U.S. medical eligibility criteria for contraceptive use, 2016. MMWR Recomm Rep. 2016;65(3):1–103.
47. Sachdeva M. Contraception in kidney disease. Adv Chronic Kidney Dis. 2020;27(6):499–505.
48. Burgner A, et al. Contraception and CKD. Clin J Am Soc Nephrol. 2020;15(4):563–5.
49. Sammaritano LR. Contraception and preconception counseling in women with autoimmune disease. Best Pract Res Clin Obstet Gynaecol. 2020;64:11–23.
50. Sammaritano LR. Contraception in patients with systemic lupus erythematosus and antiphospholipid syndrome. Lupus. 2014;23(12):1242–5.

4 Considerations for Pediatric Rheumatology Patients with Renal Disease

Megan Mariko Perron, Jennifer C. Cooper, and Jerome C. Lane

4.1 INTRODUCTION

Because of the rarity of pediatric rheumatologic disease and the difficulty in conducting pediatric randomized trials, there is a relative lack of evidence for treating children compared to adults. Guidelines are often extrapolated from adult studies, as well as expert opinions, case reports, or observational studies (1). This chapter will attempt to address the unique challenges and features of pediatric rheumatologic kidney disease. Children physiologically are not simply "small adults," and pediatric patients often have manifestations of disease that are different from, and in some cases, more severe than, those found in adults. The measurement of kidney function in children is a more complex endeavor than in adults due to the range of sizes in children. Because children are a vulnerable population and are subject to the effects of their environment, social determinants of health are of particular concern in the assessment and management of pediatric rheumatologic and kidney disease. Vaccinations are an important part of routine pediatric primary care and are of particular importance in pediatric kidney disease, in which patients are likely to be treated with immunosuppression. Lastly, children, with their inherent longer lifespan, have a greater potential lifetime exposure to the toxicities of medications.

4.2 SYSTEMIC LUPUS ERYTHEMATOSUS

Systemic lupus erythematosus (SLE) is a systemic autoimmune disease characterized by auto-antibodies and multi-organ system involvement. The childhood-onset SLE (cSLE) incidence rate is estimated to be ~1 per 100,000 children, with a greater incidence in girls compared to boys (2). cSLE accounts for ~10–20% of all SLE cases and tends to be associated with worse disease severity compared with adult-onset SLE (2, 3). The mean age of onset in cSLE is 11 years old, compared with 32 years for adult-onset lupus (4). Pediatric lupus nephritis (pLN) occurs in 50–82% of children with SLE, compared with 20–40% of adults, and is associated with significant morbidity and mortality (5–7). Kidney involvement in cSLE is most commonly seen within the first 2 years of primary disease (8), and it is estimated that 15% of patients with pLN will progress to chronic kidney disease stage 5 (CKD5, or end stage kidney disease [ESKD]) (7).

The clinical presentation of pLN can range from asymptomatic hematuria or non-nephrotic proteinuria to acute nephritic syndrome, to nephrotic syndrome, to CKD (9). The lupus nephritis (LN) class is determined by biopsy and ranges from class I to VI. Proliferative LN (class III and IV) traditionally has been associated with high mortality and progression to ESKD. Class V (membranous) LN can sometimes be managed with an ACE inhibitor alone or may require more aggressive therapy if associated with nephrotic syndrome.

The Childhood Arthritis and Rheumatology Research Alliance (CARRA) published a consensus treatment plan (CTP) for pLN, recommending the initial treatment of proliferative pLN with either intravenous (IV) cyclophosphamide (CYC) or oral mycophenolate mofetil (MMF) for the first 6 months, along with corticosteroids (10). The Single Hub and Access point for pediatric Rheumatology in Europe (SHARE) published similar evidence-based guidelines (11). IVC treatment may follow either standard "NIH" monthly IV dosing (500–1000 mg/m^2 titrated up to 1500 mg/dose) up to 6 months, or the lower-dose "Euro-Lupus" protocol of 500 mg IV every 2 weeks for six doses. Although outcome data of the Euro-Lupus CYC regimen are limited in pediatrics, a multisite retrospective cohort study of 145 pediatric patients with proliferative LN treated with either the Euro-Lupus or modified NIH IVC regimens failed to demonstrate a difference in 12-month response outcomes between the groups (12). In addition, the 2023 EULAR Update on the Management of SLE, a primarily adult-based guideline, recommends the consideration of combination strategies that include a backbone of either MMF or CYC (Euro-Lupus or NIH regimen) in conjunction with glucocorticoids and other immunosuppressants such as calcineurin inhibitors (CNI) or belimumab (BEL) (13). Target treatments for proteinuria reduction at key time points are recommended. The development of international consensus-based treatment targets for pLN is underway (14).

After the initial "induction" phase aimed at inducing a complete renal response, long-term maintenance treatment for class III and IV pLN consists of MMF or azathioprine (AZA) for a minimum of 3 years (11). Evidence for the treatment of pure class V pLN (i.e., with no features of proliferative disease) is even more limited. The SHARE guidelines recommend MMF and low-dose

DOI: 10.1201/9781003438373-5

oral prednisone (0.5 mg/kg/day) for the initial treatment of class V pLN, followed by maintenance treatment with MMF or AZA. For refractory or relapsing disease, therapy should be switched to a different agent, such as changing MMF to IVC or vice versa, and consideration can be given to other agents, such as rituximab (RTX) or a CNI (11).

Although the LUNAR trial failed to show significant benefit from adding RTX to standard MMF and steroid treatment, a secondary analysis demonstrated a significant relationship between peripheral B-cell depletion and complete renal response (15). Additional retrospective studies have suggested that RTX can be an effective add-on agent (16, 17). Small, non-randomized pediatric studies and systematic reviews have reported favorable outcomes with RTX in pLN (17, 18).

Belimumab (BEL), a newer B-cell-depleting monoclonal antibody that inhibits the activity of BAFF (B-cell activating factor), was approved by the FDA for the treatment of non-renal SLE in 2011. The pivotal, large BLISS-LN trial demonstrated that the combination of belimumab with either MMF or Euro-Lupus CYC improved renal response compared to the placebo (19). A secondary analysis of BLISS-LN revealed a decreased risk of flares and improved preservation of kidney function in the belimumab treatment group (20). Crucially, a phase 2, randomized, placebo-controlled, double-blind *pediatric* study demonstrated the safety and efficacy of BEL in cSLE; however, although an improvement in proteinuria was seen, the study excluded patients with severe LN (21). Because of these studies, the FDA has approved BEL for the treatment of cSLE and pLN in children 5 years and older. However, further studies are still required to determine the best use of BEL in pLN.

Regarding CNIs, tacrolimus (TAC) is preferred over cyclosporine (CSA) due to the latter drug's higher rate of side effects such as hypertension, kidney impairment, dyslipidemias, tremor, hirsutism, and gum hyperplasia (22, 23). A meta-analysis of 45 randomized trials with 4222 patients with LN (mostly with class 3 and 4 LN, some with class 5), including pediatric patients, demonstrated similar efficacy of TAC and MMF and higher efficacy of TAC compared to IVC (24). Voclosporin (VOC) is a cyclosporine analog that not only seems to have greater potency than cyclosporine but also appears to have fewer side effects associated with other CNIs. VOC does not require the careful monitoring of drug levels required of other CNIs, which makes VOC an attractive candidate for the pediatric population (23). Phase 3 RCTs (AURORA 1 and 2) demonstrated higher rates of complete renal response for VOC compared to a placebo at 52 weeks, with continued safety and efficacy after 3 years of follow-up (25, 26). It is unclear at this time what role voclosporin has to play in pLN.

A number of other biological agents are under investigation for the treatment of SLE and LN and are beyond the scope of this chapter. These drugs include the novel anti-CD20 drugs atacicept and telitacicept, anti-interferon therapies such as sifalimumab and anifrolumab, and others (18). Obinutuzumab, a fully-humanized anti-CD20 monoclonal antibody, shows promise compared to rituximab and, in the NOBILITY study, when added to standard MMF treatment, was demonstrated to result in increased rates of complete remission compared to the placebo (23). The phase II POSTERITY (NCT 05039619) study of obinutuzumab in pLN patients is currently underway. Cell-based therapies are another area of excitement; the single-center case series of anti-CD19 chimeric antigen receptor T-cell (CAR-T) therapy in six young adult patients with refractory LN leading to drug-free remission is especially promising; however, large multicenter trials are needed (27).

As in adult LN, treatment with ACE inhibitors (ACE-I) or angiotensin II receptor blockers (ARB) should be considered in pLN, especially in patients with proteinuria and/or hypertension. ACE-I and ARB have an antiproteinuric and renoprotective effect. This is especially important, since proteinuria is a strong predictor of renal outcomes (18). Patients with cSLE and pLN should also be treated with hydroxychloroquine (11).

Patient outcomes have improved with advances in the early detection and treatment of LN. One retrospective study from 1980–2010 showed an improvement in 5-year pediatric patient survival from 83% to 91% and an improvement in kidney survival from 52% to 88%. Predictors of poor outcome included African-American race, low GFR, and nephrotic-range proteinuria at presentation (28). Another study found that African-American children with ESKD have double the mortality rate compared to Caucasian children (29). Once ESKD develops, treatment options include dialysis and transplant.

4.3 VASCULITIDES

4.3.1 ANCA Associated Vasculitis

ANCA-associated vasculitis (AAV) is a group of small- to medium-size vessel vasculitides that consists of granulomatosis with polyangiitis (GPA), microscopic polyangiitis (MPA), and eosinophilic granulomatosis with polyangiitis (EGPA). These disorders typically involve the upper and lower respiratory tracts as well as the kidneys, and kidney involvement can be associated with long-term morbidity and mortality. Pediatric AAV is rare, with an estimated prevalence of childhood-onset AAV of 3.41–4.28 per million children (30); in the same study, 78% had GPA and 18% had MPA, while EGPA was only present in 2%. It has a higher female predominance and is often diagnosed in the second decade of life (31).

In GPA, kidney involvement is characterized by proteinuria (>0.3 g/24 hours), hematuria/red blood cell casts (>5 RBCs per HPF), and necrotizing pauci-immune glomerulonephritis on biopsy (32). The SHARE initiative has treatment recommendations for induction and maintenance therapy. For severe disease, induction treatment typically consists of corticosteroids and IV CYC, with consideration of plasma exchange and rituximab. Maintenance therapy is typically recommended with azathioprine, methotrexate, MMF, or rituximab (33).

Regarding outcomes, a systematic review and meta-analysis of childhood GPA and MPA reported a 7% overall mortality rate in a follow-up period of 4–55 months (34). Relapses are common in children and can range between 24% and 100% (34–36).

4.3.2 IgA Vasculitis

IgA vasculitis (IgAV), formerly known as Henoch–Schönlein purpura, is a small-vessel vasculitis that is typically characterized by the presence of palpable purpuric rash, arthritis, abdominal pain, and kidney inflammation. It is the most common vasculitis of childhood, with an estimated annual incidence of 20.4 per 100,000, primarily affecting children 4–6 years old (37). Up to ~50% of patients may have kidney involvement at disease onset (38). If nephritis develops (IgAV), it occurs most commonly within the first 4–6 weeks, with 97% of cases developing within 6 months (39). Therefore, frequent monitoring with blood pressure and urinalysis is warranted soon after the diagnosis of IgAV.

Most cases of IgAV are self-limited and resolve within 4 weeks. Management for IgAV depends on severity. If patients develop severe or persistent proteinuria, pediatric nephrologists should be involved and a biopsy should be performed. Treatment depends on the severity of nephritis and can include glucocorticoids, azathioprine, MMF, or IV CYC (40). One study found that 3% of patients with IgAV progressed to ESKD requiring dialysis (41). Kidney transplant is an option for these patients, although the recurrence of disease can occur post-transplant.

4.3.3 Tubulo-Interstitial Nephritis with Uveitis Syndrome

Tubulo Interstitial Nephritis with Uveitis (TINU) is a rare syndrome characterized by the concomitant presentation of acute interstitial nephritis (AIN) and bilateral anterior uveitis. The median age of diagnosis is 15 years old, and it is thought to have a female predominance (42). Presentation typically consists of acute bilateral (although can be unilateral or alternating) eye pain and redness with anterior uveitis (43). Kidney manifestations can consist of flank pain, sterile pyuria, hematuria, proteinuria, azotemia, and acute kidney injury. However, urine in interstitial nephritis is often "bland" and normal appearing, which distinguishes AIN from acute glomerulonephritis. The only clue to kidney disease in AIN may be an elevated serum creatinine, and biopsy is often required to establish the diagnosis. While there are no specific laboratory findings for TINU, patients may have leukocyturia, eosinophilia, anemia, abnormal liver function tests, elevated erythrocyte sedimentation rate, and c-reactive protein. The Standardization of Uveitis Nomenclature (SUN) working Group published classification criteria for TINU in 2021, which consist of anterior chamber inflammation and evidence of tubulointerstitial nephritis with either (1) a positive biopsy or (2) evidence of nephritis and an elevated urine beta-2 microglobulin (44).

Kidney disease in patients with TINU is often self-limited (45). Patients who do develop kidney impairment are most often treated with prednisone as first-line therapy, and steroid-sparing agents such as MMF have also been used.

4.3.4 Anti-GBM (Goodpasture's) Disease

Anti-GBM disease is a small-vessel vasculitis characterized by circulating autoantibodies directed against the glomerular and alveolar basement membrane, resulting in glomerulonephritis and/or alveolar hemorrhage. While very rare in children, it accounts for ~0.4% of all pediatric CKD5 (46) and up to 3% of crescentic glomerulonephritis in children (47). In children, there is a female:male predominance of 2:1 (48). Treatment can include plasma exchange, corticosteroids, and CYC (49). Up to 91% of children survived acute illness, although 52% ultimately progressed to ESKD. Of those patients, five received kidney transplant and two were awaiting transplant. None of the patients demonstrated relapse after remission (48).

4.4 PEDIATRIC CONSIDERATIONS FOR DRUG TOXICITIES
4.4.1 Glucocorticoids

Children are particularly vulnerable to the adverse effects of glucocorticoids (GCs), and therefore treatment dose and duration should be limited when possible. Growth impairment in 23.6% of patients with pSLE correlated with cumulative GC dose (among other factors) (50). A large study that compared disease-related and steroid-related damage between adult- and childhood-onset SLE found that childhood-onset disease predicted an increased risk of steroid-related damage (cataracts, avascular necrosis, osteoporosis resulting in fracture, and diabetes). Since the risk of steroid-related damage increases with disease duration, although adults and children accrue disease-related damage at similar rates, the earlier onset and longer duration of disease in children leads to greater accumulated damage (51).

Since peak bone mass is formed by the late teens to early 20s, GC-induced osteoporosis is of particular concern in pediatrics. The American College of Rheumatology (ACR) guidelines regarding GC-induced osteoporosis recommend that children on chronic GCs have fracture risk assessed at baseline and then annually and should have an intake of calcium of 1000 mg/day and vitamin D of 600 IU/day. For children with osteoporotic fracture(s), treatment with an oral or IV bisphosphonate can be considered (52).

4.4.2 Cyclophosphamide

Although it has been proposed that pre-pubertal children are relatively protected against the gonadal toxicity of alkylating agents, studies of boys and girls have not uniformly shown this to be the case (53). In general, males are more susceptible to gonadal toxicity from alkylating agents at any age, whereas pre-pubertal girls seem to be less vulnerable (54). For women <25 years of age, the risk of amenorrhea has been reported to be 5–10%. Furthermore, cumulative dose is a major risk factor determining gonadal toxicity. For men, there is also risk of azoospermia with CYC use; this was increased with increasing cumulative dose (55).

Fertility preservation options should be discussed for all patients undergoing treatment with CYC. The cryopreservation of sperm is available for pubertal/post-pubertal boys who are willing and able to provide ejaculate through masturbation. Alternatively, though not as widely available, testicular sperm extraction can be performed under sedation. For pre-pubertal males, the only option available is testicular tissue cryopreservation, which is experimental at this time. For pubertal/post-pubertal females, options include ovarian stimulation with oocyte retrieval and cryopreservation and ovarian tissue cryopreservation (OTC). However, despite the availability of fertility preservation methods, multiple barriers still exist, including cultural/religious and societal factors, insurance coverage, and a lack of counseling by providers regarding available options (56).

The use of GnRH agonists (GnRHAs) such as leuprolide for the suppression of ovarian function and protection against gonadal toxicity can be considered. A systematic review concluded in favor of using GnRHAs for protection against gonadal toxicity; however, the evidence was considered "low quality." The American Society of Clinical Oncology recommends caution in relying upon GnRHAs over OTCue. Though studies in rheumatologic patients are limited, they have tended to show favorable results for GnRHA protection (57). A meta-analysis of 218 female SLE patients treated with CYC showed that the preservation of ovarian function occurred in 94.6% (125/132) of women who received concurrent GnRH as compared to 58% (50/86) of women who did not receive a GnRHa (OR 10.3, CI 4.83–36.29) (58). More studies are needed in the rheumatologic population, especially regarding children and adolescents.

4.5 KIDNEY TRANSPLANT IN PEDIATRIC RHEUMATOLOGIC DISEASE

About 20% of children with IgAVN will develop CKD, and about 2% will progress to ESKD and kidney transplantation. The optimal timing for transplant in IgAVN is unclear. Although current guidelines do recommend a period of disease quiescence before transplantation, preemptive transplantation as a risk factor for recurrent disease. Therefore, a period of quiescence might be prudent prior to transplant in IgAVN. Studies report recurrence rates of 13–25% at 5 years and 60% at 15 years. The risk of recurrence increases with younger age, longer time on dialysis, preemptive transplant, preformed donor-specific antibodies, and rapid progression to ESKD. Fortunately, despite the high risk of recurrence, patient and allograft survival are equal to or exceed rates in other causes of ESKD (59).

In childhood AAV with kidney involvement, approximately 30% of cases will progress to ESKD. Transplantation should be delayed until there has been clinical remission for at least 6 months, though isolated positive serology should not delay transplantation. Rates of recurrence post-transplant range from 1.2% to 9%. As with IgAVN, rates of patient and allograft survival in AAV equal or exceed those for other diseases (59).

About 10–30% of patients with LN progress to ESKD within 15 years. Higher disease activity scores are associated with lower patient and allograft survival; therefore, transplantation should be delayed until there is minimal disease activity and minimal immunosuppression. However, increased wait time on dialysis has been correlated with higher graft loss, so preemptive transplantation prior to dialysis is recommended when possible. Disease may recur in up to 30% of children post-transplantation. In adults, SLE allograft survival is similar to that in other diseases. However, in childhood LN, allograft survival is significantly lower. Several studies have demonstrated 1.4–3-fold increased risk of graft loss and increased mortality in children with SLE undergoing transplant compared to those with other causes of ESKD (59).

4.6 MEASUREMENT OF KIDNEY FUNCTION IN CHILDREN

The measurement of kidney function is a complex matter in both adults and children. Although the kidney has multiple functions (synthesis of renin, calcitriol, and erythropoeitin; regulation of blood pressure; acid–base balance; etc.), the term "kidney function" generally refers to the filtration capacity of the kidneys as reflected by the glomerular filtration rate (GFR). GFR is defined as the plasma volume per unit of time that is entirely cleared from a marker molecule; it is expressed as milliliters per minute and standardized to 1.73 m^2 body surface area (60).

GFR may be estimated (eGFR) via endogenous markers, such as creatinine and cystatin C, or it can be directly measured (mGFR) by the clearance of exogenous markers, such as inulin, iohexol, EDTA, and others. The most widely used method for mGFR at the moment involves the infusion of iohexol and repeated measurement of blood levels to calculate plasma clearance and hence mGFR (61). Though mGFR is more precise than eGFR, which can be influenced by various conditions, methods for determining mGFR are impractical for routine use and are usually limited to research studies or cases in which eGFR is inconclusive. GFR may also be determined from creatinine clearance via 24-hour urine collection. However, due to inaccuracies from imprecise urine collection, as well as the difficulties of collecting urine for an extended period of time in children, urine creatinine clearance has largely been replaced by the eGFR formulas mentioned herein (60).

The two most commonly used endogenous plasma markers for eGFR are creatinine and cystatin C. Creatinine is a by-product of muscle metabolism and is filtered by the glomeruli and, in smaller part, excreted by the renal tubules. Since the tubular excretion of creatinine becomes a larger part of total excretion as GFR falls in chronic kidney disease, this tubular excretion may lead creatinine-based formulas to overestimate GFR. Creatinine may also be affected by unusually high or low muscle mass, severe liver disease, and certain drugs such as trimethoprim. Creatinine also is a relatively insensitive surrogate for GFR, and there may be large changes in GFR before changes in creatinine are observed. Cystatin C is a low-molecular-weight protein produced by all nucleated cells. Unlike creatinine, cystatin C levels are not influenced by muscle mass. Cystatin C may be affected by thyroid disease, obesity, and glucocorticoids (60).

A large number of formulas exist for calculating eGFR in adults and children and can use either creatinine, cystatin C, or a combination of the two. The most commonly used formulas for eGFR in children include the "bedside Schwartz," the CKiD U25 formulas, and the "full age spectrum" (FAS) equations. For practical purposes, the bedside Schwartz formula, which uses creatinine alone, is the most common method used by non-nephrologists and is determined by the formula: eGFR = 0.413 X (height/serum creatinine), with height in cm and creatinine in mg/dL (62).

However, as mentioned before, creatinine is a relatively insensitive marker for GFR and can sometimes overestimate kidney function. Given the different characteristics of creatinine and cystatin C, formulas that combine the two markers have been shown to have a higher accuracy than either marker in isolation. Online calculators exist for the complex equations, such as the CKiD U25 and FAS formulas, that combine both creatinine and cystatin C (60).

4.7 VACCINATIONS

Vaccinations are a key adjunct for patients with autoimmune kidney disease to reduce the risk of serious infections. For patients that do not require systemic immunosuppression, the routine Centers for Disease Control (CDC) immunization schedules can be followed. However, there are special considerations for immunosuppressed children and adolescents, namely, to avoid live vaccinations, but also regarding whether to hold immunosuppression or postpone vaccination to optimize the immune response to the vaccine. Live attenuated vaccines to be avoided while

Table 4.1: Recommended Timing of Vaccinations Depending on Phase of Immunosuppression for Pediatric Rheumatic Disease Patients

Patients initiating immunosuppression	• CDC guidelines recommend waiting 4 weeks after a live vaccine and 2 weeks after a non-live vaccine. • Therapy should not be delayed if urgent treatment is needed.
Patients already on immunosuppression	• Live vaccines should be avoided but routine *non-live* vaccinations can generally be given on schedule. • ACR guidelines recommend waiting to give non-live vaccines until a patient is on less than 10 mg per day of prednisone. • For patients on B-cell-depleting agents such as rituximab that impair the humoral response to vaccines, it is recommended to wait 6 months after the last dose and give the vaccine 2 weeks prior to the next rituximab infusion. • A "catch-up" vaccination schedule can be followed per CDC guidance. • Live vaccines should be withheld for: • 1 month after the discontinuation of high-dose steroid therapy (≥ 2 mg/kg of body weight or > 20 mg of prednisone or equivalent for ≥ 14 days) • 3 months after discontinuation of other systemic immunosuppression (CYC, methotrexate, MMF, tacrolimus, etc.) • 6 months after B-cell depleting agents.

Table 4.2: Specific Vaccine Recommendations for Pediatric Rheumatic Disease Populations

Vaccine Target	Recommendations for Vaccination
Pneumococcal pneumonia	Both CDC and ACR strongly recommend vaccination against *Streptococcus pneumoniae* for patients under age 65 years. CDC and American Academy of Pediatrics recommend the primary PCV13 series to all children <2 years of age and a PPSV23 vaccination to children ≥2 years old that are immunosuppressed or have another qualifying medical condition. PCV20 may decrease the need for PPSV23.
Influenza	Annual influenza vaccination is recommended. If disease activity allows, ACR guidelines recommend holding methotrexate for 2 weeks post-vaccination; other immunosuppression can be continued uninterrupted.
Shingles	Zoster vaccination using the recombinant inactivated form (Shingrix) is recommended for immunocompromised persons ≥18 years.

Abbreviations: CDC, Centers for Disease Control; ACR, American College of Rheumatology; CYC, Cyclophosphamide; MMF, mycophenolate mofetil

immunosuppressed include those for intranasal influenza, MMR, varicella, MMRV, LAIV, yellow fever, oral typhoid, BCG, rotavirus, and smallpox. Both the CDC immunization schedules and the 2022 ACR Guideline for Vaccinations in Patients with Rheumatic and Musculoskeletal Diseases include relevant information for pediatrics (63, 64). A systematic review examined the safety and efficacy of vaccinations in pediatric patients with systemic inflammatory rheumatic diseases, including 28 articles and data from almost 2100 children and adolescents (65). Although antibody titers were often lower in the patients with systemic inflammatory rheumatic diseases, most patients had seroconversion and achieved seroprotection. There were no serious adverse events nor worsening of their underlying rheumatic disease. Table 4.1 describes the timing of administration of vaccinations relative to immunosuppression. Table 4.2 lists recommendations for specific vaccines.

4.8 SUPPORTING SELF-MANAGEMENT EFFICACY AND TRANSITION TO ADULT CARE

The period of transfer from pediatric-centered to adult-centered care is a vulnerable period and often associated with long gaps in care, a loss of access to prescription medications, disease flares, and worsening psychosocial outcomes for young adults with chronic illnesses, including kidney disease. Studies have shown that the highest rate of kidney transplant loss occurs during the transition years and immediately following the transfer of care (66). The successful transfer of care requires a purposeful structured approach to facilitate communication and clinical care among providers as well as self-management efficacy from the young adult. Supporting the development of self-management efficacy begins in childhood and adolescence with the purposeful incorporation of transition readiness assessments and skill building that a young adult will need to manage their own care into routine clinical care. Many academic centers are now developing formal multidisciplinary transition programs and clinics for adolescents and young adults. The Got Transition website (gottransition.org), has many resources available to assist clinicians, patients, and caregivers with evaluating transition readiness and navigating the transition process.

4.9 CONCLUSION

Children with pediatric rheumatologic kidney disease are a vulnerable population that require considerations that are often different from adults with the same conditions. Children may have more serious morbidities from these diseases, and treatments that affect not only their present health but also their psychosocial and physical health as they grow into adulthood. The care of pediatric patients with complex disease requires the coordination of care and a unified long-term vision by patients, their families, and their healthcare team. A child with rheumatologic kidney disease, in particular, who may progress to kidney failure, dialysis, and kidney transplantation, requires the attention of dozens of individual care providers across multiple specialties, all of whom need to provide care that will assist an ill child to grow and thrive to the best of that child's potential. Social determinants of health and the transition of healthcare from pediatrics to adult medicine are particularly difficult topics that continue to require more research and attention. The development of self-management strategies is vital as these patients transition from childhood to adolescence and into adulthood, with the end goal that patients can manage their own care.

REFERENCES

1. Ogbu EA, et al. Treatment guidelines in pediatric rheumatic diseases. Rheum Dis Clin North Am. 2022;48(3):725–46.
2. Valenzuela-Almada MO, et al. Epidemiology of childhood-onset systemic lupus erythematosus: A population-based study. Arthritis Care Res (Hoboken). 2022;74(5):728–32.
3. Aggarwal A, et al. Childhood onset systemic lupus erythematosus: How is it different from adult SLE? Int J Rheum Dis. 2015;18(2):182–91.
4. Font J, et al. Systemic lupus erythematosus (SLE) in childhood: Analysis of clinical and immunological findings in 34 patients and comparison with SLE characteristics in adults. Ann Rheum Dis. 1998;57(8):456–9.
5. Hersh AO, et al. Differences in long-term disease activity and treatment of adult patients with childhood- and adult-onset systemic lupus erythematosus. Arthritis Rheum. 2009;61(1):13–20.
6. Samanta M, et al. Childhood lupus nephritis: 12 years of experience from a developing country's perspective. Eur J Rheumatol. 2017;4(3):178–83.
7. Oni L, et al. Kidney outcomes for children with lupus nephritis. Pediatr Nephrol. 2021;36(6):1377–85.
8. Hafeez F, et al. Lupus nephritis in children. J Coll Physicians Surg Pak. 2008;18(1):17–21.
9. Klein-Gitelman M, Beresford M. Chapter 23: Systemic lupus erythematosus, mixed connective tissue disease, and undifferentiated connective tissue disease. In: [book auth.], Laxer R, Lindsley C, Wedderbum L, Mellins E, Fuhlbrigge R, editors. *Petty. Textbook of Pediatric Rheumatology.* 8th ed. Philadelphia: Elselvier; 2021.
10. Mina R, et al. CARRA SLE Subcommittee. Consensus treatment plans for induction therapy of newly diagnosed proliferative lupus nephritis in juvenile systemic lupus erythematosus. Arthritis Care Res (Hoboken). 2012;64(3):375–83.
11. Groot N, et al. European evidence-based recommendations for the diagnosis and treatment of childhood-onset lupus nephritis: The SHARE initiative. Ann Rheum Dis. 2017;76(12):1965–73.
12. Wang CS, et al. Renal response outcomes of the EuroLupus and NIH cyclophosphamide dosing regimens in childhood-onset proliferative lupus nephritis. Arthritis Rheumatol. 2024;76(3):469–78.

13. Fanouriakis A, et al. EULAR recommendations for the management of systemic lupus ery-thematosus: 2023 update. Ann Rheum Dis. 2024;83(1):15–29.

14. Smith EMD, et al. Towards development of treat to target (T2T) in childhood-onset systemic lupus erythematosus: PReS-endorsed overarching principles and points-to-consider from an international task force. Ann Rheum Dis. 2023;82(6):788–98.

15. Gomez Mendez LM, et al. Peripheral blood B cell depletion after rituximab and complete response in lupus nephritis. Clin J Am Soc Nephrol. 2018;13(10):1502–9. Erratum in: Clin J Am Soc Nephrol. 2019;14(1):111.

16. Rovin BH, et al. Efficacy and safety of rituximab in patients with active proliferative lupus nephritis: The Lupus Nephritis Assessment with Rituximab study. Arthritis Rheum. 2012;64(4):1215–26.

17. Sinha R, et al. Use of rituximab in paediatric nephrology. Arch Dis Child. 2021;106(11):1058–65.

18. Trindade VC, et al. An update on the management of childhood-onset systemic lupus erythe-matosus. Paediatr Drugs. 2021;23(4):331–47.

19. Furie R, et al. Two-year, randomized, controlled trial of belimumab in lupus nephritis. N Engl J Med. 2020;383(12):1117–28.

20. Rovin BH, et al. A secondary analysis of the belimumab international study in lupus nephri-tis trial examined effects of belimumab on kidney outcomes and preservation of kidney function in patients with lupus nephritis. Kidney Int. 2022;101(2):403–13.

21. Brunner HI, et al. Safety and efficacy of intravenous belimumab in children with systemic lupus erythematosus: Results from a randomised, placebo-controlled trial. Ann Rheum Dis. 2020;79(10):1340–8.

22. Houssiau FA, et al. Current management of lupus nephritis. Best Pract Res Clin Rheumatol. 2013;27(3):319–28.

23. Kaneko M, et al. Recent advances in immunotherapies for lupus nephritis. Pediatr Nephrol. 2023;38(4):1001–12.

24. Palmer SC, et al. Induction and maintenance immunosuppression treatment of prolifera-tive lupus nephritis: A network meta-analysis of randomized trials. Am J Kidney Dis. 2017;70(3):324–36.

25. Rovin BH, et al. Efficacy and safety of voclosporin versus placebo for lupus nephritis (AURORA 1): A double-blind, randomised, multicentre, placebo-controlled, phase 3 trial. Lancet. 2021;397(10289):2070–80. Erratum in: Lancet. 2021;397(10289):2048.

26. Saxena A, et al. Safety and efficacy of long-term voclosporin treatment for lupus nephritis in the phase 3 AURORA 2 clinical trial. Arthritis Rheumatol. 2024;76(1):59–67.

27. Mackensen A, et al. Anti-CD19 CAR T cell therapy for refractory systemic lupus erythemato-sus. Nat Med. 2022;28(10):2124–32. Erratum in: Nat Med. 2022 Nov 3.

28. Pereira T, et al. Three decades of progress in treating childhood-onset lupus nephritis. Clin J Am Soc Nephrol. 2011;6(9):2192–9.

29. Hiraki LT, et al. End-stage renal disease due to lupus nephritis among children in the US, 1995–2006. Arthritis Rheum. 2011;63(7):1988–97.

30. Hirano D, et al. Epidemiology and clinical features of childhood-onset anti-neutrophil cytoplasmic antibody-associated vasculitis: A clinicopathological analysis. Pediatr Nephrol. 2019;34(8):1425–33.

31. Cabral DA, et al. Comparing presenting clinical features in 48 children with microscopic polyangiitis to 183 children who have granulomatosis with polyangiitis (Wegener's): An ARChiVe cohort study. Arthritis Rheumatol. 2016;68(10):2514–26.

32. Ruperto N, et al. EULAR/PRINTO/PRES criteria for Henoch-Schönlein purpura, childhood polyarteritis nodosa, childhood Wegener granulomatosis and childhood Takayasu arteritis: Ankara 2008. Part I: Overall methodology and clinical characterisation. Ann Rheum Dis. 2010;69(5):790–7. Erratum in: Ann Rheum Dis. 2011;70(2):397.

33. de Graeff N, et al. European consensus-based recommendations for the diagnosis and treatment of rare paediatric vasculitides—the SHARE initiative. Rheumatology (Oxford). 2019;58(4):656–71. Erratum in: Rheumatology (Oxford). 2020;59(4):919.

34. Iudici M, et al. Childhood-onset granulomatosis with polyangiitis and microscopic polyangi-itis: Systematic review and meta-analysis. Orphanet J Rare Dis. 2016;11(1):141.

35. Sacri AS, et al. Clinical characteristics and outcomes of childhood-onset ANCA-associated vasculitis: A French nationwide study. Nephrol Dial Transplant. 2015;30(Suppl 1):i104–12.

36. Morishita KA, et al. ARChiVe investigators network within the PedVas initiative. Early outcomes in children with antineutrophil cytoplasmic antibody-associated vasculitis. Arthritis Rheumatol. 2017;69(7):1470–9.
37. Gardner-Medwin JM, et al. Incidence of henoch-schönlein purpura, Kawasaki disease, and rare vasculitides in children of different ethnic origins. Lancet. 2002;360(9341):1197–202.
38. Trapani S, et al. Henoch Schonlein purpura in childhood: Epidemiological and clinical analysis of 150 cases over a 5-year period and review of literature. Semin Arthritis Rheum. 2005;35(3):143–53.
39. Narchi H. Risk of long term renal impairment and duration of follow up recommended for Henoch-Schonlein purpura with normal or minimal urinary findings: A systematic review. Arch Dis Child. 2005;90(9):916–20.
40. Ozen S, et al. European consensus-based recommendations for diagnosis and treatment of immunoglobulin A vasculitis-the SHARE initiative. Rheumatology (Oxford). 2019;58(9):1607–16.
41. Counahan R, et al. Prognosis of henoch-schönlein nephritis in children. Br Med J. 1977;2(6078):11–14.
42. Mandeville JT, et al. The tubulointerstitial nephritis and uveitis syndrome. Surv Ophthalmol. 2001;46(3):195–208.
43. Rosenbaum JT. Bilateral anterior uveitis and interstitial nephritis. Am J Ophthalmol. 1988;105(5):534–7.
44. Standardization of Uveitis Nomenclature (SUN) Working Group. Classification criteria for tubulointerstitial nephritis with uveitis syndrome. Am J Ophthalmol. 2021;228:255–61.
45. Takemura T, et al. Course and outcome of tubulointerstitial nephritis and uveitis syndrome. Am J Kidney Dis. 1999;34(6):1016–21. Erratum in: Am J Kidney Dis 2000 Mar;35(3):572.
46. Bakris GL, et al. Executive summary: Kidney Early Evaluation Program (KEEP) 2008 annual data report. Am J Kidney Dis. 2009;53(4 Suppl 4):S1–2.
47. Maliakkal JG, et al. Renal survival in children with glomerulonephritis with crescents: A pediatric nephrology research consortium cohort study. J Clin Med. 2020;9(8):2385.
48. Bayat A, et al. Characteristics and outcome of Goodpasture's disease in children. Clin Rheumatol. 2012;31(12):1745–51.
49. Lockwood CM, et al. Immunosuppression and plasma-exchange in the treatment of Goodpasture's syndrome. Lancet. 1976;1(7962):711–15.
50. Ponin L, et al. Long-term growth and final adult height outcome in childhood-onset systemic lupus erythematosus. Pediatr Rheumatol Online J. 2022;20(1):4.
51. Heshin-Bekenstein M, et al. Longitudinal disease- and steroid-related damage among adults with childhood-onset systemic lupus erythematosus. Semin Arthritis Rheum. 2019;49(2):267–72.
52. Buckley L, et al. 2017 American college of rheumatology guideline for the prevention and treatment of glucocorticoid-induced osteoporosis. Arthritis Rheumatol. 2017;69(8):1521–37. Epub 2017 Jun 6. Erratum in: Arthritis Rheumatol. 2017;69(11):2246.
53. Dooley MA, et al. Therapy insight: Preserving fertility in cyclophosphamide-treated patients with rheumatic disease. Nat Clin Pract Rheumatol. 2008;4(5):250–7.
54. Brungardt JG, et al. Fertility preservation in children and young adults with cancer. Curr Opin Pediatr. 2022;34(1):48–52.
55. Wetzels JF. Cyclophosphamide-induced gonadal toxicity: A treatment dilemma in patients with lupus nephritis? Neth J Med. 2004;62(10):347–52.
56. Nelson M, et al. Current issues in fertility preservation among pediatric and adolescent cancer patients. Curr Oncol Rep. 2023;25(7):793–802.
57. Kado R, et al. Ovarian protection with gonadotropin-releasing hormone agonists during cyclophosphamide therapy in systemic lupus erythematosus. Best Pract Res Clin Obstet Gynaecol. 2020;64:97–106.
58. Ejaz K, et al. Use of gonadotropin-releasing hormone agonists for ovarian preservation in patients receiving cyclophosphamide for systemic lupus erythematosus: A meta-analysis. Lupus. 2022;31(14):1706–13.
59. Cody E, et al. Kidney transplantation in pediatric patients with rheumatologic disorders. Curr Opin Pediatr. 2022;34(2):234–40.
60. den Bakker E, et al. Assessment of kidney function in children. Pediatr Clin North Am. 2022;69(6):1017–35.

61. Jančič SG, et al. Glomerular filtration rate assessment in children. Children (Basel). 2022;9(12):1995.

62. Schwartz GJ, et al. New equations to estimate GFR in children with CKD. J Am Soc Nephrol. 2009;20(3):629–37.

63. Centers for Disease Control and Prevention. (2023, August 1). *ACIP Altered Immunocompetence Guidelines for Immunizations.* Centers for Disease Control and Prevention. Available from: www.cdc.gov/vaccines/hcp/acip-recs/general-recs/immunocompetence.html.

64. Bass AR, et al. 2022 American college of rheumatology guideline for vaccinations in patients with rheumatic and musculoskeletal diseases. Arthritis Care Res (Hoboken). 2023;75(3):449–64.

65. Sousa S, et al. Efficacy and safety of vaccination in pediatric patients with systemic inflammatory rheumatic diseases: A systematic review of the literature. Acta Reumatol Port. 2017;42(1):8–16.

66. Foster BJ. Heightened graft failure risk during emerging adulthood and transition to adult care. Pediatr Nephrol. 2015;30(4):567–76.

PART II

KIDNEY DISEASE IN SPECIFIC RHEUMATIC DISEASES

5 Lupus Nephritis

Brian J. Skaggs, David Kellner, Jose M. Monroy Trujillo, and Maureen McMahon

5.1 INTRODUCTION

Lupus nephritis (LN), occurring in 50% of patients with systemic lupus erythematosus (SLE) and usually characterized as glomerulonephritis, is defined by immune complex deposition in glomeruli and tubules and often leads to the disruption and loss of kidney function. LN is observed in close to half of SLE patients and, as would be expected by the vital functions the kidneys perform, is a major contributor to SLE morbidity and mortality. We will discuss LN epidemiology, pathogenesis, LN classification, biomarkers, and current and future therapeutic options herein.

5.2 EPIDEMIOLOGY AND RISK FACTORS

LN is a frequent manifestation of systemic lupus erythematosus (SLE) that carries significant morbidity and mortality, requiring early recognition and treatment to improve outcomes. Renal involvement occurs in about 50% of patients with SLE (1). LN tends to occur early in the disease course, within 6 to 36 months of diagnosis, and may be the initial presentation of SLE (2). However, it can occur at any point in the disease. In a prospective cohort study of 1827 SLE patients, LN occurred in 38.3% of patients, with 80.9% of LN diagnoses occurring at enrollment and the remaining 19.1% of diagnoses occurring during follow-up (mean duration 4.6 years) (3). LN is more commonly diagnosed in childhood-onset SLE than adult-onset SLE, and risk decreases with age (4).

There is a higher incidence of LN in Black, Hispanic, and Asian patients compared to white patients, with incidences of 34–51%, 31–43%, 33–55%, and 14–23% respectively (5–8). This is due to a combination of genetic and socioeconomic factors (9, 10). Polymorphisms at several genetic loci have been implicated in LN risk, including *HLA-DRB1*, *PDGFRA*, *SLC5A11*, and *FcγRIIIa* (11–13). Some studies have associated increased risk of LN in Black patients with lower-binding-affinity alleles encoding the immunoglobulin Fc receptor FcγRIIIa; a proposed mechanism is that the lower binding affinity of this receptor results in the inadequate clearance of circulating immune complexes by macrophages (13, 14). In addition to having higher incidence of LN, Black and Hispanic patients present with more severe disease (as evidenced by renal pathology, serum creatinine, and proteinuria) and are at greater risk for disease progression than white patients (15). Risk factors for developing LN earlier in disease course include younger age at diagnosis, male sex, and non-white ethnicity (16).

Mortality is significantly higher in SLE patients with LN. In a large prospective cohort study, the age- and sex-adjusted hazard ratio of mortality in SLE patients with renal disease was 2.23 as compared to those without; this increased to 9.20 in patients with end-stage kidney disease (ESKD) (17). LN is also associated with significant morbidity—progression to ESKD occurs in 11%, 17%, and 22% of patients at 5, 10, and 15 years after diagnosis in developed countries, with higher rates in developing countries (18). The risk of progression to ESKD is highest in patients with class IV LN, with a 15-year risk of 44% in a meta-analysis of patients in the 2000s (18). Other patient characteristics associated with poor renal outcome include Black or Hispanic ancestry, pediatric onset, male sex, incomplete remission, relapsing disease, and proteinuria >4 g/day at diagnosis (19). Unfortunately, despite advances in treatments of LN, rates of complete remission are still relatively low (20, 21). Patients with complete renal response (CRR) have a better long-term prognosis than those with partial (PRR) or non-response; in one study, patients with CRR had 92% 10-year survival without ESKD, compared to 43% in those with PRR and only 13% in non-responders (22).

5.2.1 Clinical Presentation and Diagnosis

Abnormal proteinuria (>0.5 g per day) in a patient with SLE is the hallmark manifestation of LN, although it is neither sensitive nor specific on its own (23). The analysis of urine sediment can also support the diagnosis of LN. Specifically, the presence of red blood cell casts, white blood cell casts, dysmorphic red blood cells (acanthocytes), hematuria (>5 RBC/hpf), or leukocyturia (>5 WBC/hpf) in the absence of infection—collectively referred to as "active urinary sediment"—should raise suspicion for LN in a patient with SLE, especially if combined with the finding of abnormal proteinuria (23).

LN may present as a nephritic syndrome, nephrotic syndrome, or an overlap of the two. It can also be clinically silent, as evidenced by studies in which SLE patients without clinical signs of LN have undergone renal biopsy revealing LN activity (24). The true prevalence of silent LN is not

DOI: 10.1201/9781003438373-7

known but is thought to be common and may represent the earliest stage of LN that will subsequently become clinically manifest (24–26). Nephritic syndrome tends to present with hypertension, hematuria, and AKI, whereas nephrotic syndrome tends to present with nephrotic-range proteinuria (>3.5 g/day), peripheral edema, hypoalbuminemia, and hyperlipidemia (27). Nephrotic syndrome can also be caused by lupus podocytopathy, a nonimmune-complex-mediated process distinct from LN that is characterized by the effacement of podocyte foot processes on electron microscopy and tends to respond to corticosteroid monotherapy (28).

Acute kidney injury (AKI) is a common manifestation of LN, but the differential for AKI in a patient with SLE is broad. This includes volume depletion, sepsis, thrombosis (including thrombotic microangiopathy), nephrotoxin exposure (including iodinated contrast and medications such as nonsteroidal anti-inflammatory drugs, angiotensin-converting enzyme inhibitors/angiotensin receptor blockers, and calcineurin inhibitors), and non-SLE glomerular diseases (29). These causes should be excluded prior to attributing AKI to LN.

While the clinical diagnosis of LN requires only the presence of abnormal proteinuria or urinary casts in a patient with SLE, renal biopsy is the gold standard of diagnosis and is recommended for the confirmation of disease in all patients with clinical evidence of active LN that was previously untreated (23). Renal biopsy is necessary to verify LN, determine its class, and develop an appropriate treatment plan. In patients with a history of biopsy-proven LN, repeat renal biopsy may be indicated in several clinical situations. These include: 1) patients with a history of non-proliferative (class II or V) LN with clinically active LN, as recurrent disease commonly presents with a more aggressive LN class, necessitating a change in management; 2) patients with long-standing LN with ongoing proteinuria and/or AKI, as renal biopsy can differentiate active LN from chronic damage and thereby change management; 3) patients treated for LN who are in complete or partial remission, as renal biopsy can determine whether to continue or taper maintenance therapy (30). Renal biopsy may not be necessary in patients with active LN and a history of biopsy-proven proliferative (class III or IV) LLN, as recurrent LN is likely to be proliferative (31).

Current serum biomarkers used to aid in the detection of active LN include complement levels (decreased in active LN) and anti-double-stranded DNA (anti-dsDNA) antibodies (elevated in active LN) (32–34). Several studies have shown that elevated dsDNA antibody titers and low C3 and C4 can precede a flare of LN (34, 35). While these markers do correlate with renal disease activity, their sensitivity and specificity are poor to modest (36). There are ongoing efforts to develop more sensitive and specific non-invasive biomarkers for LN, but validation in prospective patient cohorts has proven challenging (37).

5.3 PATHOGENESIS OF LN

Immune complex deposition in glomeruli is generally considered the hallmark of LN. Autoantibodies that recognize DNA or other common nuclear proteins are retained by kidneys, whether by autoantibodies binding nuclear components directly, cross reacting with kidney specific autoantigens, or arriving in the kidney as large protein complexes already crosslinked with other autoantibodies through Fc receptor binding and/or complement. Before discussing mechanisms of immune complex-driven LN, however, other factors that predispose SLE patients to developing LN will be addressed.

5.3.1 Epidemiology

In the USA, males and Black, Hispanic, and Asian women are at a higher risk of developing LN than Caucasian patients, and worse outcomes such as increased proteinuria and renal failure are associated with the Black race and Hispanic ethnicity (15, 38–42). Patients diagnosed with SLE at younger ages are also at higher risk for developing LN (16, 41, 43). The risk of developing renal failure, not surprisingly, increases over time, with a recent study by Petri et al. showing a 20-year risk of renal failure at 8.4% with for SLE patients without renal failure at diagnosis and this risk is increased in patients who have a history of proteinuria at initial diagnosis, with a 20-year risk of renal failure of 20% (41, 44–46).

5.3.2 Genetics

A simple, linear genetic cause for a complex multiorgan disease such as SLE is improbable. Indeed, more than 100 risk loci for SLE have been identified by genome-wide association studies performed by many groups (47–49), with most risk alleles outside of HLA genes showing modest risk when analyzed independently. LN-specific risk alleles have been identified in recent years, and most have already been implicated in general SLE, whether as associated SNPs, relevant proteins, or both:

BAFF/BLyS (50, 51), apolipoprotein L1 (52), PDGFRα (12), ITGAM/CD11b (53–55), STAT4 (56), neutrophil cytosolic factor 2 (57), IRF5-TNPO3 (57, 58), TNIP/ABIN1 (59), and Fcγ receptors (60, 61).

Epigenetic changes are associated with SLE, with many differences noted in DNA methylation and histone methylation/acetylation across the genome (62). Studies focusing on DNA methylation in patients with LN suggest that type 1 interferon-regulated genes (including IFI44 and IFIT1) as well as HIF3A, a key hypoxia regulator, have differentially methylated promoters and/or genes in LN (63). Decreases in histone methylation are associated with early LN, while global dendritic cell hypermethylation was observed in advanced LN (64). Lower methylation levels around type 1 interferon-regulated genes distinguished LN patients of European ancestry from SLE patients without LN; although Black patients also had these epigenetic changes, they did not correlate with LN (65).

Alterations of noncoding RNA (ncRNA) levels, including microRNA (miRNA), long noncoding RNA (lncRNA), ribosomal RNA (rRNA), and piwi-interacting RNA (piRNA), have also been noted in both SLE and LN-specific contexts in recent years. Standard qPCR as well as next-generation sequencing studies have pointed to multiple altered ncRNA molecules in LN patients, including but not limited to miR124–3p, miR126, miR132, miR-146a, miR148a, LINC01015, LINC01986, NRIR, and TUG1 (66–74). Mechanistic studies of ncRNA affecting LN appear to be in their infancy, although TGFβ (70) and TLR4 (75) have been suggested as possible targets for ncRNA regulation as well as for therapeutics.

5.3.3 Immune Cells

Myeloid cell and lymphocyte infiltrations of kidney tissue are also considered hallmarks of LN pathogenesis. Immune cell infiltrates are frustratingly heterogenic in LN patients, preventing a unified therapeutic approach. There are multiple ways in which immune cells promote LN, including cytotoxicity, increased immune responses such as local autoantibody production, and the secretion of effector molecules.

5.3.3.1 Lymphocytes

T cells are more commonly observed than B cells and are found in various stages of organization in kidney biopsies (76–79). Most B and T cell subtypes infiltrate tissue, although specific functionalities are not clear. Increased CD8+ T cells are associated with more severe nephritis as well as positive treatment response (80). B cells isolated from LN kidneys sometimes show clonal expansion, possibly due to autoantigens present in the kidney (81), and CD27-IgD-T-bet+ B cells appear to be common in LN (77).

5.3.3.2 Myeloid Cells

Monocyte and macrophage kidney infiltration is associated with LN initiation and progression. Proinflammatory macrophages, usually identified by high transcript levels of inflammatory cytokines, are present in LN biopsies (77, 82). Various macrophage phenotypes appear to exist on a proinflammatory continuum from anti-inflammatory macrophage to proinflammatory myofibroblast, and these phenotypes probably reflect their local cytokine environment in the kidney and correlate with sclerosis and fibrosis (83–86).

Dendritic cells (DCs) in the kidney are also a heterogeneous resident cell population in normal kidneys that mature to proinflammatory cells in the context of LN (87). Plasmacytoid DCs (pDCs) are known to produce IFNα in SLE, and high systemic IFNα correlates with LN severity (88, 89). Work by the Clark lab illustrates that pDCs are important antigen-presenting cells in LN (90). A recent study suggests that pDCs in the kidney do not colocalize with a specific IFNα-induced transcript, suggesting but not confirming that renal resident pDCs might not be the main source of LN-driving IFNα (89).

Neutrophils, the most abundant white blood cell type, are known to infiltrate kidneys in LN and release both IFNα and neutrophil extracellular traps (NETs) (91, 92). Recent work identified elevated levels of the NET component defensin-α3 in LN kidneys (93). In addition, serum levels of the NET-associated protein–DNA complexes elastase–DNA and HMGB1–DNA were significantly higher in patients with proliferative LN and correlated with LN progression (94), suggesting that neutrophils and NETs contribute to LN through multiple mechanisms (79).

5.3.4 Endoplasmic Reticulum Stress

The endoplasmic reticulum (ER) is, in addition to being the largest eukaryotic organelle, the center for multiple crucial processes, including the synthesis, folding, and transport of proteins, lipids, and steroids (95). ER stress is induced in SLE, often through the production of autoantibodies, and appears to be an underappreciated driver of multiple SLE comorbidities (96, 97). ER stress has been observed in all immune cell types mentioned earlier, as well as in glomerular, tubular, and podocyte kidney cells (98), suggesting that ER stress inhibitors could be other pathways to target when treating LN.

5.3.5 Immune Complex Deposition

5.3.5.1 Glomerulonephritis

Traditionally, LN and glomerulonephritis have been treated as interchangeable terms. As stated earlier, glomeruli-deposited immune complexes and mesangial cell proliferation essentially define LN (42). Mesangial cells also produce TGFβ1-induced metalloproteinases and extracellular matrix proteins that are believed to contribute to chronic glomerulonephritis (99). Immune complex deposits in glomerular podocytes are the major cause of proteinuria through basement membrane alterations, in part due to aberrant nestin, nephrin, and IFNα expression (100, 101) and inflammasome activation (102).

5.3.5.2 Tubulointerstitial Inflammation

Tubulointerstitial immune complexes are noted in about 30 percent of LN patients and are often associated with more advanced disease (103). In contrast to glomerulonephritis, tubulointerstitial inflammation resembles germinal centers and other secondary lymphoid organ structures (104). Most B cells in the interstitial space appear to recognize the structural filament protein vimentin, and these anti-vimentin antibodies correlate with increased tubulointerstitial disease and a poor response to mycophenolate (MMF)/MMF plus rituximab (105). In addition, T follicular helper cells provide help to B cells and can cause full costimulatory activation and differentiation in the interstitium (42, 106), suggesting that tubulointerstitial inflammation also significantly contributes to LN.

5.3.5.3 Immune Complexes

Autoantibody immune complexes that recognize multiple antigens are deposited in the kidneys, and a full understanding of pathogenic immune complexes in LN eludes researchers at this time (107). Although anti-dsDNA immune complexes are commonly observed in both glomeruli and in the circulation, these autoantibodies are not universally observed in LN (108, 109). Autoantibody cross reactivity to glomerular basement membrane components such as chromatin, collagen, heparan sulfate proteoglycan, laminin, fibronectin, and alpha-actinin also occurs in murine and human LN (110–112).

Immune complex deposition can be initiated and compounded by a multitude of factors. Large renal capillary beds and direct blood flow from the heart to the kidneys increase immune complex presence. A variety of proinflammatory cytokines are also upregulated in the serum, including IFNα, IL-1B, IL-6, IL-8, IL-37, and IL-17A (113). Autoantibodies with positively charged amino acids (arginine, lysine, histidine) in their antigen-binding regions, class-switched autoantibodies that bind Fc receptors, the physical size of the immune complex, and resistance to proteases and nucleases all contribute to increased deposition (114–116). Antibodies to complement components also alter complement cascades, leading to higher autoantigen presence, excessive uncontrolled inflammation, and breaks in tolerance. Autoantibodies against C1q, the first component of the classical complement pathway, are associated with LN severity, and anti-C1q antibodies are directly involved in renal damage, whether due to C1q binding in the circulation or direct anti-C1q binding in glomerular tissue after C1q is recruited to the kidneys to clear initial damage (117–119). Further discussion of anti-C1q antibodies continues in the Biomarkers section 2.5.

5.4 BIOPSY CLASSIFICATION AND HISTOPATHOLOGY

LN can be the initial manifestation of SLE. In a recent study, renal involvement occurred in about 38% of SLE patients (3). LN carries significant morbidity and mortality, with a 10-year survival of 70% and 13% of patients progressing to ESKD (120). A kidney biopsy is necessary to establish the diagnosis of LN. While it is an invasive procedure, major complications defined as bleeding requiring intervention, hypotension requiring vasopressors, and upgrading the patient to a higher level of care, occurred only in 2.7% of patients (121).

One of the first LN pathological classifications was the World Health Organization (WHO) classification in 1974 (122). This classification was based only on glomerular lesions. In the following years, the International Society of Nephrology/Renal Pathology Society (ISN/RPS) introduced changes to the original classification (123).

The ISN/RPS classification includes six classes based on histopathology:

(1) *Minimal mesangial lupus nephritis (class I)*: Normal light microscopy. There are mesangial immune deposits but no mesangial cell hypercellularity. No incursion of leukocytes in mesangium. Not seen often, as patients may have a low degree of proteinuria and kidney biopsy may not be considered. It is mostly treated with steroids.

(2) *Mesangial proliferative lupus nephritis (class II)*: Mesangial immune deposits associated with mesangial hypercellularity defined as 4 cells, excluding and perihilar areas. No incursion of leukocytes. There are no subendothelial deposits. Usually associated with subnephrotic-range proteinuria and carries a good prognosis most of the time.

(3) *Focal lupus nephritis (class III)*: Less than 50% of the glomeruli seen are affected. It is associated with endocapillary hypercellularity. There are immune deposits in the subendothelial and mesangial region. Crescents and fibrinoid necrosis can be present. There are parameters to establish activity and chronicity (124, 125).

   a. *Modified NIH activity index (0–24)*: 1) Endocapillary hypercellularity, 2) neutrophils/karyorrhexis, 3) fibrinoid necrosis, 4) hyaline deposits, 5) cellular/fibrocellular crescents, 6) interstitial inflammation.

   b. *Modified NIH chronicity index (0–12)*: 1) Total glomerulosclerosis score, 2) fibrous crescents, 3) tubular atrophy, 4) interstitial fibrosis.

(4) *Diffuse lupus nephritis (class IV)*: Similar findings as class III but more than 50% of the glomeruli are involved. This represents the most active form of lupus nephritis and carries the worst prognosis. Class III and class IV lupus nephritis are treated similarly. They represent aggressive forms of lupus nephritis. Same classification for activity and chronicity index.

(5) *Lupus membranous nephropathy (class V)*: Accounts for 10–20% of cases. It is characterized by subepithelial immune deposits and podocyte foot process effacement. It can be seen in combination with class III or class IV. The main difference between primary membranous nephropathy and class V lupus nephritis is that primary can be positive for PLA2R antibody, and IgG subclasses are typically predominant for IgG4. In addition, there are usually no mesangial deposits. In class V lupus nephritis, it is common to see mesangial deposits in addition to subepithelial (126). More recently, circulating antibodies against exostosin 1 and exostosin 2 (EXT1/EXT2) have been associated with membranous LN. They were linked to good prognosis (127, 128).

(6) *Advanced sclerosis lupus nephritis (class VI)*: When global sclerotic glomeruli are seen. It may be removed in future classifications.

One of the most recent revisions occurred in 2018 (129). This classification had the following updates: 1) The term endocapillary proliferation was removed, and endocapillary hypercellularity was introduced. 2) Active lesions for class III and IV now include an activity and chronicity score. It is important to mention that there can be a switch in the class of LN—in up to 55% of cases—and repeat kidney biopsies may be necessary (30).

An important characteristic of the immunofluorescence pattern seen across all LN classes is that it is usually positive for the immunoglobulin (IgG, IgM, IgA) and for the complement proteins (C3 and C1q) (130). A "full-house pattern" is commonly used to describe this phenomenon (123, 131). Additional common features found in kidney biopsies in LN patients include tubular reticular inclusion bodies in endothelial cells (132). They are seen in about 50% of patients with LN, particularly those with anti-SSB antibodies.

5.5 BIOMARKERS OF LUPUS NEPHRITIS

Given the poor long-term outcomes in many patients with LN, there is a need for early biomarkers to help predict which patients are at risk for poor response. Traditional biomarkers of disease activity such as C3, C4, and proteinuria can be useful for predicting outcomes. For example, several studies have shown that a reduction in proteinuria to 0.7 or 0.8 g/day by the end of 1 year of treatment is associated with good long-term kidney outcomes (133–135). In one study by Dall'Era et al., the normalization of C3 and/or C4, and/or a reduction in proteinuria by ≥25%, by week 8 was predictive of renal response at week 24 (OR 3.2, $P < 0.05$) (136). However, current markers of renal response are sometimes disconnected from underlying histopathology. Urine sediment can be helpful for monitoring renal disease in SLE patients; renal inflammation, suggested by the presence of white blood cell casts and red blood cell casts, can indicate glomerular bleeding. However, the identification of cellular casts depends upon the quality and freshness of the urine sample as well as the skill of the reader, and results can be inconsistent (137). The inclusion of urinary RBCs was found to decrease the predictive value of trial data; therefore, this is no longer recommended as a trial outcome (133, 134)

Proteinuria can reflect active renal inflammation but can also occur with chronic damage (138). In one study comparing serial renal biopsies to biomarkers of response, 62% of patients with complete histologic remission after induction therapy still had persistent proteinuria. Conversely, nearly one-third of patients who achieved a clinical complete renal response after induction treatment still had high histologic activity on repeat biopsy (139). Thus, there is an unmet need for non-invasive LN biomarkers that can more accurately predict disease activity and outcomes. Although numerous serum and urinary biomarkers have been studied, there are currently no novel biomarkers of nephritis that are widely clinically available. While more research in this area is clearly needed, some of the more promising biomarkers will be highlighted herein.

5.5.1 Serum Biomarkers

5.5.1.1 Autoantibodies

C1q is the first component of the classic complement system and is instrumental for the clearance of immune complexes and apoptotic bodies. Anti-C1q antibodies have been identified in several studies and meta-analyses as potential biomarkers for the diagnosis of nephritis in patients with SLE (140, 141). Multiple studies have found an association between C1q antibodies and the presence of nephritis in SLE patients (142–144). The presence of anti-C1q antibodies 3–6 months prior was also found in one study to predict nephritis flares (145). Another longitudinal study found that the combination of anti-C1q and anti-dsDNA antibodies predicted poor renal outcomes (146). One systematic review by Wang et al. included only studies conducted in the Chinese population and found the summary receiver operating characteristic curve (SROC-AUC) for anti-C1q antibodies to be 0.749 (147).

5.5.1.2 Cytokines

A high type I IFN gene signature has been implicated in the pathogenesis of SLE and LN (88, 148, 149). Single-cell RNAseq performed on renal biopsies of patients with LN found that a high IFN responsive signature and a fibrotic signature in renal tubular cells were both associated with poor response to therapy (82). Surrogate markers of IFN response have also been studied as potential biomarkers for LN. CXC-motif chemokine ligand 10 has been shown to correlate with both SLE disease activity and nephritis flares (150). B-cell activating factor (BAFF/BLyS) is important for B-cell differentiation and is also regulated by types I and II IFN. The high expression of BAFF in kidney biopsies was associated with proliferative GN and was correlated with disease activity index (151). Reduced serum baseline levels of BAFF were associated with clinical response in proliferative LN, with a 92% PPV (152). Urinary levels of BAFF were also higher in patients with proliferative LN than in lupus patients with no renal involvement, with an AUC of 0.825 (153).

5.5.2 Urinary Biomarkers

Monocyte chemoattractant protein-1 (MCP1) is a chemokine that functions to recruit leukocytes (113). Urinary levels of MCP1 (uMCP1) have been found to differentiate between active LN and non-nephritis and to correlate with the activity index on renal biopsy (154, 155). In one longitudinal study, uMCP1 was a better predictor of active nephritis than serum MCP-1, anti-dsDNA antibodies, C3, and C4 (156). Levels of uMCP1 also appear to rise 2–4 months prior to the clinical onset of LN (157). In a meta-analysis, uMCP1 levels had a sensitivity of 89% and a specificity of 63% in differentiating active LN from inactive disease, and the SROC-AUC was 0.90 (158).

Tumor necrosis factor-like weak inducer of apoptosis (TWEAK) is a proinflammatory cytokine and member of the tumor necrosis factor family. TWEAK is secreted primarily by monocytes and macrophages and has been found in several studies to be involved in the pathogenesis of auto-immune diseases, including those with neurological, vascular, and renal involvement (147, 159). Several studies have demonstrated higher uTWEAK levels in patients with active vs. inactive LN (160–162). Another longitudinal study found that when combined with proteinuria, uTWEAK levels at 3 months predicted complete response at 6 months, with an ROC-AUC of 0.83 (163). In one systematic review, Wang et al. found a pooled sensitivity for the role of uTWEAK in diagnosing

LN of 55%, with a specificity of 92%, and SROC-AUC of 0.822. They also examined the role of uTWEAK in the detection of LN and found a sensitivity of 91%, specificity of 70%, and SROC-AUC of 0.813 (164).

Neutrophil gelatinase-associated lipocalin (NGAL) is an acute-phase glycoprotein secreted by neutrophils, macrophages, hepatocytes, adipocytes, neurons, and epithelial cells. In one longitudinal study of childhood SLE, uNGAL was useful for predicting the worsening of LN (165). A recent systematic review and meta-analysis by Gao et al. (166) found that for the diagnosis of LN, uNGAL had a pooled sensitivity of 84% and a specificity of 91%, with an SROC-AUC of 0.92 (95% CI 0.90–0.94). For the detection of active nephritis, the sensitivity of uNGAL was 72% and the specificity was 71%, with an SROC-AUC of 0.77 (95% CI 0.74–0.81). For predicting renal flare, uNGAL had a sensitivity of 80% and a specificity of 67% (160), with an AUC value of 0.74 (95% CI 0.70–0.78) (166).

Multiple adhesion molecules have been associated with LN, including vascular cell adhesion molecule (VCAM) and activated leukocyte cell adhesion molecule (ALCAM). Both uVCAM 1 and uALCAM have been able to distinguish SLE patients with active LN from those with no disease activity (154, 167), and uVCAM-1 had a 91% sensitivity and 76% specificity for the prediction of renal function deterioration within 10 years of follow-up (167).

There has been some interest in combining biomarkers into panels that may be more predictive than individual biomarkers alone. In a pediatric LN a panel of six urinary biomarkers named the RAIL panel (NGAL, MCP-1, ceruloplasmin, adiponectin, hemopexin, and KIM-1) was associated with histologic renal activity, with an AUC of 0.92 (168). The RAIL panel was also used in a longitudinal pediatric study to predict the response to therapy at 3 months, with an AUC of 0.92 (169). In addition, RAIL scores decreased in complete responders to induction therapy but did not change or increased in partial responders and non-responders, respectively (170). One study also validated the use of RAIL as a biomarker panel for the prediction of LN in an adult cohort, although the predictive value was improved with the alternative weighting of the biomarkers (171).

As technology and the ability to perform multiomics improves, it is likely that additional biomarkers for nephritis will be identified. Recently, the Accelerating Medicines Partnership in RA/SLE multicenter cohort study examined the urinary proteome from over 220 SLE subjects. They found that urinary biomarkers of monocyte/neutrophil degranulation (i.e., PR3, S100A8, azurocidin, catalase, cathepsins, MMP8), macrophage activation (i.e., CD163, CD206, galectin-1), wound healing/matrix degradation (i.e., nidogen-1, decorin), and IL-16 were significantly correlated with proliferative LN and histological activity on renal biopsy. A decline in these biomarkers after three months of treatment predicted the 1-year response more robustly than proteinuria, including CD206 (AUC 0.91), EGFR (AUC 0.9), and CD163 (AUC 0.89) compared to proteinuria (AUC 0.8) (172). As these and other biomarkers are validated in future studies, they will hopefully become widely available for use in the clinic, but at the present time, these biomarkers and panels are only used in research studies.

5.6 TREATMENT OF LN

5.6.1 Mycophenolate Mofetil

Mycophenolate (MMF, CellCept) acts as an immunosuppressant in LN by blocking guanosine synthesis in lymphoid cells after conversion to the active metabolite mycophenolic acid (173). MMF also inhibits renal mesangial/smooth muscle/fibroblast cell proliferation as well as preventing dendritic cell maturation (174).

Data from the Aspreva Lupus Management Study (ALMS) trial illustrated that MMF was not inferior to cyclophosphamide therapy (175). The ALMS trial, it is worth noting, was only powered to prove non-inferiority (not superiority) to cyclophosphamide. Subgroup post-hoc analysis, however, did show the superiority of MMF over cyclophosphamide (61% to 39%) in self-described Hispanic and Black patients (176). These results are similar to an earlier study by the Hong Kong-Guangzhou Nephrology Study Group (177) but differ from the 2005 Ginzler et al. study in a smaller cohort that suggested that MMF was superior in efficacy and side effect profile to cyclophosphamide, although superiority was not the specified endpoint (178).

Even though cyclophosphamide has documented side effects such as premature ovarian failure, bladder toxicity, and hair loss, the ALMS trial failed to show significant differences in MMF adverse events versus cyclophosphamide. Gastrointestinal complaints and anemia were issues in patients taking MMF (179, 180). In addition, MMF was shown to be superior to azathioprine in maintenance therapy/preventing the relapse of LN (21), although it is worth keeping in mind that azathioprine is safe to use during pregnancy, but MMF is not (181).

5.6.2 Cyclophosphamide

Phosphoramide mustard, the active form of cyclophosphamide (Cytoxan), alkylates nucleic acids and prevents the proliferation of white blood cells. The initial longitudinal report illustrating that cyclophosphamide plus glucocorticoid treatment was superior to glucocorticoids alone in reducing end-stage renal disease in LN was published in 1986 and included patients followed since the late 1960s (182). Subsequent reports utilizing the same cohort established at the National Institutes of Health suggested that the enhanced benefits of cyclophosphamide plus glucocorticoids over steroids alone takes a number of years to observe (183–185).

European medical centers in the 1990s began using lower doses of cyclophosphamide (3 g cumulative dose administered IV; referred to as "Euro-Lupus") in combination with azathioprine. Data suggest that in the Euro-Lupus Nephritis Trial (ELNT), Euro-Lupus was just as effective at achieving remission and preventing LN flares as higher doses used previously in the NIH studies (186). Longitudinal results in the same ELNT cohort confirmed Euro-Lupus was effective long-term in preventing LN in patients that responded early in treatment as measured by lower proteinuria (133, 187).

Concerns about the mostly Caucasian ethnic and racial makeup of the original ELNT cohort were somewhat alleviated with slightly differently designed studies successfully using Euro-Lupus to treat LN in Southeast Asian patients (188–190) and the North American ACCESS study with high percentages of Hispanic (41%) and Black (37%) patients (191). A Japanese study did not note any differences in complete renal response rates in ELNT cyclophosphamide-treated patients versus high-dose cyclophosphamide, MMF, or tacrolimus (192).

5.6.3 Belimumab

In 2011, belimumab (Benlysta) became the first medication approved for the treatment of SLE since the approval of hydroxychloroquine in 1958. Belimumab targets the B-cell survival cytokine BAFF, resulting in autoreactive B-cell apoptosis (193). As noted earlier, the increased expression of BAFF has also been seen in renal biopsy tissue from LN patients, and high levels are associated with LN activity (194, 195)

The BLISS-LN trial was a phase III, multinational, multicenter, randomized, double-blind, placebo-controlled, 104-week trial of 448 LN patients designed to assess the efficacy and safety of belimumab plus standard therapy with either MMF or Euro-Lupus for induction therapy, followed by azathioprine for maintenance (196). Patients with SLE were included in the trial if they had a urine protein/creatinine ratio of ≥1 and biopsy-confirmed ISN/RPS 2003 (197) class III or IV LN with or without coexisting class V LN or pure class V LN within 6 months before or during screening. High-dose glucocorticoids were administered as part of the induction regimen but had to be tapered to ≤10 mg/day by week 24 (196). The study met its primary endpoint, the primary efficacy renal response (PERR), at week 104, as significantly more patients in the belimumab group than in the placebo group demonstrated a PERR (43% vs. 32%; odds ratio, 1.6; 95% confidence interval [CI], 1.0 to 2.3). Patients in the belimumab arm were also more likely to have a complete renal response (30% vs. 20%; odds ratio [OR], 1.7; 95% CI, 1.1 to 2.7), and the risk of a renal-related event or death was lower among patients who received belimumab than among those who received standard therapy alone (hazard ratio (HR), 0.51; 95% CI, 0.34 to 0.77). The safety profile of belimumab was consistent with that in previous trials (196). In a post-hoc analysis of the BLISS-LN trial data, Rovin et al. found that belimumab reduced the risk of an LN flare by 55% relative to standard therapy alone (hazard ratio [95% confidence interval] 0.45 [0.28–0.72]). Belimumab also significantly reduced the risk of a sustained 30% or 40% decline in estimated glomerular filtration rate (eGFR) versus standard treatment alone and attenuated the annual rate of eGFR decline in patients. Interestingly, belimumab was found to be most effective in achieving PERR and CRR in patients with proliferative LN and in those with a baseline urine protein/creatinine ratio under 3 g/g. There was no observed improvement in the renal response with belimumab treatment in patients with LN and subepithelial deposits or with a baseline protein/creatinine ratio of 3 g/g or more (197).

5.6.4 Calcineurin Inhibitors

Voclosporin (Lupkynis) is the first calcineurin inhibitor that is FDA approved for the treatment of LN. Voclosporin is structurally similar to cyclosporine, with a methyl group added to the amino acid 1 residue. The addition of the methyl group results in a molecule that has a stable pharmacodynamic and pharmacokinetic profile and does not require drug level monitoring (198). In addition, voclosporin does not interact with MMF and has a lower risk of glucose intolerance and lipid disorders than cyclosporine (199).

Voclosporin was studied in the AURORA trial, a multicenter, randomized, double- blinded, placebo-controlled trial of voclosporin 23.7 mg BID or placebo on a background of MMF 1 g BID (200). All patients were administered a pulse of IV steroids as part of their induction regimen, but this was followed by a rapid taper of oral corticosteroids to 2.5 mg by week 16. Patients with SLE were included in the trial if they had biopsy-confirmed ISN/RPS 2003 (197) class III or IV LN with or without coexisting class V LN or pure class V LN within 2 years before or during screening and a urine protein/creatinine ratio of ≥1.5 mg/mg (or ≥2 mg/mg if pure class V). Patients who had a kidney biopsy more than 6 months before screening were required to have at least a doubling in uPCR in the 6 months before screening. Patients were excluded if their eGFR was 45 mL/minute per 1.73 m^2 or less at screening (200).

The study met its primary end point, complete renal response at 52 weeks, in 41% of the voclosporin group vs. 23% in the MMF group (OR 2.65; 95% CI 1.64–4.27). The secondary endpoint of partial renal response at 52 weeks was also met (70% vs. 52%, OR 2.26 (95% CI 1.45–3.51). The mean time to reduction in proteinuria to ≤0.5 mg/mg was 169 days in the voclosporin group compared to 372 days in the MMF group (HR 2.02, 95% CI 1.51–2.7) (200). Side effects were balanced between the groups. There was a slight decrease in mean eGFR seen in the voclosporin group, consistent with the known effects of calcineurin inhibitors (201), but this reduction was mild and occurred soon after the initiation of voclosporin, without further decreases.

The calcineurin inhibitor tacrolimus (Prograf, Advagraf, Envarsus) has also been studied in LN, primarily in studies performed in Asian cohorts. In one randomized trial, tacrolimus induction therapy was compared to MMF. All responders were switched to azathioprine for maintenance therapy. At 1 year, nearly 60% of patients in both groups achieved the primary endpoint of renal response defined as <1 g/day of proteinuria (202). In this study, 12% of tacrolimus patients (and none of the MMF treated patients) had a transient increase in SCr and no improvement of CrCl at 6 months, raising some concern for nephrotoxicity, which has previously been associated with calcineurin inhibitors (202). In the 10-year follow-up of the study participants, rates of overall renal flare and the progression of renal disease were similar between the two groups, although rates of "proteinuric flare" were higher in the tacrolimus group (203). Another open label non-inferiority trial in 314 Chinese LN patients compared tacrolimus to IV cyclophosphamide (204). The overall response rates at 6 months were similar in both groups (83% vs. 75%), but the rate of serious adverse events was lower in the tacrolimus group (204).

5.6.5 Rituximab

Rituximab (Rituxan) is a mouse/human chimeric type I anti-CD20 monoclonal antibody that induces B-cell lysis mediated by complement and Fc receptor-bearing cytotoxic cells and by induced programmed cell death (205). Rituximab did not meet its primary endpoint in the phase III LUNAR trial in LN patients (206). However, several case series and small randomized trials demonstrated that rituximab has some efficacy in treating refractory LN, especially cases resistant to cyclophosphamide and MMF (207). There has also been some interest in combining rituximab with belimumab, with the goal of preventing the expansion of autoreactive B cells by high levels of BAFF resulting from B-cell depletion (208). The phase II CALIBRATE trial studied 43 patients with recurrent or refractory LN at 24–48 weeks of treatment with cyclophosphamide, prednisone, and rituximab, followed by maintenance therapy with or without belimumab. The trial was powered to be a safety trial, and no significant differences in adverse outcomes were noted between the groups. Clinical efficacy was not different between the groups but reduced the maturation of transitional to naïve B cells and enhanced censoring of autoreactive B cells were noted in the belimumab group (209).

5.6.6 Novel Therapeutics on the Horizon

There are multiple new therapies currently being studied in LN, targeting many novel relevant pathways, including co-stimulation pathways, complement inhibition, plasma cell inhibition, and antibody clearance (210, 211). Several molecules highlighted herein are currently in phase III trials.

B-cell targets continue to be attractive for the treatment of LN. Obinutuzumab is a type II anti-CD20 humanized monoclonal antibody that targets CD20 with better antibody-dependent cellular cytotoxicity and phagocytosis than rituximab (212). The phase II NOBILITY trial was designed to evaluate the safety and efficacy of obinutuzumab in 125 participants with active LN who received 1000 mg obinutuzumab or placebo in combination with MMF and corticosteroids. More patients treated with obinutuzumab achieved a complete renal response (CRR) at week 52 (primary endpoint: 22 [35%] vs. 14 [23%] with placebo; 95% confidence interval [CI] −3.4% to 28%; $p = 0.115$) and at week 104 (213). Because of these promising and encouraging outcomes in phase II, the phase III trials are ongoing (NCT04221477).

Ianalumab, an anti-BAFF receptor mAb, is also currently in phase III (SIRIUS-LN) trials (NCT05126277). It is a human IgG1/κ monoclonal antibody with dual mechanisms of action, including competitive inhibition of BAFF:BAFFR signaling and antibody-dependent cellular cytotoxicity (214). It has also shown promise in phase II trials in Sjögren's syndrome (215).

As noted earlier, type I IFN has been implicated in the pathogenesis of LN and SLE. Anifrolumab is a human monoclonal antibody targeting the type I IFN receptor (IFNAR) (216). Anifrolumab was approved for the treatment of moderate to severe SLE in 2021 (217). The phase II TULIP LN trial examined the efficacy and safety of anifrolumab plus MMF at a standard dose (300 mg IV monthly) or intensive dose (900 mg IV · 3, then 300 mg IV monthly) vs. MMF alone. Although none of the arms reached the primary endpoint, the intensive anifrolumab was numerically superior to the MMF alone group (218). Anifrolumab is currently being further studied in the IRIS phase III LN trial (NCT05138133).

5.7 GUIDELINES FOR LN

The American College of Rheumatology has not published guidelines for LN since 2012 (23) and does not include many of the newer medications that have subsequently been approved for LN (Table 5.1). However, the backbone of induction and maintenance therapy that is proposed for LN is still relevant today. For patients with proliferative nephritis, the ACR guidelines recommend that all patients receive an IV steroid pulse, followed by 0.5–1 mg/kg prednisone. Induction therapy recommendations include either MMF 2000–3000 mg daily or cyclophosphamide (either higher dose or Euro-Lupus regimen), followed by maintenance therapy. For maintenance therapy, MMF is superior to azathioprine (21), and should be continued for at least 2–3 years. For patients with pure class V LN and with nephrotic-range proteinuria, the ACR guidelines recommended that patients be started on prednisone (0.5 mg/kg/day) plus MMF 2–3 g total daily dose.

Adjunctive treatments recommended for all patients with proteinuria >500 mg/24 hours include a blockade of the renin–angiotensin system with ACE inhibitors or angiotensin receptor blockers, which reduces proteinuria by approximately 30% and significantly delays the doubling of serum creatinine and progression to ESKD in patients with chronic renal disease (but should not be used in pregnant patients) (219). All patients should have blood pressure controlled, with a target blood pressure of <130/80 (220). Statin therapy is recommended in patients with low-density lipoprotein cholesterol >100 mg/dL (23). It is also recommended that all patients take hydroxychloroquine unless contraindicated (221).

The new 2024 EULAR guidelines for the management of SLE recommend similar induction therapy to the ACR guidelines (glucocorticoids plus either MMF or monthly IV or Euro-Lupus cyclophosphamide). The guidelines also recommend that combination therapy with belimumab (either with cyclophosphamide or MMF) or calcineurin inhibitors (especially voclosporin or tacrolimus, combined with MMF) should be considered (222). The EULAR treatment guidelines also recommend a therapeutic target of at least 25% proteinuria reduction within 3 months and at least 50% reduction by 6 months after initiating treatment, with a target proteinuria ratio of <0.5–0.7 mg/mg within the first year of treatment (222).

Similar to the 2024 EULAR guidelines, the Kidney Disease–Improving Global Outcomes (KDIGO) guidelines recommend that for induction therapy for patients with proliferative nephritis, patients should be treated with glucocorticoids at lower doses than traditional regimens (0.25–0.5 g/day IV for 1–3 days, then prednisone 0.35–1 mg/kg/day and taper over a few months) plus either mycophenolic acid analogs alone or in combination with either belimumab or a calcineurin inhibitor (voclosporin or tacrolimus), cyclophosphamide (either IV monthly or Euro-Lupus regimen), or Euro-Lupus plus belimumab (223). The guidelines strongly recommend tapering corticosteroids to <7.5 mg/day by 3–6 months (223).

Table 5.1: Factors to Consider When Using US FDA-Approved Drugs in LN

Clinical Attributes	Voclosporin	Belimumab
Kidney function	Use cautiously if GFR <45 mL/ minute per 1.73 m²	May be used if GFR is at least 30 mg/ minute per 1.73 m²; may slow decline of GFR (200)
Kidney histology	Use cautiously if widespread sclerotic and/or fibrotic changes occur	-
Proteinuria	Effective at any level of proteinuria; may be especially effective in patients with severe proteinuria with significant podocyte damage	More effective if proteinuria is <3 g/day
High risk of disease flare	No effect on flare rate	May decrease risk of severe flares
Background immunosuppression	Not tested in combination with cyclophosphamide	Effective in combination with MMF; uncertain effectiveness in combination with cyclophosphamide
Need for parenteral therapy	Oral only	IV/SC
Significant extrarenal lupus	Efficacy to be determined	Long track record of efficacy
Safety	Add-on therapy did not increase incidence of adverse events; monitor acute GFR variations with voclosporin	Add-on therapy did not increase incidence of adverse events
Pregnancy	Use not recommended (consider tacrolimus)	Use not recommended

Source: Adapted from (223)

REFERENCES

1. Almaani S, et al. Update on lupus nephritis. Clin J Am Soc Nephrol. 2017;12(5):825–35.
2. Parikh SV, et al. Update on lupus nephritis: Core curriculum 2020. Am J Kidney Dis. 2020;76(2):265–81.
3. Hanly JG, et al. The frequency and outcome of lupus nephritis: Results from an international inception cohort study. Rheumatology (Oxford). 2016;55(2):252–62.
4. Hiraki LT, et al. Prevalence, incidence, and demographics of systemic lupus erythematosus and lupus nephritis from 2000 to 2004 among children in the US Medicaid beneficiary population. Arthritis Rheum. 2012;64(8):2669–76.
5. Lim SS, et al. The incidence and prevalence of systemic lupus erythematosus, 2002–2004: The Georgia lupus registry. Arthritis Rheumatol. 2014;66(2):357–68.
6. Somers EC, et al. Population-based incidence and prevalence of systemic lupus erythematosus: The Michigan lupus epidemiology and surveillance program. Arthritis Rheumatol. 2014;66(2):369–78.
7. Izmirly PM, et al. The incidence and prevalence of systemic lupus erythematosus in New York County (Manhattan), New York: The Manhattan lupus surveillance program. Arthritis Rheumatol. 2017;69(10):2006–17.
8. Dall'Era M, et al. The incidence and prevalence of systemic lupus erythematosus in San Francisco County, California: The California lupus surveillance project. Arthritis Rheumatol. 2017;69(10):1996–2005.
9. Feldman CH, et al. Epidemiology and sociodemographics of systemic lupus erythematosus and lupus nephritis among US adults with Medicaid coverage, 2000–2004. Arthritis Rheum. 2013;65(3):753–63.

10. Alarcon GS, et al. Systemic lupus erythematosus in a multiethnic cohort: LUMINA XXXV. Predictive factors of high disease activity over time. Ann Rheum Dis. 2006;65(9):1168–74.
11. Niu Z, et al. Value of HLA-DR genotype in systemic lupus erythematosus and lupus nephritis: A meta-analysis. Int J Rheum Dis. 2015;18(1):17–28.
12. Chung SA, et al. Lupus nephritis susceptibility loci in women with systemic lupus erythematosus. J Am Soc Nephrol. 2014;25(12):2859–70.
13. Dong C, et al. Fcgamma receptor IIIa single-nucleotide polymorphisms and haplotypes affect human IgG binding and are associated with lupus nephritis in African Americans. Arthritis Rheumatol. 2014;66(5):1291–9.
14. Salmon JE, et al. Fc gamma RIIA alleles are heritable risk factors for lupus nephritis in African Americans. J Clin Invest. 1996;97(5):1348–54.
15. Contreras G, et al. Outcomes in African Americans and Hispanics with lupus nephritis. Kidney Int. 2006;69(10):1846–51.
16. Seligman VA, et al. Demographic differences in the development of lupus nephritis: A retrospective analysis. Am J Med. 2002;112(9):726–9.
17. Mok CC, et al. Effect of renal disease on the standardized mortality ratio and life expectancy of patients with systemic lupus erythematosus. Arthritis Rheum. 2013;65(8):2154–60.
18. Tektonidou MG, et al. Risk of end-stage renal disease in patients with lupus nephritis, 1971–2015: A systematic review and bayesian meta-analysis. Arthritis Rheumatol. 2016;68(6):1432–41.
19. Rovin BH, et al. Management and treatment of glomerular diseases (part 2): Conclusions from a kidney disease: Improving global outcomes (KDIGO) controversies conference. Kidney Int. 2019;95(2):281–95.
20. Asif S, et al. A review of the AURORA and BLISS trials: Will it revolutionize the treatment of lupus nephritis? Curr Opin Nephrol Hypertens. 2022;31(3):278–82.
21. Dooley MA, et al. Mycophenolate versus azathioprine as maintenance therapy for lupus nephritis. N Engl J Med. 2011;365(20):1886–95.
22. Chen YE, et al. Value of a complete or partial remission in severe lupus nephritis. Clin J Am Soc Nephrol. 2008;3(1):46–53.
23. Hahn BH, et al. American college of rheumatology guidelines for screening, treatment, and management of lupus nephritis. Arthritis Care Res (Hoboken). 2012;64(6):797–808.
24. Zabaleta-Lanz M, et al. Silent nephritis in systemic lupus erythematosus. Lupus. 2003;12(1):26–30.
25. Ishizaki J, et al. Low complements and high titre of anti-Sm antibody as predictors of histopathologically proven silent lupus nephritis without abnormal urinalysis in patients with systemic lupus erythematosus. Rheumatology (Oxford). 2015;54(3):405–12.
26. Wakasugi D, et al. Frequency of class III and IV nephritis in systemic lupus erythematosus without clinical renal involvement: An analysis of predictive measures. J Rheumatol. 2012;39(1):79–85.
27. Khanna R. Clinical presentation & management of glomerular diseases: Hematuria, nephritic & nephrotic syndrome. Mo Med. 2011;108(1):33–6.
28. Hu W, et al. Clinical-morphological features and outcomes of lupus podocytopathy. Clin J Am Soc Nephrol. 2016;11(4):585–92.
29. Esson GA, et al. Cutaneous manifestations of acute kidney injury. Clin Kidney J. 2022;15(5):855–64.
30. Greloni G, et al. Value of repeat biopsy in lupus nephritis flares. Lupus Sci Med. 2014;1(1):e000004.
31. Parikh SV, et al. The kidney biopsy in lupus nephritis: Past, present, and future. Semin Nephrol. 2015;35(5):465–77.
32. Moroni G, et al. Are laboratory tests useful for monitoring the activity of lupus nephritis? A 6-year prospective study in a cohort of 228 patients with lupus nephritis. Ann Rheum Dis. 2009;68(2):234–7.
33. Steiman AJ, et al. Anti-dsDNA and antichromatin antibody isotypes in serologically active clinically quiescent systemic lupus erythematosus. J Rheumatol. 2015;42(5):810–16.
34. Singh S, et al. Lupus nephritis. Am J Med Sci. 2009;337(6):451–60.
35. Yurkovich M, et al. Overall and cause-specific mortality in patients with systemic lupus erythematosus: A meta-analysis of observational studies. Arthritis Care Res (Hoboken). 2014;66(4):608–16.

36. Kostopoulou M, et al. The association between lupus serology and disease outcomes: A systematic literature review to inform the treat-to-target approach in systemic lupus erythematosus. Lupus. 2022;31(3):307–18.

37. Birmingham DJ, et al. Biomarkers of lupus nephritis histology and flare: Deciphering the relevant amidst the noise. Nephrol Dial Transplant. 2017;32(suppl_1):i71–9.

38. Franco C, et al. Predictors of end stage renal disease in African Americans with lupus nephritis. Bull NYU Hosp Jt Dis. 2010;68(4):251–6.

39. Adler M, et al. An assessment of renal failure in an SLE cohort with special reference to ethnicity, over a 25-year period. Rheumatology (Oxford). 2006;45(9):1144–7.

40. Barr RG, et al. Prognosis in proliferative lupus nephritis: The role of socio-economic status and race/ethnicity. Nephrol Dial Transplant. 2003;18(10):2039–46.

41. Petri M, et al. Risk of renal failure within 10 or 20 years of systemic lupus erythematosus diagnosis. J Rheumatol. 2021;48(2):222–7.

42. Chang A, et al. Cellular aspects of the pathogenesis of lupus nephritis. Curr Opin Rheumatol. 2021;33(2):197–204.

43. Bastian HM, et al. Systemic lupus erythematosus in three ethnic groups. XII. Risk factors for lupus nephritis after diagnosis. Lupus. 2002;11(3):152–60.

44. Lin WH, et al. Incidence of progression from newly diagnosed systemic lupus erythematosus to end stage renal disease and all-cause mortality: A nationwide cohort study in Taiwan. Int J Rheum Dis. 2013;16(6):747–53.

45. Iseki K, et al. An epidemiologic analysis of end-stage lupus nephritis. Am J Kidney Dis. 1994;23(4):547–54.

46. Plantinga L, et al. Incidence of end-stage renal disease among newly diagnosed systemic lupus erythematosus patients: The Georgia lupus registry. Arthritis Care Res (Hoboken). 2016;68(3):357–65.

47. Deng Y, et al. Updates in lupus genetics. Curr Rheumatol Rep. 2017;19(11):68.

48. Iwamoto T, et al. Genetics of human lupus nephritis. Clin Immunol. 2017;185:32–9.

49. Ortiz-Fernandez L, et al. A Summary on the genetics of systemic lupus erythematosus, rheumatoid arthritis, systemic sclerosis, and Sjogren's syndrome. Clin Rev Allergy Immunol. 2023;64(3):392–411.

50. Gonzalez-Serna D, et al. Association of a rare variant of the TNFSF13B gene with susceptibility to rheumatoid arthritis and systemic lupus erythematosus. Sci Rep. 2018;8(1):8195.

51. Friebus-Kardash J, et al. Susceptibility of BAFF-var allele carriers to severe SLE with occurrence of lupus nephritis. BMC Nephrol. 2019;20(1):430.

52. Freedman BI, et al. End-stage renal disease in African Americans with lupus nephritis is associated with APOL1. Arthritis Rheumatol. 2014;66(2):390–6.

53. Yang W, et al. ITGAM is associated with disease susceptibility and renal nephritis of systemic lupus erythematosus in Hong Kong Chinese and Thai. Hum Mol Genet. 2009;18(11):2063–70.

54. Kim-Howard X, et al. ITGAM coding variant (rs1143679) influences the risk of renal disease, discoid rash and immunological manifestations in patients with systemic lupus erythematosus with European ancestry. Ann Rheum Dis. 2010;69(7):1329–32.

55. Li C, et al. Association of the CD11b rs1143679 polymorphism with systemic lupus erythematosus in the Han Chinese population. J Int Med Res. 2018;46(3):1008–14.

56. Bolin K, et al. Association of STAT4 polymorphism with severe renal insufficiency in lupus nephritis. PLoS ONE. 2013;8(12):e84450.

57. Leffers HCB, et al. Established risk loci for systemic lupus erythematosus at NCF2, STAT4, TNPO3, IRF5 and ITGAM associate with distinct clinical manifestations: A Danish genome-wide association study. Joint Bone Spine. 2022;89(4):105357.

58. Qin L, et al. Association of IRF5 gene polymorphisms and lupus nephritis in a Chinese population. Nephrology (Carlton). 2010;15(7):710–13.

59. Brady MP, et al. TNIP1/ABIN1 and lupus nephritis: Review. Lupus Sci Med. 2020;7(1).

60. Xu Y, et al. Association of FcgammaRIIA-R/H131 polymorphism and systemic lupus erythematosus lupus nephritis risk: A meta-analysis. Int J Rheum Dis. 2020;23(7):853–67.

61. Tsang ASMW, et al. Fc-gamma receptor polymorphisms differentially influence susceptibility to systemic lupus erythematosus and lupus nephritis. Rheumatology (Oxford). 2016;55(5):939–48.

62. Araki Y, et al. Epigenetic dysregulation in the pathogenesis of systemic lupus erythematosus. Int J Mol Sci. 2024;25(2).

63. Mok A, et al. Genome-wide profiling identifies associations between lupus nephritis and differential methylation of genes regulating tissue hypoxia and type 1 interferon responses. Lupus Sci Med. 2016;3(1):e000183.
64. Wardowska A, et al. Transcriptomic and epigenetic alterations in dendritic cells correspond with chronic kidney disease in lupus nephritis. Front Immunol. 2019;10:2026.
65. Allen PC, et al. Genome-wide DNA methylation analysis implicates enrichment of interferon pathway in African American patients with systemic lupus erythematosus and European Americans with lupus nephritis. J Autoimmun. 2023;139:103089.
66. Somparn P, et al. Potential involvement of circulating exosomal miRNA-146a in disease activity and TRAF6 gene expression in juvenile proliferative lupus nephritis. Lupus Sci Med. 2024;11(1).
67. Ahmed RF, et al. Role of micro-RNA132 and its long non coding SOX2 in diagnosis of lupus nephritis. Lupus. 2022;31(1):89–96.
68. Pan X, et al. HOXA11-OS participates in lupus nephritis by targeting miR-124–3p mediating Cyr61 to regulate podocyte autophagy. Mol Med. 2022;28(1):138.
69. Ye H, et al. Full high-throughput sequencing analysis of differences in expression profiles of long noncoding RNAs and their mechanisms of action in systemic lupus erythematosus. Arthritis Res Ther. 2019;21(1):70.
70. Flores-Chova A, et al. Plasma exosomal non-coding RNA profile associated with renal damage reveals potential therapeutic targets in lupus nephritis. Int J Mol Sci. 2023;24(8).
71. Omidi F, et al. Comparison of circulating miR-148a and miR-126 with autoantibodies as biomarkers of lupus nephritis in patients with SLE. J Immunoassay Immunochem. 2022;43(6):634–47.
72. Abdelsalam M, et al. Study of MicroRNA-124 in patients with lupus nephritis. Endocr Metab Immune Disord Drug Targets. 2024. http://doi.org/10.2174/0118715303250919231010073608
73. Sentis G, et al. A network-based approach reveals long non-coding RNAs associated with disease activity in lupus nephritis: Key pathways for flare and potential biomarkers to be used as liquid biopsies. Front Immunol. 2023;14:1203848.
74. Tawfeek GA, et al. Long non-coding RNA TUG1 gene polymorphism and TUG1 expression level as molecular biomarkers of systemic lupus erythematosus and lupus nephritis. Noncoding RNA. 2023;9(5).
75. Hsieh YT, et al. Long noncoding RNA SNHG16 regulates TLR4-mediated autophagy and NETosis formation in alveolar hemorrhage associated with systemic lupus erythematosus. J Biomed Sci. 2023;30(1):78.
76. Suarez-Fueyo A, et al. T cells and autoimmune kidney disease. Nat Rev Nephrol. 2017;13(6):329–43.
77. Arazi A, et al. Publisher correction: The immune cell landscape in kidneys of patients with lupus nephritis. Nat Immunol. 2019;20(10):1404.
78. Bhat P, et al. B lymphocytes and lupus nephritis: New insights into pathogenesis and targeted therapies. Kidney Int. 2008;73(3):261–8.
79. Bhargava R, et al. Pathogenesis of lupus nephritis: The contribution of immune and kidney resident cells. Curr Opin Rheumatol. 2023;35(2):107–16.
80. Horisberger A, et al. Blood immunophenotyping identifies distinct kidney histopathology and outcomes in patients with lupus nephritis. bioRxiv. 2024.
81. Chang A, et al. In situ B cell-mediated immune responses and tubulointerstitial inflammation in human lupus nephritis. J Immunol. 2011;186(3):1849–60.
82. Der E, et al. Author correction: Tubular cell and keratinocyte single-cell transcriptomics applied to lupus nephritis reveal type I IFN and fibrosis relevant pathways. Nat Immunol. 2019;20(11):1556.
83. Ginhoux F, et al. Editorial: Monocyte heterogeneity and function. Front Immunol. 2020;11:626725.
84. Hsieh C, et al. Predicting outcomes of lupus nephritis with tubulointerstitial inflammation and scarring. Arthritis Care Res (Hoboken). 2011;63(6):865–74.
85. Meng XM, et al. Inflammatory macrophages can transdifferentiate into myofibroblasts during renal fibrosis. Cell Death Dis. 2016;7(12):e2495.
86. Wang YY, et al. Macrophage-to-myofibroblast transition contributes to interstitial fibrosis in chronic renal allograft injury. J Am Soc Nephrol. 2017;28(7):2053–67.
87. Tucci M, et al. Glomerular accumulation of plasmacytoid dendritic cells in active lupus nephritis: Role of interleukin-18. Arthritis Rheum. 2008;58(1):251–62.

88. Oke V, et al. High levels of circulating interferons type I, type II and type III associate with distinct clinical features of active systemic lupus erythematosus. Arthritis Res Ther. 2019;21(1):107.

89. Iwamoto T, et al. High systemic type I interferon activity is associated with active class III/IV lupus nephritis. J Rheumatol. 2022;49(4):388–97.

90. Liarski VM, et al. Quantifying in situ adaptive immune cell cognate interactions in humans. Nat Immunol. 2019;20(4):503–13.

91. Hakkim A, et al. Impairment of neutrophil extracellular trap degradation is associated with lupus nephritis. Proc Natl Acad Sci U S A. 2010;107(21):9813–18.

92. Nishi H, et al. Neutrophils in lupus nephritis. Curr Opin Rheumatol. 2019;31(2):193–200.

93. Mavragani CP, et al. Type I interferon and neutrophil transcripts in lupus nephritis renal biopsies: Clinical and histopathological associations. Rheumatology (Oxford). 2023;62(7):2534–8.

94. Whittall-Garcia LP, et al. Circulating neutrophil extracellular trap remnants as a biomarker to predict outcomes in lupus nephritis. Lupus Sci Med. 2024;11(1).

95. Schwarz DS, et al. The endoplasmic reticulum: Structure, function and response to cellular signaling. Cell Mol Life Sci. 2016;73(1):79–94.

96. Miglioranza Scavuzzi B, et al. Endoplasmic reticulum stress, oxidative stress, and rheumatic diseases. Antioxidants (Basel). 2022;11(7).

97. Sule G, et al. Endoplasmic reticulum stress sensor IRE1alpha propels neutrophil hyperactivity in lupus. J Clin Invest. 2021;131(7).

98. Li HY, et al. Endoplasmic reticulum stress in systemic lupus erythematosus and lupus nephritis: Potential therapeutic target. J Immunol Res. 2023;2023:7625817.

99. Wright RD, et al. Mesangial cells are key contributors to the fibrotic damage seen in the lupus nephritis glomerulus. J Inflamm (Lond). 2019;16:22.

100. Tian Y, et al. Nestin protects podocyte from injury in lupus nephritis by mitophagy and oxidative stress. Cell Death Dis. 2020;11(5):319.

101. Qi YY, et al. Increased autophagy is cytoprotective against podocyte injury induced by antibody and interferon-alpha in lupus nephritis. Ann Rheum Dis. 2018;77(12):1799–809.

102. Fu R, et al. Podocyte activation of NLRP3 inflammasomes contributes to the development of proteinuria in Lupus Nephritis. Arthritis Rheumatol. 2017;69(8):1636–46.

103. Wang H, et al. Tubular basement membrane immune complex deposition is associated with activity and progression of lupus nephritis: A large multicenter Chinese study. Lupus. 2018;27(4):545–55.

104. Clark MR, et al. The pathogenesis and therapeutic implications of tubulointerstitial inflammation in human lupus nephritis. Semin Nephrol. 2015;35(5):455–64.

105. Kinloch AJ, et al. Vimentin is a dominant target of in situ humoral immunity in human lupus tubulointerstitial nephritis. Arthritis Rheumatol. 2014;66(12):3359–70.

106. Liarski VM, et al. Cell distance mapping identifies functional T follicular helper cells in inflamed human renal tissue. Sci Transl Med. 2014;6(230):230ra46.

107. Sterner RM, Hartono SP, Grande JP. The pathogenesis of lupus nephritis. J Clin Cell Immunol. 2014;5(2).

108. Gatto M, et al. Clinical and pathologic considerations of the qualitative and quantitative aspects of lupus nephritogenic autoantibodies: A comprehensive review. J Autoimmun. 2016;69:1–11.

109. Mannik M, et al. Multiple autoantibodies form the glomerular immune deposits in patients with systemic lupus erythematosus. J Rheumatol. 2003;30(7):1495–504.

110. Liang Z, et al. Pathogenic profiles and molecular signatures of antinuclear autoantibodies rescued from NZM2410 lupus mice. J Exp Med. 2004;199(3):381–98.

111. Croquefer S, et al. The ananti-alpha-actinin test completes ananti-DNA determination in systemic lupus erythematosus. Ann N Y Acad Sci. 2005;1050:170–5.

112. Lefkowith JB, et al. Heterogeneity and clinical significance of glomerular-binding antibodies in systemic lupus erythematosus. J Clin Invest. 1996;98(6):1373–80.

113. Alduraibi FK, et al. Lupus nephritis biomarkers: A critical review. Int J Mol Sci. 2024;25(2).

114. Madaio MP. The role of autoantibodies in the pathogenesis of lupus nephritis. Semin Nephrol. 1999;19(1):48–56.

115. Van Bavel CC, et al. Glomerular targets of nephritogenic autoantibodies in systemic lupus erythematosus. Arthritis Rheum. 2008;58(7):1892–9.

116. Davidson A. What is damaging the kidney in lupus nephritis? Nat Rev Rheumatol. 2016;12(3):143–53.
117. Pickering MC, et al. Are anti-C1q antibodies different from other SLE autoantibodies? Nat Rev Rheumatol. 2010;6(8):490–3.
118. Mannik M, et al. Deposition of antibodies to the collagen-like region of C1q in renal glomeruli of patients with proliferative lupus glomerulonephritis. Arthritis Rheum. 1997;40(8):1504–11.
119. Tsirogianni A, et al. Relevance of anti-C1q autoantibodies to lupus nephritis. Ann N Y Acad Sci. 2009;1173:243–51.
120. Hocaoglu M, et al. Incidence, prevalence, and mortality of lupus nephritis: A population-based study over four decades using the lupus midwest network. Arthritis Rheumatol. 2023;75(4):567–73.
121. Chen TK, et al. Predictors of kidney biopsy complication among patients with systemic lupus erythematosus. Lupus. 2012;21(8):848–54.
122. Andres GA, et al. Tubular and interstitial renal disease due to immunologic mechanisms. Kidney Int. 1975;7(4):271–89.
123. Weening JJ, et al. The classification of glomerulonephritis in systemic lupus erythematosus revisited. J Am Soc Nephrol. 2004;15(2):241–50.
124. Bajema IM, et al. Update on scoring and providing evidence basis for assessing pathology in lupus nephritis. Kidney Int. 2023;103(5):813–16.
125. Bajema IM, et al. The European vasculitis society 2016 meeting report. Kidney Int Rep. 2017;2(6):1018–31.
126. Ward F, et al. Membranous lupus nephritis: The same, but different. Am J Kidney Dis. 2016;68(6):954–66.
127. Sethi S, et al. Proteomic analysis of complement proteins in glomerular diseases. Kidney Int Rep. 2023;8(4):827–36.
128. Ravindran A, et al. In Patients with membranous lupus nephritis, exostosin-positivity and exostosin-negativity represent two different phenotypes. J Am Soc Nephrol. 2021;32(3):695–706.
129. Bajema IM, et al. Revision of the international society of nephrology/renal pathology society classification for lupus nephritis: Clarification of definitions, and modified national institutes of health activity and chronicity indices. Kidney Int. 2018;93(4):789–96.
130. Javeed S, et al. Spectrum of morphological and immunofluorescence patterns in lupus nephritis: A single institutional study. Cureus. 2022;14(5):e25363.
131. Parodis I, et al. Prediction of prognosis and renal outcome in lupus nephritis. Lupus Sci Med. 2020;7(1):e000389.
132. Nossent J, et al. The importance of tubuloreticular inclusions in lupus nephritis. Pathology. 2019;51(7):727–32.
133. Tamirou F, et al. A proteinuria cut-off level of 0.7 g/day after 12 months of treatment best predicts long-term renal outcome in lupus nephritis: Data from the MAINTAIN nephritis trial. Lupus Sci Med. 2015;2(1):e000123.
134. Dall'Era M, et al. Predictors of long-term renal outcome in lupus nephritis trials: Lessons learned from the Euro-Lupus Nephritis cohort. Arthritis Rheumatol. 2015;67(5):1305–13.
135. Ugolini-Lopes MR, Seguro LPC, Castro MXF, et al. Early proteinuria response: A valid real-life situation predictor of long-term lupus renal outcome in an ethnically diverse group with severe biopsy-proven nephritis? Lupus Sci Med. 2017;4(1):e000213.
136. Dall'Era M, et al. Identification of biomarkers that predict response to treatment of lupus nephritis with mycophenolate mofetil or pulse cyclophosphamide. Arthritis Care Res (Hoboken). 2011;63(3):351–7.
137. Bose B, et al. Ten common mistakes in the management of lupus nephritis. Am J Kidney Dis. 2014;63(4):667–76.
138. Alforaih N, et al. A review of lupus nephritis. J Appl Lab Med. 2022;7(6):1450–67.
139. Malvar A, et al. Histologic versus clinical remission in proliferative lupus nephritis. Nephrol Dial Transplant. 2017;32(8):1338–44.
140. Yin Y, et al. Diagnostic value of serum anti-C1q antibodies in patients with lupus nephritis: A meta-analysis. Lupus. 2012;21(10):1088–97.
141. Eggleton P, et al. Autoantibodies against C1q as a diagnostic measure of lupus nephritis: Systematic review and meta-analysis. J Clin Cell Immunol. 2014;5(2):210.

142. Julkunen H, et al. Nonrenal and renal activity of systemic lupus erythematosus: A comparison of two anti-C1q and five anti-dsDNA assays and complement C3 and C4. Rheumatol Int. 2012;32(8):2445–51.

143. Orbai AM, et al. Anti-C1q antibodies in systemic lupus erythematosus. Lupus. 2015;24(1):42–9.

144. Pang Y, et al. Serum A08 C1q antibodies are associated with disease activity and prognosis in Chinese patients with lupus nephritis. Kidney Int. 2016;90(6):1357–67.

145. Coremans IE, et al. Changes in antibodies to C1q predict renal relapses in systemic lupus erythematosus. Am J Kidney Dis. 1995;26(4):595–601.

146. Yang XW, et al. Combination of anti-C1q and anti-dsDNA antibodies is associated with higher renal disease activity and predicts renal prognosis of patients with lupus nephritis. Nephrol Dial Transplant. 2012;27(9):3552–9.

147. Guimaraes JAR, et al. Diagnostic test accuracy of novel biomarkers for lupus nephritis: An overview of systematic reviews. PLoS ONE. 2022;17(10):e0275016.

148. Feng X, et al. Association of increased interferon-inducible gene expression with disease activity and lupus nephritis in patients with systemic lupus erythematosus. Arthritis Rheum. 2006;54(9):2951–62.

149. Mai L, et al. The baseline interferon signature predicts disease severity over the subsequent 5 years in systemic lupus erythematosus. Arthritis Res Ther. 2021;23(1):29.

150. Bauer JW, et al. Interferon-regulated chemokines as biomarkers of systemic lupus erythematosus disease activity: A validation study. Arthritis Rheum. 2009;60(10):3098–107.

151. Schwarting A, et al. Renal tubular epithelial cell-derived BAFF expression mediates kidney damage and correlates with activity of proliferative lupus nephritis in mouse and men. Lupus. 2018;27(2):243–56.

152. Parodis I, et al. Evaluation of B lymphocyte stimulator and a proliferation inducing ligand as candidate biomarkers in lupus nephritis based on clinical and histopathological outcome following induction therapy. Lupus Sci Med. 2015;2(1):e000061.

153. Phatak S, et al. Urinary B cell activating factor (BAFF) and a proliferation-inducing ligand (APRIL): Potential biomarkers of active lupus nephritis. Clin Exp Immunol. 2017;187(3):376–82.

154. Landolt-Marticorena C, et al. A discrete cluster of urinary biomarkers discriminates between active systemic lupus erythematosus patients with and without glomerulonephritis. Arthritis Res Ther. 2016;18(1):218.

155. Lee YH, Song GG. Urinary MCP-1 as a biomarker for lupus nephritis: A meta-analysis. Z Rheumatol. 2017;76(4):357–63.

156. Gupta R, et al. Longitudinal assessment of monocyte chemoattractant protein-1 in lupus nephritis as a biomarker of disease activity. Clin Rheumatol. 2016;35(11):2707–14.

157. Rovin BH, et al. Urine chemokines as biomarkers of human systemic lupus erythematosus activity. J Am Soc Nephrol. 2005;16(2):467–73.

158. Xia YR, et al. Diagnostic value of urinary monocyte chemoattractant protein-1 in evaluating the activity of lupus nephritis: A meta-analysis. Lupus. 2020;29(6):599–606.

159. Xu WD, et al. Role of the TWEAK/Fn14 pathway in autoimmune diseases. Immunol Res. 2016;64(1):44–50.

160. Schwartz N, et al. Urinary TWEAK as a biomarker of lupus nephritis: A multicenter cohort study. Arthritis Res Ther. 2009;11(5):R143.

161. Schwartz N, et al. Urinary TWEAK and the activity of lupus nephritis. J Autoimmun. 2006;27(4):242–50.

162. Salem MN, et al. Urinary TNF-like weak inducer of apoptosis (TWEAK) as a biomarker of lupus nephritis. Z Rheumatol. 2018;77(1):71–7.

163. Suttichet TB, et al. Urine TWEAK level as a biomarker for early response to treatment in active lupus nephritis: A prospective multicentre study. Lupus Sci Med. 2019;6(1):e000298.

164. Wang ZH, et al. Urinary tumor necrosis factor-like weak inducer of apoptosis as a biomarker for diagnosis and evaluating activity in lupus nephritis: A meta-analysis. J Clin Rheumatol. 2021;27(7):272–7.

165. Hinze CH, et al. Neutrophil gelatinase-associated lipocalin is a predictor of the course of global and renal childhood-onset systemic lupus erythematosus disease activity. Arthritis Rheum. 2009;60(9):2772–81.

166. Gao Y, et al. Elevated urinary neutrophil gelatinase-associated lipocalin is a bio-marker for lupus nephritis: A systematic review and meta-analysis. Biomed Res Int. 2020;2020:2768326.

167. Parodis I, et al. ALCAM and VCAM-1 as urine biomarkers of activity and long-term renal outcome in systemic lupus erythematosus. Rheumatology (Oxford). 2020;59(9):2237–49.

168. Brunner HI, et al. Development of a novel renal activity index of lupus nephritis in children and young adults. Arthritis Care Res (Hoboken). 2016;68(7):1003–11.

169. Brunner HI, et al. Urine biomarkers to predict response to lupus nephritis therapy in children and young adults. J Rheumatol. 2017;44(8):1239–48.

170. Cody EM, et al. Urine biomarker score captures response to induction therapy with lupus nephritis. Pediatr Nephrol. 2023;38(8):2679–88.

171. Gulati G, et al. Prospective validation of a novel renal activity index of lupus nephritis. Lupus. 2017;26(9):927–36.

172. Fava A, et al. Urine proteomic signatures of histological class, activity, chronicity, and treatment response in lupus nephritis. JCI Insight. 2024;9(2).

173. Allison AC, et al. Mycophenolate mofetil and its mechanisms of action. Immunopharmacology. 2000;47(2–3):85–118.

174. Mok CC. Mycophenolate mofetil for lupus nephritis: An update. Expert Rev Clin Immunol. 2015;11(12):1353–64.

175. Appel GB, et al. Mycophenolate mofetil versus cyclophosphamide for induction treatment of lupus nephritis. J Am Soc Nephrol. 2009;20(5):1103–12.

176. Isenberg D, et al. Influence of race/ethnicity on response to lupus nephritis treatment: The ALMS study. Rheumatology (Oxford). 2010;49(1):128–40.

177. Chan TM, et al. Efficacy of mycophenolate mofetil in patients with diffuse proliferative lupus nephritis. Hong Kong-Guangzhou Nephrology Study Group. N Engl J Med. 2000;343(16):1156–62.

178. Ginzler EM, et al. Mycophenolate mofetil or intravenous cyclophosphamide for lupus nephritis. N Engl J Med. 2005;353(21):2219–28.

179. Yap DY, et al. Long-term data on corticosteroids and mycophenolate mofetil treatment in lupus nephritis. Rheumatology (Oxford). 2013;52(3):480–6.

180. Houssiau FA, et al. Azathioprine versus mycophenolate mofetil for long-term immunosuppression in lupus nephritis: Results from the MAINTAIN nephritis trial. Ann Rheum Dis. 2010;69(12):2083–9.

181. Saad AF, et al. Immunosuppressant medications in pregnancy. Obstet Gynecol. 2024 Apr 1;143(4):e94–e106. http://doi.org/10.1097/AOG.0000000000005512

182. Austin HA, et al. Therapy of lupus nephritis. Controlled trial of prednisone and cytotoxic drugs. N Engl J Med. 1986;314(10):614–19.

183. Gourley MF, et al. Methylprednisolone and cyclophosphamide, alone or in combination, in patients with lupus nephritis. A randomized, controlled trial. Ann Intern Med. 1996;125(7):549–57.

184. Illei GG, et al. Combination therapy with pulse cyclophosphamide plus pulse methylprednisolone improves long-term renal outcome without adding toxicity in patients with lupus nephritis. Ann Intern Med. 2001;135(4):248–57.

185. Boumpas DT, et al. Controlled trial of pulse methylprednisolone versus two regimens of pulse cyclophosphamide in severe lupus nephritis. Lancet. 1992;340(8822):741–5.

186. Houssiau FA, et al. Immunosuppressive therapy in lupus nephritis: The Euro-Lupus Nephritis Trial, a randomized trial of low-dose versus high-dose intravenous cyclophosphamide. Arthritis Rheum. 2002;46(8):2121–31.

187. Houssiau FA, et al. The 10-year follow-up data of the Euro-Lupus Nephritis Trial comparing low-dose and high-dose intravenous cyclophosphamide. Ann Rheum Dis. 2010;69(1):61–4.

188. Herath N, et al. Clinicopathological findings, treatment response and predictors of long-term outcome in a cohort of lupus nephritis patients managed according to the Euro-lupus regime: A retrospective analysis in Sri Lanka. BMC Res Notes. 2017;10(1):80.

189. Rathi M, et al. Comparison of low-dose intravenous cyclophosphamide with oral mycophenolate mofetil in the treatment of lupus nephritis. Kidney Int. 2016;89(1):235–42.

190. Prasad N, et al. Long-term outcomes of lupus nephritis treated with regimens based on cyclophosphamide and mycophenolate mofetil. Lupus. 2020;29(8):845–53.

191. Group AT. Treatment of lupus nephritis with abatacept: The abatacept and cyclophosphamide combination efficacy and safety study. Arthritis Rheumatol. 2014;66(11):3096–104.

192. Hanaoka H, et al. Comparison of renal response to four different induction therapies in Japanese patients with lupus nephritis class III or IV: A single-centre retrospective study. PLoS ONE. 2017;12(4):e0175152.

193. Wallace DJ. Advances in drug therapy for systemic lupus erythematosus. BMC Med. 2010;8:77.

194. Marin-Rosales M, et al. Renal tissue expression of BAFF and BAFF receptors is associated with proliferative lupus nephritis. J Clin Med. 2022;12(1).

195. Suso JP, et al. Profile of BAFF and its receptors' expression in lupus nephritis is associated with pathological classes. Lupus. 2018;27(5):708–15.

196. Furie R, et al. Two-year, randomized, controlled trial of belimumab in lupus nephritis. N Engl J Med. 2020;383(12):1117–28.

197. Rovin BH, et al. A secondary analysis of the belimumab international study in lupus nephritis trial examined effects of belimumab on kidney outcomes and preservation of kidney function in patients with lupus nephritis. Kidney Int. 2022;101(2):403–13.

198. Moroni G, et al. AURORA 1 reports efficacy of voclosporin in lupus nephritis. Nat Rev Nephrol. 2021;17(10):637–8.

199. Li Y, et al. Pharmacokinetic disposition difference between cyclosporine and voclosporin drives their distinct efficacy and safety profiles in clinical studies. Clin Pharmacol. 2020;12:83–96.

200. Rovin BH, et al. Efficacy and safety of voclosporin versus placebo for lupus nephritis (AURORA 1): A double-blind, randomised, multicentre, placebo-controlled, phase 3 trial. Lancet. 2021;397(10289):2070–80.

201. Hoskova L, et al. Pathophysiological mechanisms of calcineurin inhibitor-induced nephrotoxicity and arterial hypertension. Physiol Res. 2017;66(2):167–80.

202. Mok CC, et al. Tacrolimus versus mycophenolate mofetil for induction therapy of lupus nephritis: A randomised controlled trial and long-term follow-up. Ann Rheum Dis. 2016;75(1):30–6.

203. Mok CC, et al. Long-term outcome of a randomised controlled trial comparing tacrolimus with mycophenolate mofetil as induction therapy for active lupus nephritis. Ann Rheum Dis. 2020;79(8):1070–6.

204. Zheng Z, et al. Effect of tacrolimus vs intravenous cyclophosphamide on complete or partial response in patients with lupus nephritis: A randomized clinical trial. JAMA Netw Open. 2022;5(3):e224492.

205. Neves A, et al. Promising experimental treatments for lupus nephritis: Key talking points and potential opportunities. Res Rep Urol. 2023;15:333–53.

206. Rovin BH, et al. Efficacy and safety of rituximab in patients with active proliferative lupus nephritis: The lupus nephritis assessment with rituximab study. Arthritis Rheum. 2012;64(4):1215–26.

207. Weidenbusch M, et al. Beyond the LUNAR trial. Efficacy of rituximab in refractory lupus nephritis. Nephrol Dial Transplant. 2013;28(1):106–11.

208. Kraaij T, et al. The NET-effect of combining rituximab with belimumab in severe systemic lupus erythematosus. J Autoimmun. 2018;91:45–54.

209. Atisha-Fregoso Y, et al. Phase II randomized trial of rituximab plus cyclophosphamide followed by belimumab for the treatment of lupus nephritis. Arthritis Rheumatol. 2021;73(1):121–31.

210. Mejia-Vilet JM, et al. Kidney involvement in systemic lupus erythematosus: From the patient assessment to a tailored treatment. Best Pract Res Clin Rheumatol. 2023:101925.

211. Mejia-Vilet JM, et al. The lupus nephritis management renaissance. Kidney Int. 2022;101(2):242–55.

212. Marinov AD, et al. The type II anti-CD20 antibody obinutuzumab (GA101) is more effective than rituximab at depleting B cells and treating disease in a murine lupus model. Arthritis Rheumatol. 2021;73(5):826–36.

213. Furie RA, et al. B-cell depletion with obinutuzumab for the treatment of proliferative lupus nephritis: A randomised, double-blind, placebo-controlled trial. Ann Rheum Dis. 2022;81(1):100–7.

214. Desai SB, et al. New guidelines and therapeutic updates for the management of lupus nephritis. Curr Opin Nephrol Hypertens. 2024 May 1;33(3):344–53. http://doi.org/10.1097/MNH.0000000000000969.

215. Bowman SJ, et al. Safety and efficacy of subcutaneous ianalumab (VAY736) in patients with primary Sjogren's syndrome: A randomised, double-blind, placebo-controlled, phase 2b dose-finding trial. Lancet. 2022;399(10320):161–71.

216. Morand EF, et al. Trial of anifrolumab in active systemic lupus erythematosus. N Engl J Med. 2020;382(3):211–21.

217. Deeks ED. Anifrolumab: First approval. Drugs. 2021;81(15):1795–802.

218. Jayne D, et al. Phase II randomised trial of type I interferon inhibitor anifrolumab in patients with active lupus nephritis. Ann Rheum Dis. 2022;81(4):496–506.

219. Kunz R, et al. Meta-analysis: Effect of monotherapy and combination therapy with inhibitors of the renin angiotensin system on proteinuria in renal disease. Ann Intern Med. 2008;148(1):30–48.

220. Cheung AK, et al. Blood pressure in chronic kidney disease: Conclusions from a Kidney Disease: Improving Global Outcomes (KDIGO) controversies conference. Kidney Int. 2019;95(5):1027–36.

221. Canadian Hydroxychloroquine Study G. A randomized study of the effect of withdrawing hydroxychloroquine sulfate in systemic lupus erythematosus. N Engl J Med. 1991;324(3):150–4.

222. Fanouriakis A, et al. EULAR recommendations for the management of systemic lupus erythematosus: 2023 update. Ann Rheum Dis. 2024;83(1):15–29.

223. Rovin BH, et al. Executive summary of the KDIGO 2024 clinical practice guideline for the management of lupus nephritis. Kidney Int. 2024;105(1):31–4.

6 Kidney Involvement in Pauci-Immune Anti-Neutrophil Cytoplasmic Antibody-Mediated Small-Vessel Vasculitis

Madeline Chung, Zachary Wallace, Ashwin R. Shetty, Alana Dasgupta, Salem Almaani, Duvuru Geetha, and Anisha B. Dua

6.1 ANCA-ASSOCIATED VASCULITIS

6.1.1 Clinical Presentation

Granulomatosis with polyangiitis (GPA), microscopic polyangiitis (MPA), and eosinophilic granulomatosis with polyangiitis (EGPA) represent different phenotypes of AAV with distinct clinical and serological features. Most patients with AAV have anti-neutrophil cytoplasmic antibodies (ANCAs) targeted against one of two neutrophil granule proteins: proteinase 3 (PR3-ANCA) or myeloperoxidase (MPO-ANCA). Rarely, patients have "dual positivity" with both PR3- and MPO-ANCA, which may raise suspicion for a drug-induced process. Renal-limited vasculitis (RLV) is a term used to describe patients with vasculitis limited to the kidneys, which is often due to MPO-ANCA+ AAV and may be classified as MPA (1).

The presentation of AAV is highly variable, even among people with the same type of AAV (e.g., GPA, MPA, or EGPA) (1–3). Indeed, manifestations can range from limited forms affecting the sinonasal tract to severe life- and organ-threatening disease involving the lungs and/or kidneys. Even in the so-called "limited" forms, extensive damage can leave patients with substantial morbidity and a reduced health-related quality of life (HRQoL). Prompt recognition and treatment initiation are fundamental to improving outcomes in AAV.

Typical manifestations of GPA include upper respiratory tract involvement (e.g., sinonasal disease, subglottic stenosis, orbital disease), lower respiratory tract involvements (e.g., pulmonary nodules, alveolar hemorrhage), and/or glomerulonephritis (Table 6.1). Pathologically, GPA is distinguished from MPA because of granulomatous inflammation. GPA is most often associated with PR3-ANCA+, though a well-described subgroup of patients has MPO-ANCA+ GPA (4, 5). Up to 20% of patients with GPA are ANCA negative and tend to have manifestations limited to the head and neck. Limited GPA can be challenging to diagnose because biopsies of the upper airway tract are often nonspecific and the ANCAs may be negative.

In contrast to GPA, MPA is nearly always associated with MPO-ANCA+, and pathology shows small-to-medium-vessel vasculitis (e.g., involving capillaries, arterioles, venules) that lacks granulomatous inflammation. Glomerulonephritis is common in patients with MPA and may be the only manifestation of the disease. Like in GPA, patients with MPA may have alveolar hemorrhage. A distinguishing feature of MPA is its association with fibrotic interstitial lung disease, often usual interstitial pneumonia, which may be the presenting feature of the disease (6) and can be challenging to manage.

Though classically used to differentiate among patients with AAV, the phenotypes of GPA and MPA may not be as clinically meaningful as characterizing patients according to their ANCA type (MPO-ANCA+, PR3-ANCA+, or ANCA negative). Mounting evidence suggests that using ANCA type, rather than clinical phenotypes (i.e., GPA or MPA), better differentiates patients into groups characterized by shared genetics, manifestations, response to treatment, and natural history (e.g., relapse risk).

EGPA is unique from GPA and MPA in important ways. The hallmarks of EGPA include asthma (often adult-onset and difficult to control) and eosinophilia (both in the peripheral blood and tissue affected by the disease). Other manifestations overlap with those seen in GPA and/or MPA, including sinonasal disease, cutaneous disease, arthritis, glomerulonephritis, and neuropathy. In contrast to GPA and MPA, EGPA can cause myocarditis, which is important to recognize early given its high mortality (7, 8). Approximately 50% of patients with EGPA are ANCA negative, and those with a positive ANCA tend to be MPO-ANCA+. EGPA patients with kidney involvement are often ANCA positive. The management of EGPA tends to differ significantly from that of GPA and MPA, particularly with the use of eosinophil-targeted therapies (e.g., anti-IL-5).

DOI: 10.1201/9781003438373-8

Table 6.1: Distinguishing Clinical Features of Granulomatosis with Polyangiitis, Microscopic Polyangiitis, and Eosinophilic Granulomatosis with Polyangiitis

	Granulomatosis with Polyangiitis	Microscopic Polyangiitis	Eosinophilic Granulomatosis with Polyangiitis
ANCA associations	PR3-ANCA + >>> MPO-ANCA+	MPO-ANCA+	ANCA negative (~50%) or MPO-ANCA+
Pathology features accompanying necrotizing vasculitis	Granulomatous inflammation	No granulomatous inflammation	Eosinophilic infiltrate
Renal manifestations	Glomerulonephritis is common	Glomerulonephritis is most common in MPA than GPA or EGPA; severity may be worse though this is controversial	Glomerulonephritis is less common than in GPA and MPA but may be associated with ANCA+ disease
Eyes and ears	Common, including scleritis > uveitis, orbital disease, sensorineural and conductive hearing loss	Less common than in GPA	Less common than in GPA
Upper respiratory tract involvement	Common, including sinonasal disease, subglottic stenosis	Not common	Common, including sinonasal disease
Lower respiratory tract involvement	Common, including pulmonary nodules and cavitary lung lesions, alveolar hemorrhage	Common, including alveolar hemorrhage and fibrotic lung disease (e.g., usual interstitial pneumonitis)	Common, including characteristic asthma but also pulmonary nodules
Asthma	Not characteristic	Not characteristic	Adult-onset, worsening, and/or difficult-to-control asthma is typical
Cardiac involvement	Uncommon	Uncommon	Myocarditis is common and can be life-threatening
Neurologic involvement	Vasculitic neuropathy, typically mononeuritis multiplex, can occur but less common than in MPA and EGPA	Vasculitic neuropathy, typically mononeuritis multiplex	Vasculitic neuropathy, typically mononeuritis multiplex, common

6.1.2 Epidemiology

AAVs are rare conditions that tend to affect male and female people at equal rates. People of any age can be affected by AAV, though incidence tends to rise with age, and manifestations may vary according to age of onset (9). People with GPA tend to present between 45 and 65 years of age, whereas those with MPA tend to be, on average, about 10 years older (55–75 years of age) (10). People may present with EGPA at a younger age (38–54 years of age) (10). Patients of diverse racial and ethnic backgrounds can be affected by AAV, but the epidemiology of the disease can vary globally. In northern Europe and North America, GPA and MPA are observed at similar rates, if not with a predominance of GPA. In contrast, the vast majority of patients with AAV in East Asia have MPA/MPO-ANCA+ disease. The genetic or environmental factors driving these differences are incompletely understood.

6.1.3 Pathogenesis

The cause of AAV is unknown but likely multifactorial, including genetic predisposition (e.g., HLA-associations) (11, 12) and exposures that one accumulates in life (13). Proposed exposures contributing to AAV risk include environmental or occupational factors (e.g., silica, pollution, ultraviolet light), inhaled toxins (e.g., cigarette use), and microbes (e.g., bacteria such as *S. aureus*), though many of these remain controversial in the face of often conflicting and limited evidence. While the cause of AAV is often considered idiopathic, drug culprits have been implicated in some cases. Specifically, hydralazine, minocycline, anti-thyroid medications (i.e., propylthiouracil, methimazole), and cocaine adulterated with levamisole can be associated with a positive ANCA test with or without a clinical syndrome consistent with a small-vessel vasculitis.

GPA, MPA, and EGPA are autoimmune forms of vasculitis in which tolerance to the self is lost. While the cause of this loss of tolerance is unknown, the pathogenesis of AAV is well described (10). In GPA and MPA, neutrophils are the primary cell type responsible for tissue injury, whereas eosinophils are responsible for injury in EGPA. In addition to these innate cells, the adaptive immune response is fundamental to AAV pathogenesis, as illustrated by the role of pathogenic autoantibody formation and efficacy of B-cell depleting therapies (14, 15). One of the most important advances in our understanding of GPA/MPA pathogenesis in recent years has been the recognition of the role of alternative complement pathway activation (16), which has identified a new therapeutic target in the treatment of GPA/MPA. In EGPA, the pathogenic role of eosinophils is illustrated by the efficacy of anti-IL-5 therapies like mepolizumab (17).

6.2 KIDNEY INVOLVEMENT

Kidney involvement is highly prevalent in ANCA-associated vasculitis. In some series, rates of kidney involvement were up to 90–100% of patients diagnosed with MPA (18, 19), 70% in GPA (20, 21), and only 20–25% in EGPA. The significance of kidney involvement lies in both its frequency and its substantial impact on prognosis (22), affecting both kidney and overall patient survival. For instance, in GPA, kidney involvement at diagnosis correlates with a hazard ratio for survival of 4.45 (95% CI 1.48 to 13.65) (22). When impaired kidney function is present, the risk of death increases to a hazard ratio of 5.1 (95% CI 1.59 to 10.16), rising to 8.2 (95% CI 2.03 to 33.11) (22) in cases of dialysis dependence. In MPA, significant renal insufficiency at diagnosis serves as an adverse survival marker, with a hazard ratio of 3.69 (95% CI 1.006 to 13.4) (23).

Patients with renal AAV have a wide range of presentations, from subtle to rapidly progressive. Most patients develop an acute kidney injury with hematuria and proteinuria, usually in the subnephrotic range, with an "active sediment" on urine microscopy exam characterized by the presence of isomorphic erythrocytes, acanthocytes, dysmorphic red blood cells (RBCs), and RBC casts. In GPA and MPA, around 50–65% (24) of patients with renal involvement present with a rapidly progressive glomerulonephritis (RPGN), characterized by a rapid ≥50% decrease in the glomerular filtration rate (GFR) over a short period of time, typically days to weeks. Approximately 60% (24) of patients who present with RPGN at the time of diagnosis require kidney replacement therapy (KRT). ANCA positivity can also occur in 10 to 50% (18) of patients with anti-glomerular basement membrane antibody (anti-GBM) disease, also known as double-positive disease. Double-positive patients share features of AAV such as older age at onset and a tendency for disease relapse, as well as features of anti-GBM disease such as severe kidney failure and alveolar hemorrhage. The kidney prognosis of double-positive patients is better than that in isolated anti-GBM disease (25).

Occasionally, kidney involvement follows a more indolent course of slowly progressive dysfunction, especially in MPA or RLV (24, 26). Unfortunately, this frequently leads to a delay in diagnosis, which is reflected by the increased frequency of chronic histological lesions in these patients. In one retrospective series (27) involving 16 patients with RLV, all biopsy specimens were devoid of fibrinoid necrosis and cellular/fibrocellular crescents, with a much higher percentage of global sclerosis at 47±32%. Fibrous crescents were seen in 27±26% of glomeruli. All biopsy specimens had moderate to severe interstitial fibrosis and tubular atrophy.

6.2.1 Diagnostic Approach

Kidney biopsy remains the gold standard for diagnosis of renal AAV, aiding in assessing for both the extent of damage and kidney prognosis. Histologically, the glomerular lesion in all four types of untreated ANCA-associated vasculitis is identical. Light microscopy (LM) typically shows the segmental fibrinoid necrosis of capillary loops with or without crescent formation with the mural and perivascular infiltration of neutrophils with nuclear fragmentation due to cell death (28) (See Figures 6.1 and 6.2). Crescents can involve only a segment of the glomerular tuft or expand to involve the entire glomerulus, leading to collapse. Crescents can be cellular, fibrocellular, or fibrous depending on the stage of disease. Unaffected glomeruli appear completely normal. Within a few days to weeks, the predominant inflammatory cells in the vasculitic lesions transform from neutrophils to mononuclear leukocytes, leading to fibrosis. GPA and EGPA can be characterized by either non-granulomatous and/or granulomatous inflammation. Granulomatous lesions typically have extensive necrosis with infiltrating mononuclear and polymorphonuclear leukocytes with scattered multinucleated giant cells. Chronic damage tends to be higher with more sclerosed glomeruli, interstitial fibrosis, tubular atrophy, tubular casts, and arteriosclerosis in MPA (and/or MPO-positive patients) and RLV vs. GPA (and/or PR3-positive patients). This difference has been explained by a delayed diagnosis and/or different pathogenesis of the lesions.

In less than 20% of specimens, there is an additional renal necrotizing arteritis (22, 25), most often involving the interlobar arteries, that can accompany glomerulonephritis. While these lesions are characteristic of AAV, they are not considered pathognomonic. Very rarely, there can be a medullary angiitis, which can affect the vasa rectae, manifesting as medullary interstitial disease and, in severe cases, papillary necrosis (29).

As the name suggests, the diagnosis of pauci-immune glomerulonephritis is confirmed by finding <2+ immunoglobulin and complement staining in the glomerular capillary loops on a scale of 0–4+, which differentiates the lesions from anti-GBM disease, IgA nephropathy, and lupus nephritis (30). In a small percentage of patients diagnosed with AAV, complement deposition is seen in the kidney biopsies, which correlates with greater proteinuria, disease activity, and damage and worse kidney survival compared to pauci-immune vasculitis (31). In an observational

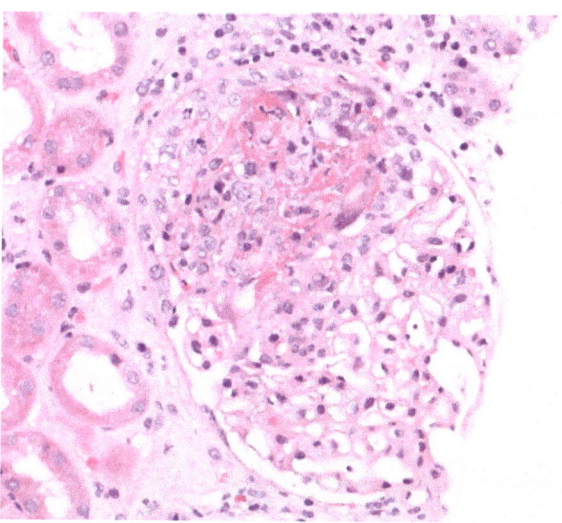

Figure 6.1 Segmental cellular crescent with fibrinoid necrosis, H&E, 200×.

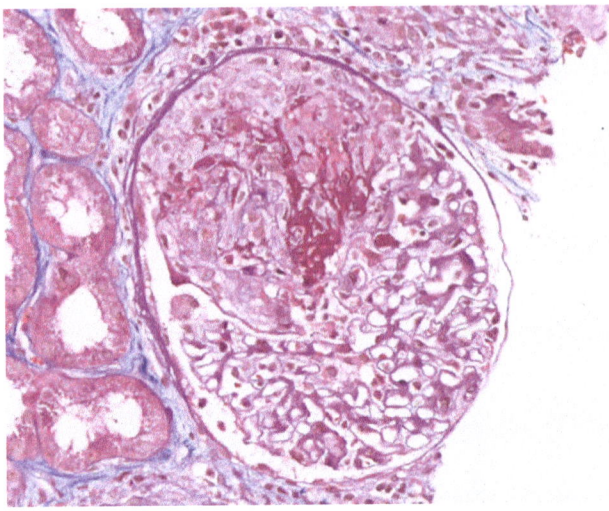

Figure 6.2   Same glomerulus with fibrinoid necrosis seen on trichrome stain, 200×.

study (32) involving 81 patients with AAV, patients who had low C3, C4, or CH50 had an increased risk of skin involvement, diffuse alveolar hemorrhage, thrombotic microangiopathy, immune complex deposition in kidney biopsy specimens, and death compared to those with normal serum complement levels. In another study involving 45 patients (33) diagnosed with AAV, low serum C3 levels were associated with worse kidney and patient survival. This has been challenged recently in a study involving 95 patients with AAV and low serum C3 levels who were found to have an increased risk of 5-year mortality, but patients with kidney deposition of C3 had a similar eGFR improvement and kidney survival at 5 years (34). Interestingly enough, in patients with MPA, higher serum levels of C4 were associated with an increased risk of end-stage kidney disease (ESKD) (35).

Rarely, interstitial nephritis can be the only lesion detected. Reported cases of AAV-interstitial nephritis were all positive for MPO with isolated interstitial inflammation and tubulitis. They had significantly fewer urinary RBCs and tended to have lower levels of serum creatinine, proteinuria, and MPO titers, although not statistically significant, and tended to respond well to immunotherapy (36, 37).

6.2.2 Relationship between Histology and Prognosis

The findings on kidney biopsy in patients with AAV have been successfully used to predict disease prognosis. The Berden Classification (30) evaluates pathologic activity and chronicity based on the presence/absence of glomerular crescents, sclerosis, and the percentage of uninvolved glomeruli observed through light microscopy. It includes four classes: focal, crescentic, sclerotic, and mixed. The focal class has the best prognosis with the least risk of progression to ESKD, while the sclerotic class has the worst prognosis. The crescentic and mixed classes fall between these extremes. However, the Berden class does not effectively predict (38) kidney outcomes in patients with an estimated glomerular filtration rate (eGFR) of less than 15 mL/minute/1.73 m². In such cases, risk factors for ESKD include having ≤10% uninvolved glomeruli (P = 0.04) and a higher overall chronicity score (P = 0.02). A meta-analysis (39) that considered >1500 patients was unable to detect different outcomes between the mixed and crescentic classes of the Berden Classification. Another prognostic tool, the ANCA Renal Risk Score (40) (ARRS), was developed utilizing the GFR at the time of diagnosis with the percentage of normal glomeruli and the degree of interstitial fibrosis and tubular atrophy to assign patients "scores" that were used to classify patients into three risk groups for developing ESKD (low/medium/high). This risk score accurately predicted ESKD at 36 months in both the training cohort of 115 patients (0%, 26%, 68% respectively) and also in an independent validation cohort of 90 patients (0%, 27%, 78% respectively).

6.3 TREATMENT

6.3.1 Microscopic Polyangiitis (MPA), Granulomatosis with Polyangiitis (GPA), and Renal-Limited Vasculitis (RLV)

6.3.1.1 Rituximab and Cyclophosphamide for Remission Induction in GPA/MPA and RLV

The treatment of pauci-immune vasculitis with kidney involvement includes the induction and maintenance of remission as well as the management of relapses and refractory disease. By definition, active renal involvement should prompt induction strategies that target severe active vasculitis. Cyclophosphamide (CYC) was shown to be effective in inducing remission in severe MPA/GPA/RLV both orally at a dose of 2 mg/kg daily or IV at a dose of 15 mg/kg every 2–3 weeks (41). However, the use of CYC is limited by known dose-dependent toxicities including myelosuppression, bladder and gonadal toxicity, and malignancy risk. As our understanding of the pathophysiology of ANCA vasculitis (AAV) advanced, rituximab (RTX) was studied as an alternative agent for induction. The efficacy of RTX (four weekly 375 mg/m² infusions) along with high-dose glucocorticoids (GCs) was demonstrated in both the RAVE (14) and RITUXIVAS (42) trials. Additionally, RTX was superior to CYC in the subset of patients with relapsing disease and PR3 positivity (43). The use of RTX over cyclophosphamide as a first-line therapy for new or relapsing severe MPA and GPA is endorsed by the ACR/VF guidelines (44). Favoring induction with RTX is primarily based on the safety profile of RTX compared to CYC. However, EULAR 2022 guidelines recommend either CYC or RTX for the induction of remission in newly diagnosed severe MPA/GPA/RLV and prefer RTX in relapsing disease (45). Because patients with a creatinine level of >4.0 mg/dL and those with rapidly deteriorating kidney function (and those on mechanical ventilation) were not included in the RAVE trial, the KDIGO guidelines recommend CYC or combination CYC/RTX as the preferred induction agent. In rare cases where RTX or CYC is unable to be used for induction, mycophenolate (46) can be considered in patients with mild to moderate impairment of kidney function, as it was shown to be non-inferior to CYC, but with significantly higher rates of relapse. Various factors influence the choice of induction therapy, including patient comorbidities, child-bearing plans, infectious risks, MPO or PR3 positivity, and new or relapsing disease, as well as cost and availability (Table 6.2 and Table 6.3).

Table 6.2: Considerations for the Treatment of Special Populations

Refractory disease	Switching induction agent to RTX if on CYC or to CYC if on RTX or combination therapy
	Combination therapies (i.e., AZA + RTX)
	Organ-targeted therapies (i.e., sinus rinses, inhalers)
Pregnancy	Consider RTX for induction > CYC
	Fertility preservation options with CYC
	Monitor neonatal B cells with RTX
	Preconception counseling to ensure disease control
	Azathioprine safe in pregnancy
End-stage kidney disease	Administer CYC or RTX after dialysis
	Dose adjustment of CYC (see Table 6.3)
	Dose adjustment of AZA: 50% normal dose and supplement 0.25 mg/kg after HD on dialysis days
Elderly	Dose adjustment of CYC (see Table 6.3)
Transplant	Ideally >12 months of stable clinical remission prior to transplant (ANCA negativity not required)
	Major relapse in transplant patient treated same as non-transplant (CYC or RTX)
Drug-induced vasculitis	Withdraw or replace triggering drug exposure (though may still require GC and immunosuppressive medication to control disease)

Abbreviations: RTX, rituximab; CYC, cyclophosphamide; AZA, azathioprine; HD, hemodialysis; GC: glucocorticoid

Table 6.3: Dose Adjustment of Cyclophosphamide Based on Age and Renal Function

Age	Creatinine (mg/dL)	
	1.7–3.4	3.4–5.6
<60	15 mg/kg	12.5 mg/kg
60–70	12.5 mg/kg	10 mg/kg
>70	10 mg/kg	7.5 mg/kg

6.3.1.2 Plasmapheresis (PLEX)

The role of plasmapheresis as part of induction in severe GPA/MPA/RLV has been evaluated in the MEPEX and PEXIVAS randomized controlled trials. The MEPEX (47) trial assessed a sick population with creatinine >5.8 mg/dL for entry and showed that PLEX decreased the risk of developing ESKD at 1 year but did not decrease mortality. The more recent PEXIVAS (48) trial enrolled patients with a median creatinine of 3.7 mg/dL with 20% requiring dialysis and demonstrated that there was no benefit to adding PLEX to standard induction therapy (with CYC/RTX and GCs) in terms of progression to ESRD or mortality. These results informed the ACR/VF recommendation against PLEX in severe GPA and MPA. Interestingly, two meta-analyses (49) demonstrated the potential benefit of PLEX in those with advanced renal involvement at presentation. The use of PLEX remains controversial and would be driven by a patient's specific clinical scenario.

6.3.1.3 Maintenance

Patients with GPA, MPA, and RLV have demonstrated high rates of relapse ranging from 21 to 89% at 5 years depending (50) on the induction and maintenance strategy used, so employing effective maintenance strategies is key in improving morbidity and mortality. Maintenance therapy for relapse prevention is indicated in all patients except for those with RLV who reach ESKD and have no extrarenal manifestations. Historically, GCs and CYC were the main options for both the induction and maintenance of remission in patients with AAV, resulting in significant toxicities. Azathioprine initiated 3 months after CYC induction was shown to be non-inferior to long-term cyclophosphamide (51) and superior to mycophenolate mofetil (52) as a maintenance agent. The duration of azathioprine use can be from 24 to 48 months based on the results of the REMAIN trial (53), which demonstrated a decreased relapse risk with an extended course of azathioprine (53). While relapses, including renal relapses, remained common, azathioprine was the preferred agent for the maintenance of remission until the demonstrated superiority of rituximab (54). Rituximab dosed at 500 mg–1 g every 4–6 months in a fixed-dose regimen is the preferred maintenance regimen in GPA/MPA and RLV (55). The length of maintenance therapy is often based on patient tolerance, risk factors for relapse, side effects, and disease course, but a minimum of 18 months after induction is recommended to decrease the risk of relapses, after which tailored regimens can be considered (with monitoring of ANCA titer, B-cell count, and clinical activity) (56). The risks of prolonged immunosuppression must be weighed against the morbidity and risks of relapsing disease while taking into account each patient's disease-specific factors.

6.3.1.4 Glucocorticoid-Sparing Strategies

The toxicity of high-dose prolonged GC use has led to important research evaluating steroid-sparing strategies in severe MPA/GPA/RLV. Either IV pulse (1 g/day × 3 days) or high-dose oral (1 mg/kg/day) glucocorticoids can be used for induction (57). In the PEXIVAS (53) trial, a reduced-dose GC regimen was compared to a standard regimen and showed that the reduced-dose regimen had equal efficacy with regard to ESRD and death, fewer infections, and 50% less GC exposure at 3 months. This resulted in the adoption of a "rapid" steroid taper as the preferred regimen for remission induction by the ACR/VF (57) as well as EULAR. It is important to note that majority of patients in PEXIVAS received CYC for induction, and hence close monitoring of kidney function is suggested when using a reduced-dose GC regimen in RTX-induced patients.

Efforts to lower GC toxicity have also resulted in the development of therapeutic agents targeting the alternative complement pathway, which plays an important role in the pathogenesis of MPA/GPA/RLV. Avacopan is an oral C5a receptor antagonist that demonstrated significant steroid-sparing capability when combined with standard-of-care induction therapy (RTX or

CYC) in achieving remission in PR3+ and MPO+ patients with AAV. In the ADVOCATE (58) trial, the use of avacopan resulted in a reduction in relapses, a decrease in GC toxicity, numeric improvements in eGFR (non-statistically significant), and improved HRQoL measures and was significantly GC sparing. Questions regarding the efficacy of avacopan in advanced renal failure, its effect on extrarenal disease manifestations, the optimal length of treatment, long-term outcomes beyond 1 year, and cost-effectiveness still remain.

6.3.2 Eosinophilic Granulomatosis with Polyangiitis (EGPA)

Kidney involvement is seen in up to 25% of EGPA (59) patients, is associated with ANCA positivity (usually MPO+), and is considered a poor prognostic factor. Recommendations are to treat EGPA based on the five-factor score, and kidney involvement is sufficient to be considered severe disease warranting aggressive therapy whether the 1996 (59, 60) or 2011 (61) criteria are utilized. Aggressive induction strategies include intravenous glucocorticoids of 500–1000 mg daily for 3 days followed by an oral GC taper starting at 1 mg/kg per day along with the use of CYC or RTX (46, 58). While studies showed a lower rate of overall relapses with the use of 12 months compared to 6 months (62) of CYC, the ability to achieve remission and major relapse rates were comparable. In clinical practice, given the poor side effect profile of CYC, switching to a maintenance agent (azathioprine, methotrexate, or mycophenolate mofetil) after 3–6 months of CYC is recommended once remission is achieved in the treatment of severe disease. RTX is another potential induction agent in EGPA with kidney involvement and has been studied in the REOVAS (63) trial, which did not show superiority compared to CYC but did show comparable outcomes overall regardless of ANCA status. The role of RTX as a maintenance agent in EGPA is being studied. In non-severe EGPA, mepolizumab is the preferred agent for the induction of remission along with GCs, though GC monotherapy can be considered in very mild presentations. Mepolizumab should be added to the treatment regimen in cases of non-severe relapse (57).

6.3.3 Assessing Treatment Response

Through all phases of induction and maintenance therapy, it is important to monitor patients for side effects from the therapies being used as well as clinically monitoring for disease activity. A thorough physical examination and lab monitoring (including a complete blood count with differential, comprehensive metabolic panel, urinalysis, inflammatory markers, and, in some cases, ANCA titers, B-cell counts, and immunoglobulin levels) should be performed. Minimizing GC doses as well as other immunosuppressive regimens has to be weighed against patient tolerance, comorbidities, and clinical status. The safety and timing of withdrawal regimens is not uniform from patient to patient and has not yet been clearly established in these diseases.

6.4 CONCLUSION

AAV is a group of challenging systemic necrotizing vasculitides with substantial disease heterogeneity with respect to disease manifestations and severity. Kidney involvement is common and severe and remains one of the most important predictors of outcome in AAV. The pathogenesis of AAV is complex, involving multiple components of the innate and adaptive immune systems in addition to genetic and environmental factors. Treatment advances have transformed AAV from a universally fatal disease to a chronic disease with a remitting and relapsing course. The goals of treatment are to provide patients with long-lasting remission, better kidney outcomes, improved HRQoL, and a decreased risk of disease relapse. Evidence for remission induction and remission maintenance therapy in AAV continues to evolve, and treatment regimens need to be tailored based on clinical manifestations, disease severity, ANCA serotype, and patient-specific factors. Current challenges in the management of AAV include identifying defined biomarkers of disease activity and risk of relapse, the uncertain duration of maintenance therapy, and the need for newer targeted and tailored therapies with a focus on faster time to remission, decreased relapse risk, and minimizing treatment-related adverse events.

REFERENCES

1. Suppiah R, et al. 2022 American college of rheumatology/European alliance of associations for rheumatology classification criteria for microscopic polyangiitis. Arthritis Rheumatol. 2022;74(3):400–6.
2. Robson JC, et al. 2022 American college of rheumatology/European alliance of associations for rheumatology classification criteria for granulomatosis with polyangiitis. Arthritis Rheumatol. 2022;74(3):393–9.

3. Grayson PC, et al. 2022 American college of rheumatology/European alliance of associations for rheumatology classification criteria for eosinophilic granulomatosis with polyangiitis. Arthritis Rheumatol. 2022;74(3):386–92.

4. Miloslavsky EM, et al. Myeloperoxidase-antineutrophil cytoplasmic antibody (ANCA)-positive and ANCA-negative patients with granulomatosis with polyangiitis (Wegener's): Distinct patient subsets. Arthritis Rheumatol. 2016;68(12):2945–52.

5. Schirmer JH, et al. Myeloperoxidase-antineutrophil cytoplasmic antibody (ANCA)-positive granulomatosis with polyangiitis (Wegener's) is a clinically distinct subset of ANCA-associated vasculitis: A retrospective analysis of 315 patients from a German vasculitis referral center. Arthritis Rheumatol. 2016;68(12):2953–63.

6. Turgeon D, Interstitial lung disease in patients with anti-neutrophil cytoplasm antibody-associated vasculitis: An update on pathogenesis and treatment. Curr Opin Pulm Med. 2023;29(5):436–42.

7. Garcia-Vives E, et al. Heart disease in eosinophilic granulomatosis with polyangiitis (EGPA) patients: A screening approach proposal. Rheumatology (Oxford). 2021;60(10):4538–47.

8. Sartorelli S, et al. Revisiting characteristics, treatment and outcome of cardiomyopathy in eosinophilic granulomatosis with polyangiitis (formerly Churg-Strauss). Rheumatology (Oxford). 2022;61(3):1175–84.

9. Bloom JL, et al. The association between age at diagnosis and disease characteristics and damage in patients with ANCA-associated vasculitis. Arthritis Rheumatol. 2023;75(12):2216–27.

10. Kitching AR, et al. ANCA-associated vasculitis. Nat Rev Dis Primers. 2020;6(1):71.

11. Lyons PA, et al. Genetically distinct subsets within ANCA-associated vasculitis. N Engl J Med. 2012;367(3):214–23.

12. Merkel PA, et al. Identification of functional and expression polymorphisms associated with risk for antineutrophil cytoplasmic autoantibody-associated vasculitis. Arthritis Rheumatol. 2017;69(5):1054–66.

13. Katz G, et al. Environmental triggers for vasculitis. Rheum Dis Clin North Am. 2022;48(4):875–90.

14. Stone JH, et al. Rituximab versus cyclophosphamide for ANCA-associated vasculitis. N Engl J Med. 2010;363(3):221–32.

15. Specks U, et al. Efficacy of remission-induction regimens for ANCA-associated vasculitis. N Engl J Med. 2013;369(5):417–27.

16. Chen M, et al. Complement in ANCA-associated vasculitis: Mechanisms and implications for management. Nat Rev Nephrol. 2017;13(6):359–67.

17. Wechsler ME, et al. Mepolizumab or placebo for eosinophilic granulomatosis with polyangiitis. N Engl J Med. 2017;376(20):1921–32.

18. Jennette JC, et al. ANCA glomerulonephritis and vasculitis. Clin J Am Soc Nephrol. 2017;12(10):1680–91.

19. Villiger PM, et al. Microscopic polyangiitis: Clinical presentation. Autoimmun Rev. 2010;9(12):812–19.

20. Holle JU, et al. Clinical manifestations and treatment of Wegener's granulomatosis. Rheum Dis Clin North Am. 2010;36(3):507–26.

21. Schilder AM. Wegener's granulomatosis vasculitis and granuloma. Autoimmun Rev. 2010;9(7):483–7.

22. Sinico RA, et al. Renal involvement in anti-neutrophil cytoplasmic autoantibody associated vasculitis. Autoimmun Rev. 2013;12(4):477–82.

23. Mukhtyar C, et al. Outcomes from studies of antineutrophil cytoplasm antibody associated vasculitis: A systematic review by the European League Against Rheumatism systemic vasculitis task force. Ann Rheum Dis. 2008;67(7):1004–10.

24. Hedger N, et al. Incidence and outcome of pauci-immune rapidly progressive glomerulonephritis in Wessex, UK: A 10-year retrospective study. Nephrol Dial Transplant. 2000;15(10):1593–9.

25. McAdoo SP, et al. Patients double-seropositive for ANCA and anti-GBM antibodies have varied renal survival, frequency of relapse, and outcomes compared to single-seropositive patients. Kidney Int. 2017;92(3):693–702.

26. D'Amico G, et al. Renal vasculitis. Nephrol Dial Transplant. 1996;11(Suppl 9):69–74.

27. Novick TK, et al. Patient outcomes in renal-limited antineutrophil cytoplasmic antibody vasculitis with inactive histology. Kidney Int Rep. 2018;3(3):671–6.

28. Fogo AB, et al. AJKD atlas of renal pathology: Pauci-immune necrotizing crescentic glomerulonephritis. Am J Kidney Dis. 2016;68(5):e31–2.

29. Klein J, et al. Medullary angiitis and pauci-immune crescentic glomerulonephritis. Proc (Bayl Univ Med Cent). 2017;30(3):351–2.

30. Berden AE, et al. Histopathologic classification of ANCA-associated glomerulonephritis. J Am Soc Nephrol. 2010;21(10):1628–36.

31. Oba R, et al. Long-term renal survival in antineutrophil cytoplasmic antibody-associated glomerulonephritis with complement C3 deposition. Kidney Int Rep. 2021;6(10):2661–70.

32. Fukui S, et al. Antineutrophilic cytoplasmic antibody-associated vasculitis with hypocomplementemia has a higher incidence of serious organ damage and a poor prognosis. Medicine (Baltimore). 2016;95(37):e4871.

33. Augusto JF, et al. Low serum complement C3 levels at diagnosis of renal anca-associated vasculitis is associated with poor prognosis. PLoS ONE. 2016;11(7):e0158871.

34. Cassard A, et al. Are serum C3 levels or kidney C3 deposits useful markers for predicting outcomes in patients with ANCA-associated vasculitis? J Transl Autoimmun. 2023;7:100217.

35. Klein J, et al. Medullary angiitis and pauci-immune crescentic glomerulonephritis. Proc (Bayl Univ Med Cent). 2017;30(3):351–2.

36. He X, et al. Interstitial nephritis without glomerulonephritis in ANCA-associated vasculitis: A case series and literature review. Clin Rheumatol. 2022;41(11):3551–63.

37. Muhammad A, et al. Acute interstitial nephritis caused by ANCA-associated vasculitis: A case based review. Clin Rheumatol. 2024;43(3):1227–44.

38. Lee T, et al. Predictors of treatment outcomes in ANCA-associated vasculitis with severe kidney failure. Clin J Am Soc Nephrol. 2014;9(5):905–13.

39. Chen YX, et al. Histopathological classification and renal outcome in patients with antineutrophil cytoplasmic antibodies-associated renal vasculitis: A study of 186 patients and metaanalysis. J Rheumatol. 2017;44(3):304–13.

40. Brix SR, et al. Development and validation of a renal risk score in ANCA-associated glomerulonephritis. Kidney Int. 2018;94(6):1177–88.

41. de Groot K, et al. Pulse versus daily oral cyclophosphamide for induction of remission in antineutrophil cytoplasmic antibody-associated vasculitis: A randomized trial. Ann Intern Med. 2009;150(10):670–80.

42. Jones RB, et al. Rituximab versus cyclophosphamide in ANCA-associated renal vasculitis. N Engl J Med. 2010;363(3):211–20.

43. Unizony S, et al. Clinical outcomes of treatment of anti-neutrophil cytoplasmic antibody (ANCA)-associated vasculitis based on ANCA type. Ann Rheum Dis. 2016;75(6).1166–9.

44. Chung SA, et al. 2021 American college of rheumatology/vasculitis foundation guideline for the management of antineutrophil cytoplasmic antibody-associated vasculitis. Arthritis Rheumatol. 2021;73(8):1366–83.

45. Hellmich B, et al. EULAR recommendations for the management of ANCA-associated vasculitis: 2022 update. Ann Rheum Dis. 2024;83(1):30–47.

46. Jones RB, et al. Mycophenolate mofetil versus cyclophosphamide for remission induction in ANCA-associated vasculitis: A randomised, non-inferiority trial. Ann Rheum Dis. 2019;78(3):399–405.

47. Jayne DR, et al. Randomized trial of plasma exchange or high-dosage methylprednisolone as adjunctive therapy for severe renal vasculitis. J Am Soc Nephrol. 2007;18(7):2180–8.

48. Walsh M, et al. Plasma exchange and glucocorticoids in severe ANCA-associated vasculitis. N Engl J Med. 2020;382(7):622–31.

49. Walsh M, et al. The effects of plasma exchange in patients with ANCA-associated vasculitis: An updated systematic review and meta-analysis. BMJ. 2022;376:e064604.

50. Salama AD. Relapse in anti-neutrophil cytoplasm antibody (ANCA)-associated vasculitis. Kidney Int Rep. 2019;5(1):7–12.

51. Walsh M, et al. Long-term follow-up of cyclophosphamide compared with azathioprine for initial maintenance therapy in ANCA-associated vasculitis. Clin J Am Soc Nephrol. 2014;9(9):1571–6.

52. Hiemstra TF, et al. Mycophenolate mofetil vs azathioprine for remission maintenance in anti-neutrophil cytoplasmic antibody-associated vasculitis: A randomized controlled trial. JAMA. 2010;304(21):2381–8.

53. Karras A, et al. Randomised controlled trial of prolonged treatment in the remission phase of ANCA-associated vasculitis. Ann Rheum Dis. 2017;76(10):1662–8.

54. Guillevin L, et al. Rituximab versus azathioprine for maintenance in ANCA-associated vasculitis. N Engl J Med. 2014;371(19):1771–80.

55. Smith RM, et al. Rituximab versus azathioprine for maintenance of remission for patients with ANCA-associated vasculitis and relapsing disease: An international randomised controlled trial. Ann Rheum Dis. 2023;82(7):937–44.

56. Charles P, et al. Comparison of individually tailored versus fixed-schedule rituximab regimen to maintain ANCA-associated vasculitis remission: Results of a multicentre, randomised controlled, phase III trial (MAINRITSAN2). Ann Rheum Dis. 2018;77(8):1143–9. Erratum in: Ann Rheum Dis. 2019;78(9):e101.

57. Chung SA, et al. 2021 American college of rheumatology/vasculitis foundation guideline for the management of antineutrophil cytoplasmic antibody-associated vasculitis. Arthritis Rheumatol. 2021;73(8):1366–83.

58. Jayne DRW, et al. Avacopan for the treatment of ANCA-associated vasculitis. N Engl J Med. 2021;384(7):599–609. Erratum in: N Engl J Med. 2024;390(4):388.

59. Reggiani F, et al. Renal involvement in eosinophilic granulomatosis with polyangiitis. Front Med (Lausanne). 2023;10:1244651.

60. Guillevin L, et al. Prognostic factors in polyarteritis nodosa and Churg-Strauss syndrome. A prospective study in 342 patients. Medicine (Baltimore). 1996;75:17–28.

61. Guillevin L, et al. The five-factor score revisited: Assessment of prognoses of systemic necrotizing vasculitides based on the French Vasculitis Study Group (FVSG) cohort. Medicine (Baltimore). 2011;90(1):19–27.

62. Cohen P, et al. Churg-Strauss syndrome with poor-prognosis factors: A prospective multicenter trial comparing glucocorticoids and six or twelve cyclophosphamide pulses in forty-eight patients. Arthritis Rheum. 2007;57(4):686–93.

63. Mohammad AJ, et al. Rituximab for the treatment of eosinophilic granulomatosis with polyangiitis (Churg-Strauss). Ann Rheum Dis. 2016;75(2):396–401.

7 Renal Involvement in Immune Complex Vasculitides

Margaret A. Deoliveira, Desh Nepal, Michael Putman, and Abdallah S. Geara

7.1 IMMUNE COMPLEX VASCULITIS

Immune complex (IC) vasculitis is an inflammatory disease of the vessel walls associated with the perivascular deposition of ICs (immunoglobulin and complement components). Based on the 2012 International Chapel Hill Consensus Conference Nomenclature of Vasculitides, IC vasculitis includes the following: Anti-glomerular basement membrane (anti-GBM) disease, cryoglobulinemic vasculitis, IgA vasculitis (IgAV), and hypocomplementemic urticarial vasculitis syndrome (HUVS) (1). Other forms of IC vasculitis can be associated with drug exposure, serum sickness, infection, paraproteins, or autoimmune systemic diseases, such as systemic lupus erythematosus (SLE), Sjögren's syndrome (SJS), or rheumatoid arthritis (RA). The Chapel Hill Consensus Conference continued the trend of the preferential use of new names that reflect our evolving understanding of the pathophysiology of these conditions: IgAV for Henoch–Schönlein purpura, anti-C1q vasculitis for hypocomplementemic urticarial vasculitis, and anti-GBM vasculitis for Goodpasture's disease. Depending on the extent of involvement, these conditions can be classified as skin-limited or cutaneous versus systemic vasculitides. This chapter aims to describe kidney involvement in immune complex vasculitis and less common small-vessel vasculitis (SVV).

7.2 COMMON FEATURES OF IC VASCULITIS

Each of these conditions has a unique pathogenesis, but they all share pathologic deposition into the small-vessel walls (venules, capillaries, arterioles, small arteries), which results in tissue ischemia and necrosis (1). Except for anti-GBM disease, which does not involve the skin, dermatologic manifestations are the most common presenting features (2). Biopsies of these lesions typically reveal leukocytoclastic vasculitis (LCV) (2, 3).

The clinical presentation differs depending on the organ involved. When approaching differential diagnosis, vasculitis mimickers should be considered, including infections (endocarditis, syphilis, rickettsial diseases), malignancies (lymphoma and paraneoplastic syndromes), thrombotic or hypercoagulable conditions, amyloidosis, and sarcoidosis. In addition to a detailed history and physical examination, laboratory evaluations help narrow the differential diagnosis. A tissue biopsy is needed to confirm the diagnosis and exclude mimickers. Table 7.1 summarizes recommended investigations.

7.3 CRYOGLOBULINEMIC VASCULITIS

Cryoglobulins are proteins that precipitate at temperatures less than 37 degrees Celsius in vitro and dissolve after rewarming; the precipitate is composed of immunoglobulins (Igs) with or without complement components (4). Cryoglobulinemia is the presence of circulating cryoglobulins in the serum, which may be symptomatic or asymptomatic. Cryoglobulinemic vasculitis is a systemic inflammatory response due to the deposition of cryoglobulins in the capillaries and arterioles (5).

Based on the Ig composition on immunoelectrophoresis, cryoglobulins can be grouped into three types: cryoglobulin type I, II, or III (Table 7.2). Cryoglobulin types II and III (also called mixed cryoglobulinemia since it contains more than one type of immunoglobulin) account for 85–90% of all cases (4, 5). They result from an imbalance between the endogenous production of ICs and their clearance from circulation by immunoglobulins. The endogenous production is accelerated either by chronic immune stimulation, such as hepatitis C virus (HCV) or autoimmune diseases, or by a lymphoproliferative disorder, such as lymphoma (6).

Clinical features of cryoglobulinemic vasculitis (7, 8, 9, 10) (reviewed in Table 7.3) can wax and wane over weeks to months, which may delay diagnosis. Renal involvement with glomerulonephritis can occur (Figure 7.1). Laboratory evaluation includes testing for cryoglobulins and evaluating for the underlying etiology (Table 7.2) (11). The detection of cryoglobulins requires a specific collection technique with prewarming the syringes and/or collection tubes to 37 degrees Celsius since colder temperatures will cause the cryoglobulins to precipitate and result in false negative results (11). In cases where the initial evaluation is negative but suspicion remains high, retesting should be conducted. In a large French cohort, 9% of patients who initially tested negative became positive on repeat testing (12). Testing for viral infections in general and HCV in particular—which occurs in 60–90% of patients—is required (13). In 10% of cases of mixed cryoglobulinemia where

DOI: 10.1201/9781003438373-9

Table 7.1: Laboratory Evaluation for Vasculitis*

Nonspecific inflammatory laboratory and extension of organ involvement	CBC, ESR, CRP Urinalysis, microscopy, and urine protein/creatinine ratio Liver function tests Creatinine Blood culture
Antibody, complement components, and other laboratory tests in search for a diagnosis	C3, C4, ANA, anti-DS-DNA ANCA serology Cryoglobulins HBV, HCV, HIV, syphilis IgE Paraprotein evaluation (SPEP, IFE and serum free light chains)

Abbreviations: CBC, complete blood count; ESR, erythrocyte sedimentation rate; CRP, c-reactive protein; ANA, antinuclear antibody; anti-ds-DNA, anti-double stranded DNA; ANCA, antineutrophilic cytoplasmic antibody; HBV, hepatitis B virus; HCV, hepatitis C virus; HIV, human immunodeficiency virus; SPEP, serum protein electrophoresis; IFE, immunofixation
*The clinical scenario guides tests ordered.

Table 7.2: Different Types of Cryoglobulins

	Cryoglobulin Type I	Cryoglobulin Type II	Cryoglobulin Type III
		Mixed Cryoglobulins	
Type of Ig	Monoclonal Ig (usually IgG or IgM)	Monoclonal IgM (or IgG or IgA) and polyclonal Igs	Polyclonal IgG and IgM immune complexes
Associated diseases	MGUS, MM, Waldenstrom's macroglobulinemia, CLL, non-Hodgkin's lymphoma	Persistent HCV, SLE, Sjögren's syndrome, other viruses (HBV, HIV, EBV, CMV, human parvovirus B19)	Autoimmune or HCV
Additional laboratory findings	Complement not consumed Very high ESR Very high hypergammaglobulinemia	Low C4 C3 is normal or mildly consumed RF activity Moderate hypergammaglobulinemia of IgM, IgA, and/or IgG	Low C4 C3 is normal or mildly consumed Moderate hypergammaglobulinemia of IgM, IgA, and/or IgG

Abbreviations: Ig, immunoglobulin; MGUS, monoclonal gammopathy of undetermined significance; MM, multiple myeloma; CLL, chronic lymphocytic leukemia; HCV, hepatitis C virus; HBV, hepatitis B virus; HIV, human immunodeficiency virus; CMV, cytomegalovirus; C3, complement 3; C4, complement 4. SLE, systemic lupus erythematous; ESR, erythrocyte sedimentation rate; RF, rheumatoid factor

no underlying etiology can be found, patients are categorized as essential mixed cryoglobulinemia. Serum creatinine, urinalysis, and microscopy should be checked (7, 14). Renal biopsy is done with renal involvement (5). Nerve biopsy could be considered depending on the clinical context. Bone marrow biopsy may be needed for cryoglobulinemia type I to evaluate for plasma cell dyscrasias.

Treatment is directed at the underlying etiology; for example, antiviral therapy should be considered for HCV, clone-directed therapy for MGUS and MM, and anticancer therapy for CLL. Regardless of the underlying etiology, treatment is necessary for patients with end-organ damage, such as rapidly progressive glomerulonephritis (RPGN). For RPGN from HCV, rituximab is preferred (5, 15). In the setting of kidney involvement, the patient presents with nephritic syndrome (hematuria, proteinuria, and AKI) that requires urgent biopsy unless indicated. The renal histology shows predominantly membranoproliferative lesions with endocapillary proliferation and duplication of the basement membranes (9, 10). Eosinophilic refractile intracapillary "cryo-plugs" or pseudothrombi due to the

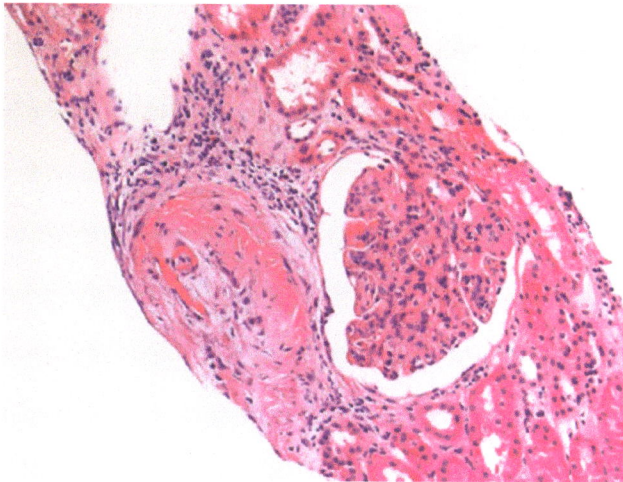

Figure 7.1 Cryoglobulin-related glomerulonephritis. The glomeruli have a lobular appearance with an endocapillary proliferative pattern of injury. The adjacent vessel shows a vasculitis lesion with cryoglobulin deposit in the vessel wall.

Table 7.3: Clinical Features of Immune Complex Small-Vessel Vasculitides (IC-SVV)

IC-SVV	Renal Manifestations	Non-Renal Manifestations
CV	Occurs in 30 % of patients. Clinical presentation includes proteinuria, hematuria, hypertension, and mild/chronic renal insufficiency. Biopsy most commonly shows MPGN; mesangioproliferative GN can be seen; abundant cells (monocytes/macrophages) and intracapillary thrombi can be seen; RPGN leading to ESRD can occur.	*CV type I*: Features of vascular occlusion and hyperviscosity such as cutaneous ulceration, livedo reticularis, necrosis, digital ischemia, blurry vision, dizziness, deafness, diplopia, ataxia, confusion, and stroke can occur. *CV type II and III*: Palpable purpura (>90%), constitutional symptoms (>70%), gastrointestinal (GI) involvement (<30%), pulmonary involvement (<5%), and peripheral neuropathy.
IgAV	Occurs in about 50% of patients. Clinical presentation includes microscopic or macroscopic hematuria, mild or no proteinuria. Nephrotic and nephritic syndromes, although less common, can occur. Most resolve spontaneously. Progression to ESRD can occur. Severity often correlates with the presence of crescents.	Skin involvement (>90%) includes purpura with lower extremity predilection; joint involvement (>75%) with arthralgia, arthritis; gastrointestinal involvement (>60%) with abdominal pain, nausea, vomiting, bleeding; neurological involvement (<10%); ENT (<5%); and pulmonary (<5%). Skin, joint, and GI involvement together constitutes the classic triad.
Anti-GBM disease	All patients have renal involvement, with glomerulonephritis with crescent formation as the most common feature. Progression to ESRD can occur.	Diffuse alveolar hemorrhage (40–60%). Cutaneous manifestations are notably absent.

(Continued)

Table 7.3: (Continued)

IC-SVV	Renal Manifestations	Non-Renal Manifestations
HUVS	Occurs in 14–50% patients. Clinical presentation varies from mild to nephrotic-range proteinuria. Nephritic syndrome can occur. Biopsy findings can vary; while MPGN is most common, membranous nephropathy, crescentic glomerulonephritis, and interstitial nephritis have been described. C1q antibody deposition is frequently observed. Progression to ESRD is rare.	Skin involvement occurs in all patients with chronic urticaria as the most common presentation. Urticarial vasculitis lesions (raised and pruritic patches associated with pain or burning) persist for more than 24 hours, often leave residual purpura or hyperpigmentation; annular lesions, palpable purpura, target lesions, livedo reticularis, vesicles, blisters, bullae can occur; no predilection for lower extremities. Angioedema (lips, tongue, periorbital tissue, or hands) seen in >50% patients; can be an initial presentation. Inflammatory eye conditions (>30%) include conjunctivitis, episcleritis, or uveitis. Pulmonary involvement (>25%) present with cough, dyspnea, moderate to severe COPD. Gastrointestinal involvement (abdominal pain, nausea, vomiting) can occur.
Drug-induced IC vasculitis	Occurs in >34% patients. Clinical presentation ranges from nephrotic syndrome to nephritic syndrome to renal insufficiency.	80% patients have cutaneous manifestations that include maculopapular rash, palpable purpura, and petechiae; ulcers, bullae, and livedo reticularis can occur too. Constitutional symptoms (fever, arthralgia), arthritis with joint effusion, and gastrointestinal involvement (abdominal pain, nausea, vomiting, GI bleeding) can occur.
Vasculitis in monoclonal gammopathy	Glomerular disease, tubulointerstitial disease, and direct tissue invasion can occur due to either the paraprotein load circulating in the kidney or secondary vasculitis due to IC formation.	Palpable and macular purpura without predilection to lower extremities can occur. Features due to occlusive vasculopathy include retiform purpura, cutaneous ulcerations, livedo reticularis, nodules, or digital ischemia. Monoclonal gammopathy can also present as erythema elevatum et diutinum.

Abbreviations: CV, cryoglobulinemic vasculitis; IgAV, IgA vasculitis; HUVS, hypocomplementemic urticarial vasculitis syndrome; GBM, glomerular basement membrane; MPGN, membranoproliferative glomerulonephritis; RPGN, rapidly progressive glomerulonephritis; ESRD, end-stage renal disease; CNS, central nervous system; RRT, renal replacement therapy

IgM component of these deposits can be seen. Immunofluorescence will show prominent IgM and C3, often with the clonal bias of κ light chain versus λ. On electron microscopy, the immune deposits may show short fibrillary substructures and are organized similar to fibrin (9, 10).

Steroids with or without high-dose pulse are recommended for moderate to severe mixed cryoglobulinemia. Very rarely, cyclophosphamide can be used as an alternative to rituximab. Plasma exchange can be used in patients with hyperviscosity syndrome, mainly in cryoglobulinemia type I, very severe RPGN, very high cryocrit level (>10%), and refractory skin lesions. Patients should be monitored clinically and with cryocrit levels to assess for relapse, in which case retreatment with rituximab with or without steroids is indicated. It should be noted that some patients with previously treated HCV have persistent cryoglobulinemia, can present with cryoglobulinemic vasculitis even after the clearance of HCV, and can be treated with rituximab (16).

7.4 IGA VASCULITIS

IgAV is an IC-SVV characterized by deposits of IgA (17). It is the most common form of vasculitis in children but is increasingly being recognized in adults, which tends to cause severe disease, especially with renal or gastrointestinal involvement (18). Its clinical presentation is noted in Table 7.3. It is characterized by the "classic triad" of purpura, arthralgia, and abdominal pain (17). Purpura and renal complications occur more frequently in older patients, while joint and gastrointestinal disease is more common in children (18).

A "multi-hit" model for pathogenesis is the most widely accepted theory for IgAV and the nephropathy that occurs with it (18). Based on common temporal and geospatial factors, including seasonality (September to April) and proximity to the course of the Drava and Danube rivers, environmental factors may trigger IgAV (18). Upper respiratory infections and antigen exposure frequently occur before IgAV onset (18).

The progression to and severity of renal involvement in adults is the primary determinant of a long-term prognosis for IgAV patients (19). Although initial disease presentation does not correlate with the clinical course of renal manifestation (17), age of onset, degree of renal impairment, and proteinuria excretion at the time of diagnosis are primary predictors of the risk of ESRD (20). Similarly, severe GI involvement may also predict prognosis, although long-term prospective studies are required (21, 22).

Adult patients frequently require corticosteroids to address inflammation, and steroid-sparing agents may be warranted up front (23). The efficacy of immunosuppressant treatment, however, warrants further exploration given the risk of progression to renal failure (23). The effectiveness of corticosteroid usage for IgAV is not well supported by data, but prescriptions for symptom management are common (23).

For persistent renal involvement, the approach to therapy is similar to that in patients with IgA nephropathy. It includes supportive care with a renin–angiotensin–aldosterone blockade used at the maximum tolerated dose +/– SGLT2 inhibitors for 3 to 6 months (24). If the proteinuria is persistently elevated (>750 mg/g of creatinine) or if the CKD is progressive, an immunosuppressive approach is considered with prednisone (dosed as per the testing trial) (25) or a targeted-release formulation of budesonide (26).

7.5 ANTI-GBM VASCULITIS

Anti-GBM vasculitis is a rare form of SVV affecting glomerular and pulmonary capillaries, caused by deposits of anti-GBM autoantibodies (27). The autoantibodies bind to basement membrane antigens, leading to the in situ formation of ICs with resultant neutrophil-dependent inflammation (27). It has a bimodal age distribution with an early peak in the third decade, where pulmonary involvement is more frequent, and a late peak in the sixth to seventh decades, where isolated glomerulonephritis is the most common presentation. The cause of anti-GBM disease is not fully understood, although a combination of environmental factors, infectious triggers, and genetic predispositions are believed to be involved (28). Specific genetic linkages to HLA-DRB1(*)1501 and DRB1(*)1502 have been observed (27).

The clinical presentation is noted in Table 7.3 (28). Anti-GBM can be diagnosed by identifying anti-GBM antibodies in circulation through rapid assay tests (29). However, in rare cases of "atypical anti-GBM nephritis", clinical presentation is mild, and circulating anti-GBM antibodies are absent (30). Kidney biopsies often reveal crescentic glomerulonephritis with linear GBM IgG deposits, differentiating it from AAV. ANCA serologies should be checked to evaluate for concomitant AAV, which has been described.

The treatment of anti-GBM disease focuses on the removal of pathologic autoantibodies with a combination of plasma exchange, steroids, and cytotoxic therapy (28). Plasma exchange is initially performed daily and continued until the improvement or normalization of anti-GBM titers. This may be cumbersome depending on the local availability of rapid testing for anti-GBM antibodies. Oral cyclophosphamide is the most commonly used immunosuppressive agent for induction therapy, although the use of rituximab has also been reported (31).

Transplantation should be delayed until anti-GBM antibodies are undetectable for more than 6 months (27). Early detection and intervention can improve outcomes; approximately one-third of patients survive with functioning kidneys (29). Renal outcomes improve if therapy is started before serum creatinine exceeds 600 micromole/L (5 mg/dL) (27).

Relapse and recurrence after kidney transplantation are rare, although post-transplant de novo anti-GBM disease has been observed among patients diagnosed with X-linked Alport syndrome (28).

7.6 HYPOCOMPLEMENTEMIC URTICARIAL VASCULITIS

Hypocomplementemic urticarial vasculitis syndrome (HUVS) was first described in 1973 (32). Patients with primary HUVS are not associated with a connective tissue disease or neoplasia (32,

33). HUVS is a rare disease characterized by antibodies to C1q that bind to C1q and form an IC that activates the classic complement pathway (34, 35). This leads to the recruitment and activation of neutrophils and macrophages. C5a also acts as an anaphylatoxin, causing mast cell recruitment and degranulation, leading to urticaria (35). Skin biopsies reveal LCV with immunoglobulin and complement deposition (35, 36)

The clinical features of HUVS (33, 37–40) are described in Table 7.3. Diseases that may mimic HUVS include chronic urticaria, SLE, mixed cryoglobulinemia, the hereditary deficiency of a complement component or C1 esterase inhibitor, normocomplementemic urticarial vasculitis, and HBV infection (33, 38, 41). Notably, 9–21% of patients with chronic urticaria will be diagnosed with HUVS (42). Proposed diagnostic criteria for HUVS, including the presence of chronic urticaria and hypocomplementemia (C1q, C4, and C3 levels) for 6 months and the presence of at least two of the additional features (dermal venulitis, arthritis, glomerulonephritis, episcleritis or uveitis, recurrent abdominal pain, or C1Q precipitin), have been proposed (33, 41). As complement level can vary with disease activity, it should be repeated 2–3 times over several months when the disease is both active and quiescent (33).

Non-steroidal anti-inflammatory drugs (NSAIDs) and symptomatic treatments (antihistamines such as cinnarazine), as outlined in Table 7.4, should be considered (43–45). Systemic glucocorticoids (prednisone at 0.5–1 mg/kg) and steroid-sparing agents (colchicine, dapsone, hydroxychloroquine), as outlined in Table 7.5, are used in cases of systemic involvement. Glucocorticoid monotherapy, with or without antihistamines, can induce remission in over 80% of patients (43). In severe or recurrent disease, azathioprine, cyclophosphamide, cyclosporin A, IVIG, and plasma exchange have been used (33, 39, 43, 45). Still, no high-quality studies have been conducted supporting any approach. One case series has reported the successful use of omalizumab in severe recurrent cases, and IL-1 inhibitors may be considered in refractory cases (43, 44). The evidentiary basis for management decisions is limited. It often is based on a very low level of evidence, but a reasonable therapeutic ladder that increases with the severity of the disease is suggested in Table 7.5 (44, 45).

7.7 DRUG-INDUCED IMMUNE COMPLEX VASCULITIS

The 2012 update on the nomenclature of vasculitis has incorporated drug-induced immune complex vasculitis when a drug is suspected as a probable etiology (1). Various drugs, including antibiotics (beta-lactams including amoxicillin [46, 47], fluoroquinolones [47]), non-steroidal

Table 7.4: Supportive Measures for IC Vasculitis

Remove trigger	Identify and stop relevant medications, treat underlying infections, oncologic management of paraproteinemia
Rest	—
Joint pain	Analgesics (NSAIDs), low-dose corticosteroids
Edema	Leg elevation, compression stockings as tolerated
Localized skin manifestations	Topical corticosteroids, emollients, antihistamines (hydroxyzine)
Ulcers	Early involvement of wound care, limiting corticosteroid exposure as able
Renal involvement	Blood pressure management—consider ACE inhibition

Abbreviations: NSAIDs, non-steroidal anti-inflammatory drugs

Table 7.5: Immunomodulatory Treatment of IC-Mediated Systemic Vasculitis

Severity	Intervention
Mild	Supportive measures alone
Moderate to severe	Systemic glucocorticoids, colchicine, dapsone
Severe, organ threatening	Rituximab, cyclophosphamide, plasma exchange
Refractory disease to glucocorticoids	Glucocorticoid-sparing agents (azathioprine, methotrexate, or mycophenolate mofetil)
Recurrent disease	Glucocorticoid-sparing agents (azathioprine, methotrexate, or mycophenolate mofetil)

anti-inflammatory drugs (46, 47), and tumor necrosis factor inhibitors (48) have been implicated in drug-induced vasculitis.

Drug-induced IC vasculitis typically occurs 1 to 9 weeks after drug exposure (49). Clinical features (47–49) can vary and are reviewed in Table 7.3. The diagnosis relies on a thorough exposure history, which includes both prescribed and illicit drugs (49). In cases where the temporal relationship between initiating therapy and the onset of symptoms has been established, suspected agents should be stopped immediately if possible. Resolution after discontinuation supports the diagnosis, but uncertainty about whether or not the offending agent caused the vasculitic symptoms frequently persists (49). Rechallenging should generally be avoided, though in cases where the suspected agent is necessary, a trial of therapy may be considered. Skin biopsies may show non-necrotizing mononuclear cells and classic necrotizing LCV (49). Lung and kidney biopsy may be required to characterize the degree of disease activity and chronicity and to differentiate from disease mimickers (49).

Recommendations to guide the management of drug-induced vasculitis are based on expert opinion; high-quality studies or consensus-based recommendations have yet to be published. The discontinuation of the offending agent (often based on the temporal association) should be done promptly (49). Early withdrawal, especially in cases of limited cutaneous vasculitis, may result in the resolution of symptoms (49). The overall prognosis of drug-induced IC vasculitis is good (49). In one study, 82–93% of patients had durable remission; the minority who developed relapsing or persistent microhematuria or proteinuria did not experience progression to ESRD (47).

7.8 VASCULITIS IN MONOCLONAL GAMMOPATHY

Monoclonal gammopathy can cause organ damage (peripheral nerves, kidneys) either by vasculitis or due to vascular occlusion due to paraprotein (non-vasculitis vasculopathy) (50). Vasculitis, when present, can occur due to IgG/IgM mediated immune complex/type 1 cryoglobulinemic vasculitis or as IgA vasculitis (2).

Clinical features in patients with vasculitis due to monoclonal gammopathy (2, 50) are described in Table 7.3. Diagnosis is established with organ biopsy. Vessel wall thrombosis without vasculitis would suggest occlusive vasculopathy; such cases should prompt investigation for alternative etiologies, including hypercoagulable states. When vasculitis is observed, the workup discussed in Table 7.1, including evaluation for paraprotein, should be performed (51). A bone marrow biopsy may be necessary if monoclonal proteins are observed (51).

Management involves treating the cause of monoclonal gammopathy. Additional measures for symptomatic management and controlling inflammation are discussed in Table 7.4 and Table 7.5. In severe cases, corticosteroids, plasmapheresis, and cyclophosphamide may be required (51). Most importantly, the successful treatment of an underlying plasma cell disorder improves prognosis.

7.9 CONCLUSION

IC-SVV includes a group of rare diseases with various underlying inciting processes that ultimately lead to IC formation, causing vasculitis. While there are similarities in the overall clinical presentation, careful evaluation can differentiate between them. The clinical course and disease progression can vary among individuals. Management is based on low-quality evidence and is typically guided by the disease severity and clinical course.

REFERENCES

1. Jennette JC, et al. 2012 Revised international Chapel Hill consensus conference nomenclature of vasculitides. Arthritis Rheum. 2013;65(1):1–11.
2. Sunderkotter CH, et al. Nomenclature of cutaneous vasculitis: Dermatologic addendum to the 2012 revised international Chapel Hill consensus conference nomenclature of vasculitides. Arthritis Rheumatol. 2018;70(2):171–84.
3. Jennette JC, et al. Small-vessel vasculitis. N Engl J Med. 1997;337(21):1512–23.
4. Silva F, et al. New insights in cryoglobulinemic vasculitis. J Autoimmun. 2019;105:102313.
5. Sethi S, et al. Acute glomerulonephritis. Lancet. 2022;399(10335):1646–63.
6. Brouet JC, et al. Biologic and clinical significance of cryoglobulins. A report of 86 cases. Am J Med. 1974;57(5):775–88.
7. Dispenzieri A, Gorevic PD. Cryoglobulinemia. Hematol Oncol Clin North Am. 1999;13(6):1315–49.
8. Dammacco F, et al. Clinical practice: Hepatitis C virus infection, cryoglobulinemia and cryoglobulinemic vasculitis. Clin Exp Med. 2019;19(1):1–21.

9. Menter T, et al. Renal disease in Cryoglobulinemia. Glomerular Dis. 2021;1(2):92–104.

10. Chen YP, et al. Cryoglobulinemic vasculitis and glomerulonephritis: Concerns in clinical practice. Chin Med J (Engl). 2019;132(14):1723–32.

11. Kolopp-Sarda MN, et al. Cryoglobulinemic vasculitis: Pathophysiological mechanisms and diagnosis. Curr Opin Rheumatol. 2021;33(1):1–7.

12. Kolopp-Sarda MN, et al. Cryoglobulins today: Detection and immunologic characteristics of 1,675 positive samples from 13,439 patients obtained over six years. Arthritis Rheumatol. 2019;71(11):1904–12.

13. Misiani R, et al. Hepatitis C virus infection in patients with essential mixed cryoglobulinemia. Ann Intern Med. 1992;117(7):573–7.

14. Terrier B, et al. The spectrum of type I cryoglobulinemia vasculitis: New insights based on 64 cases. Medicine (Baltimore). 2013;92(2):61–8.

15. Montero N, et al. Treatment for hepatitis C virus-associated mixed cryoglobulinaemia. Cochrane Database Syst Rev. 2018;5(5):CD011403.

16. Batsaikhan B, et al. Persistent cryoglobulinemia after antiviral treatment is associated with advanced fibrosis in chronic hepatitis C patients. PLoS ONE. 2022;17(5):e0268180.

17. Audemard-Verger A, et al. IgA vasculitis (Henoch-Shonlein purpura) in adults: Diagnostic and therapeutic aspects. Autoimmun Rev. 2015;14(7):579–85.

18. Song Y, et al. Pathogenesis of IgA vasculitis: An up-to-date review. Front Immunol. 2021;12:771619.

19. Neumann T. [Update on immunoglobulin A vasculitis]. Z Rheumatol. 2022;81(4):305–12.

20. Gonzalez-Gay MA, et al. IgA vasculitis: Genetics and clinical and therapeutic management. Curr Rheumatol Rep. 2018;20(5):24.

21. Castaneda S, et al. Gastrointestinal involvement in adult IGA vasculitis. Rheumatology (Oxford). 2020;59(10):2659–60.

22. Audemard-Verger A, et al. Gastrointestinal involvement in adult IgA vasculitis (Henoch–Schönlein purpura): Updated picture from a French multicentre and retrospective series of 260 cases. Rheumatology (Oxford). 2020;59(10):3050–7.

23. Delbet JD, et al. Management of IgA vasculitis with nephritis. Paediatr Drugs. 2021;23(5):425–35.

24. Wheeler DC, et al. A pre-specified analysis of the DAPA-CKD trial demonstrates the effects of dapagliflozin on major adverse kidney events in patients with IgA nephropathy. Kidney Int. 2021;100(1):215–24.

25. Lv J, et al. Effect of oral methylprednisolone on decline in kidney function or kidney failure in patients with IgA nephropathy: The TESTING randomized clinical trial. JAMA. 2022;327(19):1888–98.

26. Barratt J, et al. Results from part A of the multi-center, double-blind, randomized, placebo-controlled NefIgArd trial, which evaluated targeted-release formulation of budesonide for the treatment of primary immunoglobulin A nephropathy. Kidney Int. 2023;103(2):391–402.

27. Hellmark T, et al. Diagnosis and classification of Goodpasture's disease (anti-GBM). J Autoimmun. 2014;48–49:108–12.

28. McAdoo SP, et al. Anti-glomerular basement membrane disease. Clin J Am Soc Nephrol. 2017;12(7):1162–72.

29. Segelmark M, et al. Anti-glomerular basement membrane disease: An update on subgroups, pathogenesis and therapies. Nephrol Dial Transplant. 2019;34(11):1826–32.

30. Nasr SH, et al. The clinicopathologic characteristics and outcome of atypical anti-glomerular basement membrane nephritis. Kidney Int. 2016;89(4):897–908.

31. Uematsu-Uchida M, et al. Rituximab in treatment of anti-GBM antibody glomerulonephritis: A case report and literature review. Medicine (Baltimore). 2019;98(44):e17801.

32. McDuffie FC, et al. Hypocomplementemia with cutaneous vasculitis and arthritis. Possible immune complex syndrome. Mayo Clin Proc. 1973;48(5):340–8.

33. Khasnis A, et al. Update on vasculitis. J Allergy Clin Immunol. 2009;123(6):1226–36.

34. Kishore U, et al. C1q: Structure, function, and receptors. Immunopharmacology. 2000;49(1–2):159–70.

35. Mehregan DR, et al. Pathophysiology of urticarial vasculitis. Arch Dermatol. 1998;134(1):88–9.

36. Dincy CV, et al. Clinicopathologic profile of normocomplementemic and hypocomplementemic urticarial vasculitis: A study from South India. J Eur Acad Dermatol Venereol. 2008;22(7):789–94.

37. Ion O, et al. Kidney involvement in hypocomplementemic urticarial vasculitis syndrome: A case-based review. J Clin Med. 2020;9(7).
38. Marzano AV, et al. Urticarial vasculitis: Clinical and laboratory findings with a particular emphasis on differential diagnosis. J Allergy Clin Immunol. 2022;149(4):1137–49.
39. Corthier A, et al. Biopsy-proven kidney involvement in hypocomplementemic urticarial vasculitis. BMC Nephrol. 2022;23(1):67.
40. Marzano AV, et al. Urticarial vasculitis and urticarial autoinflammatory syndromes. G Ital Dermatol Venereol. 2015;150(1):41–50.
41. Schwartz HR, et al. Hypocomplementemic urticarial vasculitis: Association with chronic obstructive pulmonary disease. Mayo Clin Proc. 1982;57(4):231–8.
42. Puhl V, et al. A novel histopathological scoring system to distinguish urticarial vasculitis from chronic spontaneous urticaria. Clin Transl Allergy. 2021;11(2):e12031.
43. Kolkhir P, et al. Treatment of urticarial vasculitis: A systematic review. J Allergy Clin Immunol. 2019;143(2):458–66.
44. Gu SL, et al. Urticarial vasculitis. Int J Womens Dermatol. 2021;7(3):290–7.
45. Radic M, et al. Drug-induced vasculitis: A clinical and pathological review. Neth J Med. 2012;70(1):12–17.
46. Garcia-Porrua C, et al. Drug associated cutaneous vasculitis in adults in northwestern Spain. J Rheumatol. 1999;26(9):1942–4.
47. Ortiz-Sanjuan F, et al. Drug-associated cutaneous vasculitis: Study of 239 patients from a single referral center. J Rheumatol. 2014;41(11):2201–7.
48. Sokumbi O, et al. Vasculitis associated with tumor necrosis factor-alpha inhibitors. Mayo Clin Proc. 2012;87(8):739–45.
49. Calabrese LH, et al. Drug-induced vasculitis. Curr Opin Rheumatol. 1996;8(1):34–40.
50. Perazella MA, et al. Paraprotein-related kidney disease: Attack of the killer M proteins. Clin J Am Soc Nephrol. 2016;11(12):2256–9.
51. Levine SM, et al. Paraprotein and cryoglobulin-associated medium-vessel vasculitis. J Rheumatol. 2011;38(8):1697–8.

8 Large- and Medium-Vessel Vasculitis

Raisa Lomanto Silva[†], Zain M. AlShanableh[†], Syeda Behjat Ahmad[‡], and Sebastian E. Sattui[‡]
[†]These are co-first authors.
[‡]These are co-senior authors.

8.1 INTRODUCTION

Large- (LVV) and medium-vessel vasculitides (MVV) consist of a heterogenous group of diseases characterized by inflammation of the blood vessel walls. Vessel injury results in the compromise of the lumen and blood flow, leading to ischemia, necrosis, and the disruption of vessel wall integrity, increasing the risk of rupture or bleeding (1). Although less common than small-vessel vasculitides, LVV and MVV commonly affect the kidney. Giant cell arteritis and Takayasu arteritis (TAK) are the most common types of LVV, which affect large arteries, including the aorta and its major branches (2). Polyarteritis nodosa (PAN) and Kawasaki disease are the major forms of MVV, which affect the main visceral arteries and their branches (2).

This chapter will focus on TAK and PAN, as these affect the kidneys, and will review their manifestations, diagnosis, and treatment.

8.2 TAKAYASU ARTERITIS

8.2.1 Definition and Epidemiology

TAK is an inflammatory, granulomatous vasculitis that most commonly involves the aorta and its proximal branches (3). In 2022, validated international classification criteria for TAK were endorsed that include <60 years of age at the time of diagnosis and evidence of vasculitis on imaging as absolute requirements, along with additional clinical and imaging criteria (4). TAK is most often diagnosed in the third decade of life, with a female to male ratio ranging from 3:1 to 12:1 in different countries (3, 4). Although TAK has been reported globally, the highest prevalence has been reported in individuals of Asian and North African descent, with increased prevalence in Japan compared with Western countries (5, 6).

8.2.2 Pathogenesis

The precise pathogenesis is not entirely known. An intense granulomatous inflammation involving the inner wall of blood vessels with infiltrating monocytes and lymphocytes and a large population of cytotoxic CD8+ T cells is noted in the early stages of disease (7, 8). Transmural thickening with fibrosis ensues, leading to vessel narrowing, occlusion, dilation, aneurysm formation, and ischemia (7–9).

Both the innate and adaptive immune systems are involved in aberrant immunologic responses culminating in LVV. The loss of protective immune tolerance occurs via a loss of T regulatory cells, deficiencies in programmed cell death 1/programmed cell death 1 ligand 1, and reactive oxygen species-induced permeability of the endothelial barrier. Several cytokines, including interferon gamma (IFNγ), interleukin-6 (IL-6), IL-12, IL-17, IL-23, and IL-1, are produced by migrating T helper 1 and T helper 17 cells in the vessel wall, along with platelet-derived growth factors and metalloproteinases (10–12). Extravascular systemic inflammation is established, and IL-6 is further produced by hepatocytes, macrophages, endothelial cells, and fibroblasts.

8.2.3 Clinical Manifestations

The onset of symptoms in TAK is most often subacute, which often leads to a delay in diagnosis (13, 14). In early stages, weight loss, low-grade fever, and fatigue are common, along with anorexia, arthralgias, and myalgias (9, 14).

Persistent inflammation leads to structural vascular changes, with stenoses predominating over aneurysms. Severe upper extremity vessel stenosis (most commonly radial arteries) causes diminished or absent pulses, limb claudication, vascular bruits, and blood pressure discrepancies (15–17). Retinopathies occur due to retinal ischemia (18). Neurological symptoms (headaches, lightheadedness, syncope, seizures) occur due to carotid and vertebral arterial involvement (19). Other manifestations include dilated cardiomyopathy, aortic regurgitation, and carotidynia (16). Hypertension is common, reflective of renal involvement (16, 17, 20).

8.2.3.1 Renal Manifestations

The most common renal manifestation is renal artery stenosis (RAS). RAS is found in up to 65–75% of individuals with TAK (21). Stenosis results from initial inflammation leading to intimal

 DOI: 10.1201/9781003438373-10

thickening with multinucleated giant cells and infiltrating monocytes and lymphocytes. In later stages, there is a loss of vascular elastic lamina, adventitial fibrosis, and neovascularization. The resultant stenosis causes renovascular hypertension (RVH) (Figure 8.1). The diagnosis of hypertension can be challenging due to coexisting subclavian, femoral, and iliac stenoses, sometimes requiring alternative methods for blood pressure measurement such as aortic pressures by catheterization. RVH is not always the sole cause of hypertension in TAK. Multiple studies show similar prevalence of secondary hypertension in TAK. For example, in a single center study in China of 530 patients, 60% had secondary hypertension (22).

RVH specifically occurs due to increased activity of the renin–angiotensin–aldosterone system (Figure 8.1). Reduced perfusion secondary to renal artery involvement results in the release and activation of renin. Renin converts angiotensinogen to angiotensin I, which is converted to angiotensin II by angiotensin-converting enzyme (ACE). Salt and water reabsorption and volume expansion result from aldosterone release (23–25). Because RAS is usually unilateral, the contralateral kidney will have increased perfusion, resulting in compensatory "pressure natriuresis", restoring volume status. Consequently, there is chronic hypoperfusion. Hypertension is attributed to the direct effects of angiotensin II. Angiotensin II causes direct vasoconstriction, sympathetic nervous system stimulation, and vascular remodeling. When RAS is bilateral, hypertension is volume mediated due to the absence of pressure natriuresis (25, 26). Another mechanism leading to hypertension is systemic endothelial dysfunction, which results in coagulation augmentation and complement activation, leading to thrombosis and parenchymal ischemic necrosis. The decline in vasodilatory prostaglandins causes an increase in arterial blood pressure. Renal ischemia also decreases glomerular filtration and the excretion of free water, resulting in volume expansion and further hypertension (23).

Glomerulonephritis is rare in TAK (21). Mesangial glomerulonephritis has been reported along with hyaline deposits and microaneurysms. Focal and segmental lesions have been reported with membranoproliferative glomerulonephritis (21). Nephrotic syndrome and IgA nephropathy have also been reported (21).

8.2.4 Diagnosis

Conventional angiography was the gold standard for TAK diagnosis but has been replaced by non-invasive testing such as computerized tomography angiography (CTA) or magnetic resonance

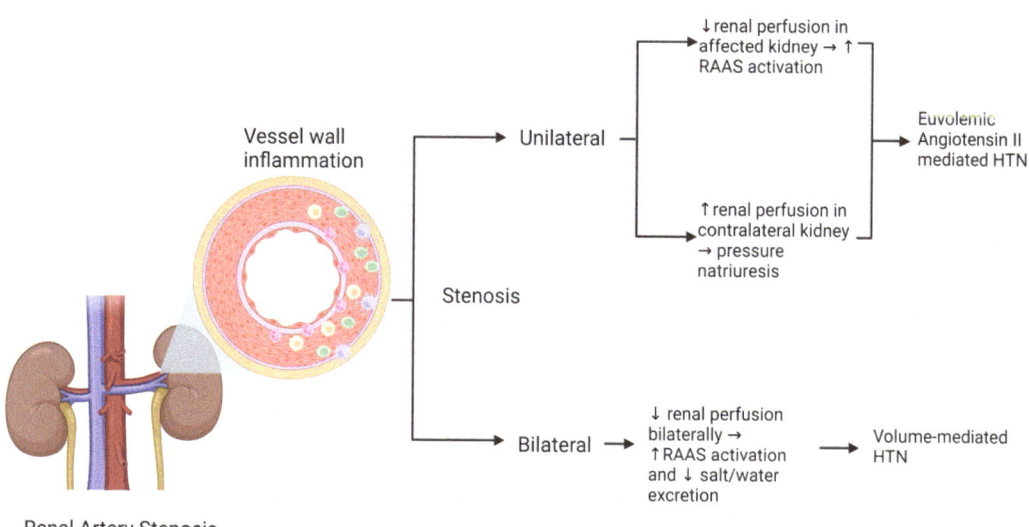

Renal Artery Stenosis

Figure 8.1 Renal artery stenosis and renovascular hypertension in Takayasu arteritis. Mechanisms of renovascular hypertension in Takayasu arteritis resulting from either unilateral or bilateral renal artery stenosis.

RAS = renal artery stenosis, RAAS = renin-angiotensin-aldosterone system, HTN = hypertension.

angiography (MRA) (27, 28). F-fluorodeoxyglucose positron emission tomography (FDG-PET) detects abnormal metabolic activity in the wall of inflamed vessels and is useful for diagnosis and disease monitoring (29–34). The cost of FDG-PET, though, is prohibitive. Ultrasound is a promising portable diagnostic tool with the potential for detecting disease activity and/or progression (35–37).

No laboratory markers are specific for TAK diagnosis. C-reactive protein (CRP) and erythrocyte sedimentation rate (ESR) can be used to monitor disease activity (17, 38). However, IL-6 inhibitors result in dampening CRP production by hepatocytes. Histopathology is seldom practical since large artery biopsy is often unnecessary. Diagnosis is based on clinical aspects and vascular imaging (4). RVH involves a demonstration of >60% RAS by imaging while other common causes such as atherosclerotic RAS, fibromuscular dysplasia, and aortic coarctation are ruled out (25, 39).

8.2.5 Treatment

Glucocorticoids (GCs) are the first line of treatment in patients with active TAK. However, due to the condition's chronic and relapsing nature, the early initiation of GC-sparing agents is imperative (40). For new and active TAK, high-dose GCs are recommended along with non-GC immunosuppressive treatments such as methotrexate, azathioprine, mycophenolate mofetil, leflunomide, or biologics. High-dose intravenous GC is recommended for life-threatening organ damage (32). Once remission occurs over 6–12 months, GC can be tapered off. If disease remains active, the use of another non-GC agent is recommended. TNF inhibitors are recommended over IL-6 inhibitors as the first biologic agent (32, 41–43). IL-6 inhibitors may be considered in cases of refractory cases (12, 44, 45). The soluble CTLA4 analog abatacept is not currently recommended due to a lack of efficacy (46). Clinical trials assessing the use of other therapies are currently underway. Cyclophosphamide may be an option in severe refractory cases; however, consideration should be taken that infertility is a side effect and is a concern in the young female-predominant population. Antiplatelet therapy is conditionally recommended in patients at higher risk for ischemic events (32, 47).

8.2.5.1 Renal Disease Management

The treatment of RVH can be challenging due to fluid retention associated with GC. ACE inhibitors or angiotensin receptor blockers are the preferred medications for medical management. These require the close monitoring of kidney function, and their use is limited due to intolerance (Figure 8.1) (14). Guidelines recommend medical management for RVH and renal artery stenosis. The 2021 ACR-VF guidelines recommend medical management for RVH and renal artery stenosis. If ineffective, surgical intervetion can be utilized (32).

Percutaneous renal artery angioplasty (PTRA) is indicated in refractory RVH (14, 48). Improvements in blood pressure after successful revascularization have been noted in patients with RVH and TAK (49, 50). Balloon angioplasty and stent placement have similar clinical efficacy. While stenting has fewer complications, higher rates of restenosis have been noted in comparison to angioplasty. Stent placement should be reserved for angioplasty failure, ostial lesion, and long segment stenosis (51, 52). Surgical bypass could be considered in long segment stenosis (48, 52). Intervention, surgical or endovascular, should be avoided in the acute phase (14, 48).

Relapses occur in as many as 50% of patients, usually occurring within 5 years of diagnosis and with male sex, carotidynia, and elevated CRP being independent risk factors (53). Clinical monitoring, including periodic non-invasive vascular imaging, is recommended.

8.3 POLYARTERITIS NODOSA

8.3.1 Definition and Epidemiology

Polyarteritis nodosa (PAN) is a rare, systemic, multi-organ, necrotizing, medium-vessel vasculitis that frequently involves the gastrointestinal, musculoskeletal, renal, and neurologic systems and is more commonly diagnosed in middle-aged and older adults with a peak in the sixth decade of life, with men more affected than women. PAN can be primary (idiopathic), or secondary, often associated with viral infections (hepatitis B [HBV], hepatitis C, parvovirus B19, cytomegalovirus, human T cell leukemia virus 1) or malignancies (hairy cell leukemia) (54–61) (Table 8.1).

8.3.2 Pathogenesis

In primary PAN, proinflammatory cytokines and antibodies cause vessel wall inflammation and endothelial cell activation with consequent dysfunction (62, 63). Elevated serum IFNγ, IL-2, and IL-8 have been noted (64–66). Wall thickening and intimal proliferation cause luminal narrowing and reduced blood flow, thus predisposing patients to thrombosis, tissue ischemia or infarction, or weakening of the vasculature and aneurysm formation (56, 67). Inflammatory infiltrates with

Table 8.1: Polyarteritis Nodosa (PAN)—Its Subtypes and Clinical Manifestations

	Primary/Idiopathic PAN	HBVa-Associated PAN	Cutaneous PAN	DADA 2b
Constitutional symptoms	+++	+++	+	++/+++
Skin	+/++	++	+++	+++
Musculoskeletal	++	++	+/++	+++
Gastrointestinal	++	++	−	+/++
Renal/urogenital	++	+	−	+
Peripheral nervous system	+++	+++	−/+	+
Central nervous system	−/+	−/+	−	++
Cardiac or vascular	+	+	−	+
Disease relapse	+/++	−/+	++	+

a HBV, hepatitis B
b Deficiency of adenosine deaminase 2 (DADA 2)

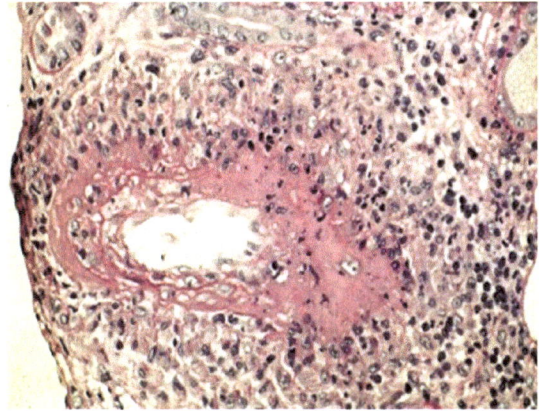

Figure 8.2 Renal biopsy in polyarteritis nodosa. Small artery with circumferential fibrinoid necrosis, loss of the endothelial cell lining, and karyorrhectic debris adjacent to the lumen. Few histiocytes seen peripherally.

polymorphonuclear leukocytes and mononuclear cells in arterial walls, along with fibrinoid necrosis, with the absence of granulomas and giant cells have been noted (Figure 8.2) (68, 69).

In HBV-associated PAN, vascular lesions result from immune complex deposition and in situ formation (70, 71), which activates the complement cascade, leading to neutrophil activation. Hypocomplementemia from complement deposition is notable.

8.3.3 Clinical Manifestations

PAN can cause single- to multi-organ failure (Table 8.1). Affected individuals present with fatigue, weight loss, weakness, fever, arthralgias, and/or signs of organ compromise. Cutaneous manifestations may occur as the sole manifestation or with systemic PAN and include palpable purpura, subcutaneous nodules, bullous eruption, or even digital infarction (72–76). Mononeuropathy multiplex occurs in up to 70% of patients (77, 78). Deficiency of adenosine deaminase 2 (DADA2), should be a concern when cerebrovascular accidents with PAN-like vasculopathy, immunodeficiency, and bone marrow failure occur (Table 8.1) (79, 80). Gastrointestinal manifestations can occur early and be the predominant symptom. Mesenteric arteritis can result in bowel infarction with perforation (77, 81). Ischemic retinopathy can also occur. Other manifestations of PAN include ischemic retinopathy, orchitis, coronary artery disease, and splenic infarction (66, 69, 82–85).

8.3.3.1 Renal Manifestations

Renal artery microaneurysms can occur in up to 66.2% of patients, and their rupture may result in hematoma, infarction, and retroperitoneal hemorrhage (24, 77). As a result, hematuria (>10 RBCs per hpf) and an elevated creatinine level has been noted in 15.2% of patients, while proteinuria (>0.4 g per 24 hours) has been noted in 21.6% (77). Multiple renal infarcts or uncontrolled hypertension can result in renal failure (77, 86). Patients >50 years of age are more likely to have kidney dysfunction (87). Progression to end-stage kidney disease, however, is rare (86).

Other histological lesions in PAN include arterial fibrinoid necrosis and membranous glomerulonephritis (24, 77). The former is associated with perivascular inflammatory infiltrates predominated by neutrophils in the early phase and mononuclear cells in the late phase and is thought to drive microaneurysm formation (24). PAN does not cause glomerulonephritis. However, membranous glomerulonephritis is seen with HBV-associated PAN and is likely due to HBV infection itself (24, 77).

RVH occurs in 34.8% of PAN cases, usually those with HBV infection (77). Following the acute arteritis phase, sclerosis ensues, resulting in intimal fibrosis, arterial narrowing and ischemia (24). The sequelae are similar to RVH in TAK.

8.3.4 Diagnosis

The diagnosis of PAN is based on clinical features along with histopathology, or angiography if biopsy cannot be obtained. There are no specific laboratory markers for PAN. Acute-phase reactants are often elevated. Screening for hepatitis and other infections is essential (88). In patients with rashes and peripheral neuropathy, a skin punch biopsy and nerve and muscle biopsy, respectively, can be informative (77, 86). Kidney and/or liver biopsy should be reserved for cases where the diagnosis is difficult, given the risk of bleeding. Segmental necrotizing transmural inflammation without granuloma formation has been noted with a predilection for bifurcations and branch points. Arterioles, capillaries, venules, and glomeruli are typically spared. Remodeling in advanced disease results in intimal hyperplasia, wall fibrosis, and microaneurysms.

Mesenteric or renal angiography are the optimal vascular studies. However, due to risks of arterial cannulation (e.g., bleeding, embolization, pseudoaneurysm), CTA and MRA can be used and can delineate arterial lesions and parenchymal lesions (e.g., renal infarcts, bowel wall thickening) and establish the extent of disease (56, 88, 89). Multiple 1–5 mm arterial saccular or fusiform microaneurysms, occlusions, irregular stenosis, and/or diffuse wall thickening of medium-sized arteries may be noted.

Tests to rule out PAN mimics and/or delineate the subtype of disease (e.g., HBV-PAN) are recommended, including tests for HIV, DADA2, and VEXAS syndrome, along with serum complements, anti-neutrophil cytoplasmic antibodies, antinuclear antibodies, cryoglobulins, and serum and urine immunofixation electrophoresis. Selection depends on the patient's clinical manifestations and local epidemiology (e.g., Lyme disease testing for polyradiculopathy in endemic areas). The identification of DADA2 is crucial given differences in treatment (i.e., TNF inhibitors preferred) (79).

8.3.5 Treatment

The treatment of PAN is guided by etiology, organ involvement, and disease progression. For HBV-PAN, the major approach is the use of antivirals with GCs (90). Prolonged GC use is cautioned against, as it can hamper immunological HBV clearance and promote seroconversion. Further immunosuppression may be considered in severe disease in cases of intolerance or inadequate response to antivirals (71, 91). Plasma exchange with antivirals has been advocated to remove circulating immune complexes, with possible reduced relapses (71, 92).

The five-factor score (FFS) is a prognostic scoring system aimed to guide therapeutic decisions regarding systemic necrotizing vasculitides (93). The 1996 score comprises the following criteria: cardiac involvement, GI involvement, serum creatinine >1.6 mg/dL, proteinuria >1 g/day, and CNS involvement. Each criterion has a value of 1 point; a score of 0, 1, or ≥2 is associated with a 12, 26, or 46% 5-year mortality, respectively. A 2011 FFS version was released, which includes different criteria, but its use and prognostication remain similar (94). For mild, non-organ/life-threatening systemic PAN (FFS 0), oral GCs alone can be considered. However, given the risks of relapse and need for a faster GC taper, GC-sparing immunosuppression should be considered early. GC-sparing agents should be considered for resistant cases or where there is GC intolerance. Eighteen months of therapy is recommended. For systemic active severe disease (FFS >1, with organ/life-threatening disease), high-dose intravenous pulse GCs are recommended over high-dose oral GCs (68). Oral or intravenous cyclophosphamide is recommended for treatment induction with high-dose GCs, offering reduced relapse rates and a decreased GC burden, but with an unclear mortality benefit (95–98). Methotrexate or azathioprine can be used for maintenance therapy for 18 months. Mycophenolate mofetil is an alternative option but requires more study. Plasmapheresis is not recommended for non-HBV-PAN (68).

8.3.5.1 Renal Disease Management

Prognosis varies due to the degree of organ involvement. For individuals with kidney involvement including hematuria and proteinuria, ACE inhibitors or angiotensin receptor blockers can be used. For individuals who develop chronic kidney disease and proteinuria, SGLT-2 inhibitors can be added (36). A low-salt diet is recommended to help control blood pressure (99).

REFERENCES

1. Jennette JC, et al. 2012 revised international Chapel Hill consensus conference nomenclature of vasculitides. Arthritis Rheum. 2013;65(1):1–11.
2. Saadoun D, et al. Medium- and large-vessel vasculitis. Circulation. 2021;143(3):267–82.
3. Onen F, et al. Epidemiology of Takayasu arteritis. Presse Med. 2017;46(7–8):e197–203.
4. Grayson PC, et al. 2022 American college of rheumatology/EULAR classification criteria for Takayasu arteritis. Ann Rheum Dis. 2022;81:1654–60.
5. Jiang Z, et al. Variations in Takayasu arteritis characteristics in a cohort of patients with different racial backgrounds. Semin Arthritis Rheum. 2022;53:151971.
6. Gudbrandsson B, et al. Prevalence, incidence, and disease characteristics of Takayasu Arteritis by ethnic background: Data from a large, population-based cohort resident in southern Norway. Arthritis Care Res (Hoboken). 2017;69(2):278–85.
7. Espinoza JL, et al. New insights on the pathogenesis of Takayasu Arteritis: Revisiting the microbial theory. Pathogens. 2018;7(3):73.
8. Arnaud L, et al Z. Pathogenesis of Takayasu's arteritis: A 2011 update. Autoimmun Rev. 2011;11(1):61–7.
9. Trinidad B, et al. Takayasu arteritis. In: *StatPearls* [Internet]. Treasure Island, FL: StatPearls Publishing; 2024.
10. Weyand CM, et al. Medium- and large-vessel vasculitis. N Engl J Med. 2003;349(2):160–9.
11. Pryshchep O, et al. Vessel-specific Toll-like receptor profiles in human medium and large arteries. Circulation. 2008;118(12):1276–84.
12. Pugh D, et al. Large-vessel vasculitis. Nat Rev Dis Primers. 2022;7(1):93.
13. Sreih AG, et al. Diagnostic delays in vasculitis and factors associated with time to diagnosis. Orphanet J Rare Dis. 2021;16(1):184.
14. Johnston SL, et al. Takayasu arteritis: A review. J Clin Pathol. 2002;55(7):481–6.
15. Serra R, et al. Updates in pathophysiology, diagnosis and management of Takayasu Arteritis. Ann Vasc Surg. 2016;35:210–25.
16. Subramanyan R, et al. Natural history of aortoarteritis (Takayasu's disease). Circulation. 1989;80(3):429–37.
17. Kerr GS, et al. Takayasu arteritis. Ann Intern Med. 1994;120(11):919–29.
18. Szydełko-Paśko U, et al. Ocular manifestations of Takayasu's arteritis: a case-based systematic review and meta-analysis. J Clin Med. 2023;12(11):3745.
19. Rodríguez-Pla A, et al. Bilateral blindness in Takayasu's disease. Scand J Rheumatol. 1996;25(6):394–5.
20. Lupi-Herrera E, et al. Takayasu's arteritis. Clinical study of 107 cases. Am Heart J. 1977;93(1):94–103.
21. Samarkos M, et al. The clinical spectrum of primary renal vasculitis. Semin Arthritis Rheum. 2005;35(2):95–111.
22. Zheng D, et al. Takayasu arteritis in China: A report of 530 cases. Heart Vessels Suppl. 1992;7:32–6.
23. Zhu Q, et al. Systemic vasculitis: An important and underestimated cause of malignant hypertension. CVIA. 2019;4(2):99–108.
24. Jennette JC, et al. The pathology of vasculitis involving the kidney. Am J Kidney Dis. 1994;24(1):130–41.
25. Herrmann SM, et al. Renovascular hypertension. Endocrinol Metab Clin North Am. 2019;48(4):765–78.

26. Herrmann SM, et al. Current concepts in the treatment of renovascular hypertension. Am J Hypertens. 2018;31(2):139–49.
27. Alibaz-Oner F, et al. Update on Takayasu's arteritis. Presse Med. 2015;44(6 Pt 2):e259–65.
28. Kato Y, et al. Vessel wall inflammation of Takayasu arteritis detected by contrast-enhanced magnetic resonance imaging: Association with disease distribution and activity. PLoS ONE. 2015;10(12):e0145855.
29. Quinn KA, et al. Comparison of magnetic resonance angiography and 18F-fluorodeoxyglucose positron emission tomography in large-vessel vasculitis. Ann Rheum Dis. 2018;77(8):1165–71.
30. Blockmans D, et al. Imaging for large-vessel vasculitis. Curr Opin Rheumatol. 2009;21(1):19–28.
31. Slart RHJA, et al. FDG-PET/CT(A) imaging in large vessel vasculitis and polymyalgia rheumatica: Joint procedural recommendation of the EANM, SNMMI, and the PET Interest Group (PIG), and endorsed by the ASNC. Eur J Nucl Med Mol Imaging. 2018;45(7):1250–69.
32. Maz M, et al. 2021 American college of rheumatology/vasculitis foundation guideline for the management of giant cell arteritis and Takayasu Arteritis. Arthritis Rheumatol. 2021;73(8):1349–65.
33. Taimen K, et al. The delay and costs of diagnosing systemic vasculitis in a tertiary-level clinic. Rheumatol Ther. 2021;8(1):233–42.
34. Quinn, KA, et al. Association of 18 F-fluorodeoxyglucose-positron emission tomography activity with angiographic progression of disease in large vessel vasculitis. Arthritis Rheumatol. 2023;75(1):98–107.
35. Li Z, et al. Contrast-enhanced ultrasonography for monitoring arterial inflammation in Takayasu Arteritis. J Rheumatol. 2019;46(6):616–22.
36. Sun Y, et al. Ultrasonographic study and long-term follow-up of Takayasu's arteritis. Stroke. 1996;27(12):2178–82.
37. Fan W, et al. Ultrasound morphological changes in the carotid wall of Takayasu's arteritis: Monitor of disease progression. Int Angiol. 2016;35(6):586–92.
38. Misra R, et al. Development and initial validation of the Indian Takayasu clinical activity score (ITAS2010). Rheumatology (Oxford). 2013;52(10):1795–801.
39. Ozen S, et al. EULAR/PRINTO/PRES criteria for Henoch-Schönlein purpura, childhood polyarteritis nodosa, childhood Wegener granulomatosis and childhood Takayasu arteritis: Ankara 2008. Part II: Final classification criteria. Ann Rheum Dis. 2010;69(5):798–806.
40. Hellmich B, et al. 2018 Update of the EULAR recommendations for the management of large vessel vasculitis. Ann Rheum Dis. 2020;79(1):19–30.
41. Aeschlimann FA, et al. Childhood Takayasu arteritis: Disease course and response to therapy. Arthritis Res Ther. 2017;19(1):255.
42. Mekinian A, et al. Efficacy of biological-targeted treatments in Takayasu Arteritis: Multicenter, retrospective study of 49 patients. Circulation. 2015;132(18):1693–700.
43. Schmidt J, et al. Tumor necrosis factor inhibitors in patients with Takayasu arteritis: Experience from a referral center with long-term followup. Arthritis Care Res (Hoboken). 2012;64(7):1079–83.
44. Mekinian A, et al. Efficacy of tocilizumab in Takayasu arteritis: Multicenter retrospective study of 46 patients. J Autoimmun. 2018;91:55–60.
45. Nakaoka Y, et al. Efficacy and safety of tocilizumab in patients with refractory Takayasu arteritis: Results from a randomised, double-blind, placebo-controlled, phase 3 trial in Japan (the TAKT study). Ann Rheum Dis. 2018;77(3):348–54.
46. Langford CA, et al. A Randomized, double-blind trial of abatacept (CTLA-4Ig) for the treatment of Takayasu Arteritis. Arthritis Rheumatol. 2017;69(4):846–53.
47. de Souza AW, et al. Antiplatelet therapy for the prevention of arterial ischemic events in Takayasu arteritis. Circ J. 2010;74(6):1236–41.
48. Keser G, et al K. Management of Takayasu arteritis: A systematic review. Rheumatology (Oxford). 2014;53(5):793–801.
49. Tyagi S, et al. Balloon angioplasty for renovascular hypertension in Takayasu's arteritis. Am Heart J. 1993;125(5):1386–93.
50. Jeong HS, et al. Endovascular balloon angioplasty versus stenting in patients with Takayasu arteritis: A meta-analysis. Medicine (Baltimore). 2017;96(29):e7558.
51. Mason JC. Takayasu arteritis: Surgical interventions. Curr Opin Rheumatol. 2015;27(1):45–52.

52. Chaudry MA, et al. Takayasu's arteritis and its role in causing renal artery stenosis. Am J Med Sci. 2013;346(4):314–18.

53. Comarmond C, et al. Long-term outcomes and prognostic factors of complications in Takayasu Arteritis: A multicenter study of 318 patients. Circulation. 2017;136(12):111422.

54. Balow JE. Renal vasculitis. Kidney Int. 1985;27(6):954–64.

55. Kallenberg CG, et al. Anti-neutrophil cytoplasmic antibodies: Current diagnostic and pathophysiological potential. Kidney Int. 1994;46(1):1–15.

56. Stanton M, et al. Polyarteritis nodosa. In: *StatPearls* [Internet]. Treasure Island, FL: StatPearls Publishing; 2023.

57. Guillevin L, et al. Hepatitis B virus-associated polyarteritis nodosa: Clinical characteristics, outcome, and impact of treatment in 115 patients. Medicine (Baltimore). 2005;84(5):313–22.

58. Hasler P, et al. Vasculitides in hairy cell leukemia. Semin Arthritis Rheum. 1995;25(2):134–42.

59. Stone JH. Polyarteritis nodosa. JAMA. 2002;288(13):1632–9.

60. Watts RA, et al. Epidemiology of vasculitis in Europe. Ann Rheum Dis. 2001;60(12):1156–7.

61. Mahr A, et al. Prevalences of polyarteritis nodosa, microscopic polyangiitis, Wegener's granulomatosis, and Churg-Strauss syndrome in a French urban multiethnic population in 2000: A capture-recapture estimate. Arthritis Rheum. 2004;51(1):92–9.

62. Filer AD, et al. Diffuse endothelial dysfunction is common to ANCA-associated systemic vasculitis and polyarteritis nodosa. Ann Rheum Dis. 2003;62(2):162–7.

63. Chanseaud Y, et al. IgM and IgG autoantibodies from microscopic polyangiitis patients but not those with other small- and medium-sized vessel vasculitides recognize multiple endothelial cell antigens. Clin Immunol. 2003;109(2):165–78.

64. De Virgilio A, et al. Polyarteritis nodosa: A contemporary overview. Autoimmun Rev. 2016;15(6):564–70.

65. Freire Ade L, Bertolo MB, de Pinho AJ Jr, Samara AM, Fernandes SR. Increased serum levels of interleukin-8 in polyarteritis nodosa and Behçet's disease. Clin Rheumatol. 2004;23(3):203–5.

66. Hughes LB, Bridges SL Jr. Polyarteritis nodosa and microscopic polyangiitis: Etiologic and diagnostic considerations. Curr Rheumatol Rep. 2002;4(1):75–82.

67. Lapiner M, et al. [Diagnosis of periarteritis nodosa (Kussmaul-Maier disease)]. Klin Med (Mosk). 1957;35(9):153–4. Russian.

68. Chung SA, et al. 2021 American college of rheumatology/vasculitis foundation guideline for the management of polyarteritis nodosa. Arthritis Rheumatol. 2021;73(8):1384–93.

69. Ng WF, et al. Localized polyarteritis nodosa of the breast—report of two cases and a review of the literature. Histopathology. 1993;23(6):535–9.

70. Guillevin L, et al. Polyarteritis nodosa related to hepatitis B virus. A prospective study with long-term observation of 41 patients. Medicine (Baltimore). 1995;74(5):238–53.

71. Trepo C, et al. Polyarteritis nodosa and extrahepatic manifestations of HBV infection: The case against autoimmune intervention in pathogenesis. J Autoimmun. 2001;16(3):269–74.

72. Nakamura T, et al. Cutaneous polyarteritis nodosa: Revisiting its definition and diagnostic criteria. Arch Dermatol Res. 2009;301(1):117–21.

73. Bauzá A, et al. Cutaneous polyarteritis nodosa. Br J Dermatol. 2002;146(4):694–9.

74. Assicot C, et al. Cutaneous polyarteritis nodosa in children: Three cases. Ann Dermatol Venereol. 2002;129(2):207–11.

75. Morgan AJ, et al. Cutaneous polyarteritis nodosa: A comprehensive review. Int J Dermatol. 2010;49(7):750–6.

76. Daoud MS, et al. Cutaneous periarteritis nodosa: A clinicopathological study of 79 cases. Br J Dermatol. 1997;136(5):706–13.

77. Pagnoux C, et al. Clinical features and outcomes in 348 patients with polyarteritis nodosa: A systematic retrospective study of patients diagnosed between 1963 and 2005 and entered into the French vasculitis study group database. Arthritis Rheum. 2010;62(2):616–26.

78. Moore PM. Neurological manifestation of vasculitis: Update on immunopathogenic mechanisms and clinical features. Ann Neurol. 1995;37(Suppl 1):S131–41.

79. Lee PY, et al. Evaluation and management of deficiency of adenosine deaminase 2: An international consensus statement. JAMA Netw Open. 2023;6(5):e2315894.

80. Fayand A, et al. DADA2 diagnosed in adulthood versus childhood: A comparative study on 306 patients including a systematic literature review and 12 French cases. Semin Arthritis Rheum. 2021;51(6):1170–9.

81. Pagnoux C, et al. Presentation and outcome of gastrointestinal involvement in systemic necrotizing vasculitides: Analysis of 62 patients with polyarteritis nodosa, microscopic polyangiitis, Wegener granulomatosis, Churg-Strauss syndrome, or rheumatoid arthritis-associated vasculitis. Medicine (Baltimore). 2005;84(2):115–28.

82. Kastner D, et al. Polyarteritis nodosa and myocardial infarction. Can J Cardiol. 2000;16(4):515–18.

83. Teichman JM, et al. Polyarteritis nodosa presenting as acute orchitis: A case report and review of the literature. J Urol. 1993;149(5):1139–40.

84. Hsu CT, et al. Choroidal infarction, anterior ischemic optic neuropathy, and central retinal artery occlusion from polyarteritis nodosa. Retina. 2001;21(4):348–51.

85. Akova YA, et al. Ocular presentation of polyarteritis nodosa. Clinical course and management with steroid and cytotoxic therapy. Ophthalmology. 1993;100(12):1775–81.

86. Hernández-Rodríguez J, et al. Diagnosis and classification of polyarteritis nodosa. J Autoimmun. 2014;48–49:84–9.

87. Adu D, et al. Polyarteritis and the kidney. Q J Med. 1987;62(239):221–37.

88. Hočevar A, et al. Clinical approach to diagnosis and therapy of polyarteritis nodosa. Curr Rheumatol Rep. 2021;23(3):14.

89. Howard T, et al. Polyarteritis nodosa. Tech Vasc Interv Radiol. 2014;17(4):247–51.

90. Farrell GC, et al. Management of chronic hepatitis B virus infection: A new era of disease control. Intern Med J. 2006;36(2):100–13.

91. Guillevin L, et al. Short-term corticosteroids then lamivudine and plasma exchanges to treat hepatitis B virus-related polyarteritis nodosa. Arthritis Rheum. 2004;51(3):482–7.

92. Guillevin L, et al. Longterm followup after treatment of polyarteritis nodosa and Churg-Strauss angiitis with comparison of steroids, plasma exchange and cyclophosphamide to steroids and plasma exchange. A prospective randomized trial of 71 patients. The Cooperative Study Group for Polyarteritis Nodosa. J Rheumatol. 1991;18(4):567–74.

93. Guillevin L, et al. Prognostic factors in polyarteritis nodosa and Churg-Strauss syndrome. A prospective study in 342 patients. Medicine (Baltimore). 1996;75(1):17–28.

94. Guilevin L, et al. The five-factor score revisited: Assessment of prognoses of systemic necrotizing vasculitides based on the French Vasculitis Study Group (FVSG) cohort. Medicine (Baltimore). 2011;90(1):19–27.

95. Samson M, et al. Microscopic polyangiitis and non-HBV polyarteritis nodosa with poor-prognosis factors: 10-year results of the prospective CHUSPAN trial. Clin Exp Rheumatol. 2017;35(1 Suppl 103):176–84.

96. Cohen RD, et al. Clinical features, prognosis, and response to treatment in polyarteritis. Mayo Clin Proc. 1980;55(3):146–55.

97. Gayraud M, et al. Treatment of good-prognosis polyarteritis nodosa and Churg-Strauss syndrome: Comparison of steroids and oral or pulse cyclophosphamide in 25 patients. French Cooperative Study Group for Vasculitides. Br J Rheumatol. 1997;36(12):1290–7.

98. Guillevin L, et al. Treatment of polyarteritis nodosa and microscopic polyangiitis with poor prognosis factors: A prospective trial comparing glucocorticoids and six or twelve cyclophosphamide pulses in sixty-five patients. Arthritis Rheum. 2003;49(1):93–100.

99. Kidney Disease: Improving Global Outcomes (KDIGO) Blood Pressure Work Group. KDIGO 2021 clinical practice guideline for the management of blood pressure in chronic kidney disease. Kidney Int. 2021;99(3S):S1–S87.

9 Scleroderma Renal Crisis and Other Renal Complications in Scleroderma

Brian S. Lee, Marissa Savoie, Andrew Z. Fenves, and Lorinda S. Chung

9.1 INTRODUCTION

Scleroderma renal crisis (SRC) is a rare, life-threatening complication of systemic sclerosis (SSc). It typically presents with an abrupt onset of severe hypertension accompanied by rapidly progressive renal failure and can present with hypertensive encephalopathy, congestive heart failure, and/or microangiopathic hemolytic anemia (1). With the advent of angiotensin-converting enzyme (ACE) inhibitors, the mortality rates from SRC have gone down significantly. However, outcomes are still poor, with over 30% mortality and over 20% remaining on dialysis at 1 year (2–4). As clinicians, it is important to understand and recognize this medical emergency so that patients can be managed and treated appropriately. In this chapter, we will first give a brief overview of SSc. Then, we will focus on SRC and discuss the epidemiology, pathophysiology, histopathology, diagnosis, differential diagnosis/non-SRC renal manifestations of SSc, and management.

9.2 BRIEF OVERVIEW OF SYSTEMIC SCLEROSIS

SSc is an autoimmune disease that causes the thickening of the skin and fibrosis of multiple internal organs. SSc is associated with substantial morbidity and mortality, without a cure. It is estimated that 2.5 million people worldwide and 100,000 people in the United States have SSc (5, 6). Every age group can be affected, but onset is most frequent between the ages of 30 and 50, and it is more common in females than males (6). While the diagnosis of SSc is ultimately made clinically, the 2013 American College of Rheumatology (ACR)/European League Against Rheumatism (EULAR) classification criteria for SSc can be used to aid in the diagnosis of the disease (Table 9.1) (7). Once diagnosed, SSc can be divided into two subtypes based on the extent of skin thickening: 1) limited cutaneous SSc (lcSSc) and 2) diffuse cutaneous SSc (dcSSc) (7, 8).

Limited cutaneous SSc can involve the face, neck, hands, forearms, and lower extremities to the level of the knees but can be limited to the fingers with sclerodactyly or even just puffy fingers. DcSSc is differentiated from lcSSc by skin thickening involving the proximal extremities and/or trunk (Figure 9.1) (9). Both subtypes of SSc may involve internal organs, with wide-ranging complications including gastrointestinal dysmotility, interstitial lung disease, pulmonary hypertension, digital ischemic ulcers, myositis, arthritis, and contractures. Scleroderma renal crisis (SRC) is an acute severe complication of SSc, which will be the focus of this chapter.

9.3 SCLERODERMA RENAL CRISIS

9.3.1 Epidemiology and Risk Factors

The prevalence of SRC among the overall SSc population is 4% (7% to 9% in the dcSSc subset, and 0.5–2% for the lcSSc subset) (10). The risk of SRC is highest in the initial years of disease, with a median of 7.5 months after initial disease diagnosis, and 66% of SRC cases develop in the first year of diagnosis (11). Patients are considered high risk if they have any of the following features: early dcSSc (less than 5 years from first non-Raynaud's symptom), rapid progression of skin thickening, RNA polymerase III antibody-positive state, tendon friction rubs, large joint contractures, and corticosteroid use >15 mg prednisone equivalence daily in the preceding 6 months (2, 11–16).

Regarding demographic factors, the black race has been described as a risk factor for SRC in one retrospective cohort study of 353 patients, which reported a 6.4 times increased odds of black patients developing SRC compared with non-black patients (17).

Pregnancy has also been evaluated as a risk factor for SRC. In a prospective study that enrolled 59 women with SSc (56% dcSSc) and observed 91 total pregnancies over a 10-year period, only two participants developed SRC during pregnancy (18). These results have led experts to conclude that pregnancy is probably not an independent risk factor for SRC (19). However, due to the life-threatening nature of SRC, many experts recommend deferring pregnancy during the first few years after the diagnosis of dcSSc is made.

9.3.2 Pathophysiology

The exact pathophysiology of SRC remains unknown. It is believed that the primary process involves a series of insults to the kidneys (4, 20–22). More specifically, initial injuries to the endothelial cells

DOI: 10.1201/9781003438373-11

Table 9.1: The American College of Rheumatology/European League Against Rheumatism Criteria for the Classification of Systemic Sclerosis (SSc)*

Items	Sub-Items	Weight/Score[#]
Skin thickening of the fingers of both hands extending proximally to the metacarpophalangeal joints (sufficient criterion)		9
Skin thickening of the fingers (only count the higher score)	Puffy fingers	2
	Sclerodactyly of the fingers (distal to the metacarpophalangeal joints but proximal to the proximal interphalangeal joints)	4
Fingertip lesions (only count the higher score)	Digital tip ulcers	2
	Fingertip pitting scars	3
Telangiectasias	-	2
Abnormal nailfold capillaries	-	2
Pulmonary arterial hypertension and/or interstitial lung disease (maximum score is 2)	Pulmonary arterial hypertension	2
	Interstitial lung disease	2
Raynaud's phenomenon		3
SSc-related autoantibodies (maximum score is 3)	Anticentromere	3
	Anti-topoisomerase I/Anti-scl-70	
	Anti-RNA polymerase III	

*These criteria are applicable to any patient considered for inclusion in an SSc study. The criteria are not applicable to patients with skin thickening sparing the fingers or to patients who have a scleroderma-like disorder that better explains their manifestations (e.g., nephrogenic sclerosing fibrosis, generalized morphea, eosinophilic fasciitis, scleredema diabeticorum, scleromyxedema, erythromyalgia, porphyria, lichen sclerosis, graft-versus-host disease, diabetic cheiroarthropathy).

[#]The total score is determined by adding the maximum weight (score) in each category. Patients with a total score of ≥9 are classified as having definite SSc.

Source: Table adapted with permission from Frank van den Hoogen et al., 2013 classification criteria for systemic sclerosis: an American college of rheumatology/European league against rheumatism collaborative initiative. Ann Rheum Dis. 2013 Nov; 72(11):1747–55.

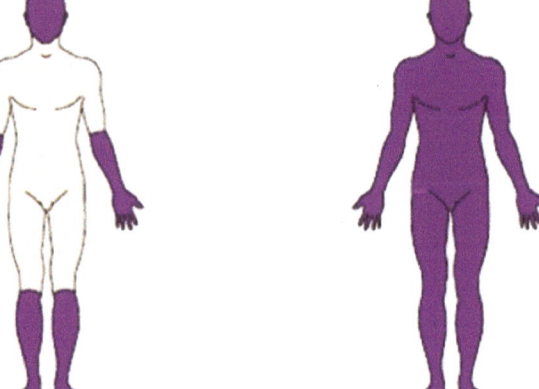

Limited Systemic Sclerosis   Diffuse Systemic Sclerosis

Figure 9.1 Two subtypes of systemic sclerosis are shown.

result in intimal thickening and proliferation of the renal interlobular and arcuate arteries (4, 20, 21, 23). Interestingly, the histology of renal biopsies taken during SRC demonstrates a notable absence of inflammatory cells (lymphocytes and monocytes) in the renal vasculature. However, platelet adhesion and aggregation take place and release platelet factors that cause increased vascular permeability, fibrin deposition, and collagen formation. This leads to the narrowing or total obliteration of the vessel lumen (4, 20, 21). The decreased renal blood flow and episodic renal vasospasm ("renal Raynaud phenomenon") cause hyperplasia of the juxtaglomerular apparatus and the release of renin (1, 2, 4, 20, 21, 24–26). Consequently, the renin–angiotensin–aldosterone system (RAAS) is activated, leading to the production of angiotensin II, resulting in hypertension. RAAS activation results in further vasoconstriction and sets up a vicious cycle of hypoperfusion and ischemia that feeds back into the pathogenic loop and leads to kidney injury (1, 4, 22).

9.3.3 Histopathology

The histology of SRC varies over the course of the disease (25, 27). Early vascular changes include the intimal accumulation of myxoid material, thrombosis, and/or fibrinoid necrosis in the interlobular and arcuate arteries, resulting in severe luminal narrowing (20, 28). As vascular lesions progress, there is smooth muscle cell infiltration and the deposition of collagen in the intima. In the later stages, there is a change from edematous mucoid intima to concentric fibrosis, resulting in an "onion-skin" appearance (1, 20, 27). In chronic stages, tubular atrophy and interstitial fibrosis that are proportional to vascular injury are frequently manifested (1, 27) (Figure 9.2) (58).

The exact event that triggers this pathogenic loop is unknown, and different factors have been proposed. Endothelin-1 (ET-1), a potent vasoconstrictor peptide, has been proposed because studies have found elevated levels of ET-1 in SRC patients (4, 23, 29, 30). Complement activation is another factor that garnered significant interest because in a subset of SSc patients, a distinct pattern of complement markers was observed (4, 23, 28, 31, 32). Genetics may also play a role. Studies have found SRC to be associated with distinct MHC class I haplotypes of HLA-DRB1*0406 and *1304 (4, 33). Two candidate proteins, GPATCH2L and CTNND2, were increased in SRC patients, and genes associated with these proteins may be implicated in SRC pathogenesis (4, 34). Yet how Endothelin-1, complement activation, and genetics fit into SRC pathophysiology remains unknown, and more research needs to be carried out.

9.3.4 Diagnosis

Currently, there are no universally accepted diagnostic criteria for SRC, and variable definitions of SRC exist (3, 11, 35, 36). Moreover, the definition of hypertension is controversial, as some patients with SRC may present with normal blood pressure, and the cut-offs for hypertension are also frequently changing (36). Therefore, updated diagnostic criteria are being developed and refined by the Scleroderma Clinical Trials Consortium Scleroderma Renal Crisis Working Group (37).

Nonetheless, most definitions share commonalities in approaches to diagnosing SRC. These include two essential components 1) hypertension as defined by >140/90, systolic blood pressure >30mmHg from baseline, or diastolic blood pressure >20mmHg from baseline and 2) acute kidney injury as defined by Kidney Disease Improving Global Outcomes (KDIGO). The diagnosis is further strengthened if there are additional findings such as microangiopathic hemolytic anemia (MAHA), retinal examination consistent with accelerated hypertension, microscopic hematuria on urine microscopy, oliguria/anuria, and flash pulmonary edema (3, 11, 24, 38, 39). Renal biopsy showing the classic histopathologic findings may also help to confirm the diagnosis.

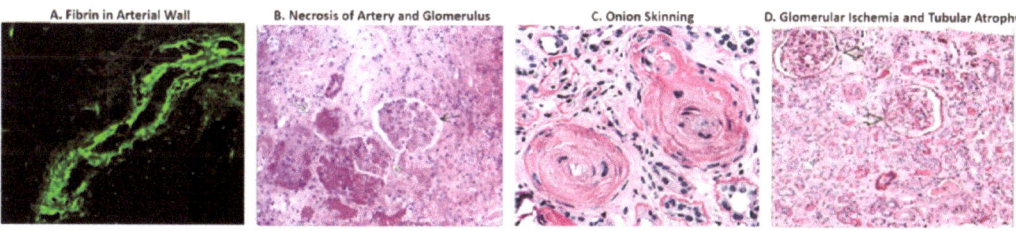

Figure 9.2   Four renal pathology images are shown.

9.3.5 Differential Diagnosis of SRC and Non-SRC Renal Manifestations of SSc

In considering the differential diagnosis of SRC, an important mimic is thrombotic thrombocytopenic purpura (TTP), in which patients also present in acute renal failure, often with hypertension and evidence of MAHA. TTP is usually distinguished from SRC by a low ADAM-TS 13 level and the presence of prominent abnormal neurologic findings. It is critical to differentiate these entities, as both are associated with high morbidity, and management is very different, with ACE inhibitors for SRC and plasma exchange for TTP.

For pregnant persons with SSc, the development of hypertension should prompt evaluation for pre-eclampsia in addition to SRC. Similarly, thrombocytopenia should prompt evaluation for HELLP syndrome (hemolysis, elevated liver enzymes, and low platelet count).

Rapidly progressive glomerulonephritis (RPGN) secondary to ANCA-associated vasculitis (AAV-RPGN) is another important mimic of SRC that has been described in patients with SSc. In contrast to SRC, which is more common in patients with dcSSc in the first 5 years since diagnosis, AAV-RPGN is more likely in patients with lcSSc after 5 years of disease (40). AAV-RPGN is distinguished from SRC by ANCA positivity (almost always myeloperoxidase antibodies) and the finding of a pauci-immune crescentic glomerulonephritis on renal biopsy. Differentiating AAV-RPGN from SRC is crucial, as the management differs completely. AAV-RPGN in patients with SSc has been managed similarly to AAV-RPGN without SSc with high doses of glucocorticoids and cyclophosphamide (40, 41).

Essential (or primary) hypertension is very common in the general population, and many patients with SSc may develop this form of hypertension. These patients are usually well controlled with standard blood pressure-lowering agents, have normal kidney function, and have no or minimal proteinuria.

9.3.6 Management and Treatment

9.3.6.1 Prevention

There are no specific preventative measures for SRC, but identifying high-risk patients and counseling them on daily home blood pressure monitoring can facilitate early detection and treatment. Patients with high-risk features as described earlier may benefit from frequent follow-up. Corticosteroids should be avoided in high-risk patients or, if absolutely necessary, should be limited to the lowest dose for the shortest possible period (2, 16).

In general, observation involves regularly measuring blood pressure. It is recommended that the patient promptly report if their blood pressure is >140/90mmHg and/or >20mmHg over baseline for 2 or more consecutive days to a healthcare provider. Patients should be counseled to check their blood pressure daily at the same time of day when they are relaxed. In addition to reporting elevated blood pressures, they should contact a provider if they develop symptoms of headache, visual changes, fatigue, or breathlessness (2, 21, 24).

While ACE inhibitors are the mainstay of treating SRC, there is no role for prophylactic ACE inhibitors to prevent SRC (2, 3, 42, 43). This is supported by a meta-analysis of nine studies (8612 patients) that showed a higher incidence of SRC after ACE inhibitor exposure compared with no ACE inhibitor exposure (relative risk: 2.05, 95% confidence interval 1.08–3.91, p = 0.03) (44). However, confounding by indication may have influenced these data, as these patients were likely at increased risk for SRC from the beginning. As a result, we favor continuing ACE inhibitors or angiotensin II receptor blockers (ARB) if clinically indicated such as to treat hypertension, diabetic nephropathy, and congestive heart failure.

9.3.6.2 ACE Inhibitors, Calcium Channel Blockers, Angiotensin Receptor Blockers, and Alpha-Blockers

Once SRC is diagnosed, the patient should immediately be hospitalized and treated with ACE inhibitors. Prompt diagnosis is critical because delayed treatment can increase SRC complications such as irreversible damage to the kidneys, hypertensive retinopathy, pulmonary edema, and even death (23, 42, 45).

ACE inhibitors remain the first-line treatment in SRC and should be continued indefinitely after the first episode of SRC. There have been no randomized controlled trials to evaluate the effect of ACE inhibitors on SRC. However, case report, observational, and uncontrolled studies continue to show favorable data with regard to survival rates, improvement in renal function, and an increased chance of eventual discontinuation of renal replacement therapy if ACE inhibitors are initiated (20, 42). Therefore, EULAR experts recommend the aggressive and early initiation of ACE inhibitors for SRC treatment (46).

ACE inhibitors are contraindicated during pregnancy due to an increased risk of oligohydramnios and fetal renal dysplasia. However, in pregnant SSc patients, ACE inhibitors are recommended during acute SRC given the life-threatening nature of SRC for the mother and fetus, as benefits outweigh the risks. For women with a history of SRC who become pregnant, it is strongly recommended that they continue ACE inhibitors in discussion with the patient (2, 4, 19).

Captopril is the preferred initial drug of choice because of its rapid onset of action and short duration. This allows for rapid titration of the dose to lower the blood pressure. The goal is to lower the systolic blood pressure by about 20mmHg and diastolic blood pressure by 10mmHg within 24 hours, with a goal blood pressure of 120/70mmHg to 120/80mmHg within 72 hours, while avoiding hypotension (1, 4, 20, 22, 23). Once the blood pressure has stabilized, captopril should be transitioned to an equivalent long-acting ACE inhibitor. Importantly, angiotensin receptor blockers (ARBs) should not replace ACE inhibitors, as they do not seem to be clinically equivalent in the treatment of SRC. The exact mechanism is unclear, but it may be that ARBs do not inhibit the degradation of bradykinin, a potent molecule that can help vasodilate renal vessels (2, 4, 21, 22, 47).

For patients whose blood pressure remains elevated despite maximum doses of ACE inhibitor, other agents should be added. Experts from the Scleroderma Clinical Trials Consortium and the Canadian Scleroderma Research group recommend adding calcium channel blockers, angiotensin receptor blockers, and alpha-blockers as second-, third-, and fourth-line treatments, respectively (4, 48). In addition, beta blockers are avoided because of the theoretical risk of decreasing cardiac output in the setting of severely increased afterload from SRC and due to the risk of renal artery vasospasm from unopposed alpha receptor agonism (2, 20, 21, 42).

9.3.6.3 Renal Replacement Therapy and Renal Transplant

If a patient with SRC develops end-stage renal disease despite medical therapy, renal replacement therapy should be initiated if it is within the patient's goals of care. Both hemodialysis and peritoneal dialysis are options for renal replacement therapy after SRC. Many nephrologists prefer hemodialysis based on reports of higher complications with peritoneal dialysis, including peritoneal fluid leakage and catheter infections. However, fistula access for hemodialysis may be difficult due to fibrosed skin in patients with SSc (20, 49, 50).

Treatment with ACE inhibitors has been associated with a 50% improvement in SRC mortality, but studies show that temporary dialysis is still needed in about a quarter of SRC patients, and permanent dialysis is needed in about 19–40% of SRC patients (4, 11, 51). Nonetheless, patients should still be continued on an ACE inhibitor indefinitely, even if they are on dialysis, especially for those who have the possibility of improvement in renal function (20, 52). Patients with SRC most often recover renal function within 12–18 months and have been reported to recover renal function even up to 3 years after initial SRC. As a result, many clinicians recommend deferring renal transplantation for up to 2 years (1, 4, 11, 20, 53, 54).

Approximately 3–17% of patients with SRC undergo renal transplantation. Prior to transplant, existing comorbidities such as pulmonary and cardiac disease and candidacy for post-transplant immunosuppression need to be considered. Post-transplant immunosuppressive medications such as calcineurin inhibitors (cyclosporine and tacrolimus) are renal vasoconstrictors and can potentially increase the risk of SRC (2, 51, 53). Renal transplant can result in improved survival compared with long-term renal replacement therapy. For example, 3-year survival rates among patients who underwent renal transplant for SRC were 54–91%, compared with rates of 31–56% among patients on renal replacement therapy (1, 23, 55). Higher rates of comorbidities and frailty in patients ineligible for transplant may contribute to this differential survival. Graft survival post-renal transplant in SSc is now similar to that of patients with other types of end-stage renal disease (2, 51). The recurrence of SRC in transplanted kidneys ranges from 2% to 9%, with a higher recurrence risk for patients who had more aggressive disease before renal transplantation (1, 2, 43, 47, 51).

9.3.6.4 Other Treatments

Endothelin-1 has been implicated in SRC pathogenesis and has been considered a therapeutic target. Bosentan, a non-selective ET-1 receptor antagonist, has been utilized in some case reports of SRC refractory to ACE inhibitors, but studies showed inconclusive results (2, 4, 21, 29, 42, 50).

Medications targeting the complement pathway have been explored. Eculizumab, a monoclonal antibody against complement factor 5, has been proposed as a possible treatment option. Case reports and case series report improvements in SRC with this medication, particularly in patients with microangiopathic hemolytic anemia (2, 23, 42, 43, 50). Based on this, it may be reasonable to treat a subset of SRC patients with eculizumab who demonstrate complement-mediated thrombotic microangiopathy and are refractory to ACE inhibitors. Randomized clinical trials are necessary to support the use of eculizumab as an adjunctive treatment in SRC.

Plasma exchange may be useful in SRC by removing autoantibodies, pro-fibrotic cytokines, vasoconstrictor factors, and factors related to the renin–angiotensin system. Case reports and retrospective studies suggest that combining ACE inhibitors and plasma exchange in SRC patients with microangiopathy may be useful (20, 23, 43, 50, 56–58). However, prospective clinical trials are necessary to support the role of plasma exchange in refractory SRC.

9.4 CONCLUSION

SSc is a rare fibrosing disorder, often with skin, pulmonary, vascular, and gastrointestinal manifestations, while renal manifestations are less common. SRC is a severe manifestation of SSc that is characterized by acute renal injury, hypertension (or relative hypertension), and often microangiopathic hemolytic anemia. SRC is more common in diffuse cutaneous systemic sclerosis and in the first 5 years after disease onset. Glucocorticoid exposure is the most important modifiable risk factor, and systemic steroids should be avoided in patients with systemic sclerosis, particularly if at high risk for SRC. While the pathophysiology of SRC is not well understood, it likely involves excessive renin–angiotensin–aldosterone activation and vascular proliferation, leading to microangiopathic hemolytic anemia. Important mimics of SRC include thrombotic thrombocytopenic purpura and AAV, which have been reported in patients with SSc. The early initiation of angiotensin-converting enzyme inhibitors is the mainstay of treatment and should be continued indefinitely after the first episode of SRC.

REFERENCES

1. Vaidya PN, Basyal B, Finnigan NA. Scleroderma and renal crisis. In: *StatPearls*. Treasure Island, FL: StatPearls Publishing; 2023.
2. Cole A, Ong VH, Denton CP. Renal disease and systemic sclerosis: An update on scleroderma renal crisis. Clin Rev Allergy Immunol. 2023;64(3):378–91.
3. Hudson M, Baron M, Tatibouet S, Furst DE, Khanna D, International Scleroderma Renal Crisis Study Investigators. Exposure to ACE inhibitors prior to the onset of scleroderma renal crisis-results from the International Scleroderma Renal Crisis Survey. Semin Arthritis Rheum. 2014;43(5):666–72.
4. Hudson M, Ghossein C, Steen V. Scleroderma renal crisis. Presse Med. 2021;50(1):104063.
5. Varga J., Loscalzo J, Fauci A, Kasper D, Hauser S, Longo D, Jameson J. *Systemic Sclerosis (Scleroderma) and Related Disorders. Harrison's Principles of Internal Medicine.* 21st ed. McGraw Hill; 2022.
6. Rodriguez-Pla A, Simms RW. Geographic disparity in systemic sclerosis mortality in the United States: 1999–2017. J Scleroderma Relat Disord. 2021;6(2):139–45.
7. van den Hoogen F, Khanna D, Fransen J, Johnson SR, Baron M, Tyndall A, et al. 2013 classification criteria for systemic sclerosis: An American college of rheumatology/European league against rheumatism collaborative initiative. Ann Rheum Dis. 2013;72(11):1747–55.
8. Wollheim FA. Classification of systemic sclerosis. Visions and reality. Rheumatology (Oxford). 2005;44(10):1212–16.
9. Knobler R, Moinzadeh P, Hunzelmann N, Kreuter A, Cozzio A, Mouthon L, et al. European dermatology forum S1-guideline on the diagnosis and treatment of sclerosing diseases of the skin, Part 1: Localized scleroderma, systemic sclerosis and overlap syndromes. J Eur Acad Dermatol Venereol. 2017;31(9):1401–24.
10. Turk M, Pope JE. The frequency of scleroderma renal crisis over time: A metaanalysis. J Rheumatol. 2016;43(7):1350–5.
11. Penn H, Howie AJ, Kingdon EJ, Bunn CC, Stratton RJ, Black CM, et al. Scleroderma renal crisis: Patient characteristics and long-term outcomes. QJM. 2007;100(8):485–94.
12. Montanelli G, Beretta L, Santaniello A, Scorza R. Effect of dihydropyridine calcium channel blockers and glucocorticoids on the prevention and development of scleroderma renal crisis in an Italian case series. Clin Exp Rheumatol. 2013;31(2 Suppl 76):135–9.
13. Steen VD. Autoantibodies in systemic sclerosis. Semin Arthritis Rheum. 2005;35(1):35–42.
14. Gordon SM, Stitt RS, Nee R, Bailey WT, Little DJ, Knight KR, et al. Risk factors for future scleroderma renal crisis at systemic sclerosis diagnosis. J Rheumatol. 2019;46(1):85–92.

15. Avouac J, Walker UA, Hachulla E, Riemekasten G, Cuomo G, Carreira PE, et al. Joint and tendon involvement predict disease progression in systemic sclerosis: A EUSTAR prospective study. Ann Rheum Dis. 2016;75(1):103–9.

16. Steen VD, Medsger TA. Case-control study of corticosteroids and other drugs that either precipitate or protect from the development of scleroderma renal crisis. Arthritis Rheum. 1998;41(9):1613–19.

17. Forman CJ, Olson SW, Gordon SM, Hughes JB, Stitt RS, Bailey WT, et al. Association of race and risk of future scleroderma renal crisis at systemic sclerosis diagnosis. Arthritis Care Res (Hoboken). 2023;75(4):801–7.

18. Steen VD. Pregnancy in women with systemic sclerosis. Obstet Gynecol. 1999;94(1):15–20.

19. Clark KE, Etomi O, Ong VH. Systemic sclerosis in pregnancy. Obstet Med. 2020;13(3):105–11.

20. Soukup T, Toms J, Honsova E, Safranek R. Renal involvement in systemic sclerosis. In: Tomcik M, editor. *New Insights into Systemic Sclerosis* [Internet]. IntechOpen; 2019 [cited 2023 Jun 29]. http://doi.org/10.5772/intechopen.87187.

21. Bose N, Chiesa-Vottero A, Chatterjee S. Scleroderma renal crisis. Semin Arthritis Rheum. 2015;44(6):687–94.

22. Steen VD. Scleroderma renal crisis. Rheum Dis Clin North Am. 2003;29(2):315–33.

23. Chrabaszcz M, Małyszko J, Sikora M, Alda-Malicka R, Stochmal A, Matuszkiewicz-Rowinska J, et al. Renal involvement in systemic sclerosis: An update. Kidney Blood Press Res. 2020;45(4):532–48.

24. Woodworth TG, Suliman YA, Li W, Furst DE, Clements P. Scleroderma renal crisis and renal involvement in systemic sclerosis. Nat Rev Nephrol. 2016;12(11):678–91.

25. Chabtini L, Mounayar M, Azzi J, Bijol V, Bastacky S, et al. Scleroderma renal crisis. In: Radstake T, editor. *Systemic Sclerosis—An Update on the Aberrant Immune System and Clinical Features.* InTech; 2012.

26. Cannon PJ, Hassar M, Case DB, Casarella WJ, Sommers SC, LeRoy EC. The relationship of hypertension and renal failure in scleroderma (progressive systemic sclerosis) to structural and functional abnormalities of the renal cortical circulation. Medicine (Baltimore). 1974;53(1):1–46.

27. Batal I, Domsic RT, Medsger TA, Bastacky S. Scleroderma renal crisis: A pathology perspective. Int J Rheumatol. 2010;2010:543704.

28. Batal I, Domsic RT, Shafer A, Medsger TA, Kiss LP, Randhawa P, et al. Renal biopsy findings predicting outcome in scleroderma renal crisis. Hum Pathol. 2009;40(3):332–40.

29. Penn H, Quillinan N, Khan K, Chakravarty K, Ong VH, Burns A, et al. Targeting the endothelin axis in scleroderma renal crisis: Rationale and feasibility. QJM. 2013;106(9):839–48.

30. Kobayashi H, Nishimaki T, Kaise S, Suzuki T, Watanabe K, Kasukawa R, et al. Immunohistological study endothelin-1 and endothelin-A and B receptors in two patients with scleroderma renal crisis. Clin Rheumatol. 1999;18(5):425–7.

31. Varga J, Trojanowska M, Kuwana M. Pathogenesis of systemic sclerosis: Recent insights of molecular and cellular mechanisms and therapeutic opportunities. JSRD. 2017;2(3):137–52.

32. Okrój M, Johansson M, Saxne T, Blom AM, Hesselstrand R. Analysis of complement biomarkers in systemic sclerosis indicates a distinct pattern in scleroderma renal crisis. Arthritis Res Ther. 2016;18(1):267.

33. Nguyen B, Mayes MD, Arnett FC, del Junco D, Reveille JD, Gonzalez EB, et al. HLA-DRB1*0407 and *1304 are risk factors for scleroderma renal crisis. Arthritis Rheum. 2011;63(2):530–4.

34. Stern EP, Guerra SG, Chinque H, Acquaah V, González-Serna D, Ponticos M, et al. Analysis of anti-RNA polymerase III antibody-positive systemic sclerosis and altered GPATCH2L and CTNND2 expression in scleroderma renal crisis. J Rheumatol. 2020;47(11):1668–77.

35. Butler E-A, Baron M, Fogo AB, Frech T, Ghossein C, Hachulla E, et al. Generation of a core set of items to develop classification criteria for scleroderma renal crisis using consensus methodology. Arthritis Rheumatol. 2019;71(6):964–71.

36. Helfrich DJ, Banner B, Steen VD, Medsger TA. Normotensive renal failure in systemic sclerosis. Arthritis Rheum. 1989;32(9):1128–34.

37. Butler EA, Baron M, Fogo AB, Frech T, Ghossein C, Hachulla E, et al. Generation of a core set of items to develop classification criteria for scleroderma renal crisis using consensus methodology. Arthritis Rheumatol. 2019;71(6):964–71.

38. Lynch BM, Stern EP, Ong V, Harber M, Burns A, Denton CP. UK Scleroderma Study Group (Ukssg) guidelines on the diagnosis and management of scleroderma renal crisis. Clin Exp Rheumatol. 2016;100(5 Suppl 34):106–9.

39. Denton, Christopher P. and Hudson, MarieMarie. Renal crisis and other renal manifestations of scleroderma. 2017. http://doi.org/10.1007/978-3-319-31407-5_21.

40. Arad U, Balbir-Gurman A, Doenyas-Barak K, Amit-Vazina M, Caspi D, Elkayam O. Anti-neutrophil antibody associated vasculitis in systemic sclerosis. Semin Arthritis Rheum. 2011;41(2):223–9.

41. Derrett-Smith EC, Nihtyanova SI, Harvey J, Salama AD, Denton CP. Revisiting ANCA-associated vasculitis in systemic sclerosis: Clinical, serological and immunogenetic factors. Rheumatology (Oxford). 2013;52(10):1824–31.

42. Nagaraja V. Management of scleroderma renal crisis. Curr Opin Rheumatol. 2019;31(3):223–30.

43. Zanatta E, Polito P, Favaro M, Larosa M, Marson P, Cozzi F, et al. Therapy of scleroderma renal crisis: State of the art. Autoimmun Rev. 2018;17(9):882–9.

44. Xiong A, Cao Y, Xiang Q, Song Z, Zhang Y, Zhou S, et al. Angiotensin-converting enzyme inhibitors prior to scleroderma renal crisis in systemic sclerosis: A systematic review and meta-analysis. J Clin Pharm Ther. 2022;47(6):722–31.

45. Denton CP, Lapadula G, Mouthon L, Müller-Ladner U. Renal complications and scleroderma renal crisis. Rheumatology (Oxford). 2009;48(Suppl 3):iii32–5.

46. Kowal-Bielecka O, Fransen J, Avouac J, Becker M, Kulak A, Allanore Y, et al. Update of EULAR recommendations for the treatment of systemic sclerosis. Ann Rheum Dis. 2017;76(8):1327–39.

47. Cheung WY, Gibson IW, Rush D, Jeffery J, Karpinski M. Late recurrence of scleroderma renal crisis in a renal transplant recipient despite angiotensin II blockade. Am J Kidney Dis. 2005;45(5):930–4.

48. Fernández-Codina A, Walker KM, Pope JE, Scleroderma Algorithm Group. Treatment algorithms for systemic sclerosis according to experts. Arthritis Rheumatol. 2018;70(11):1820–8.

49. Siriphannon Y, Foocharoen C, Ussanawarong T, Reungjui S, Mahakkanukrauh A, Suwannaroj S, Nanagara R. Poor outcome of peritoneal dialysis during scleroderma renal crisis in scleroderma patients. J Med Assoc Thai. 2018;101:235.

50. Foocharoen C, Tonsawan P, Pongkulkiat P, Anutrakulchai S, Mahakkanukrauh A, Suwannaroj S. Management review of scleroderma renal crisis: An update with practical pointers. Mod Rheumatol. 2023;33(1):12–20.

51. Kim H, Lefebvre F, Hoa S, Hudson M. Mortality and morbidity in scleroderma renal crisis: A systematic literature review. J Scleroderma Relat Disord. 2021;6(1):21–36.

52. Stern EP, Steen VD, Denton CP. Management of renal involvement in scleroderma. Curr Treatm Opt Rheumatol. 2015;1(1):106–18.

53. Lynch BM, Stern EP, Ong V, Harber M, Burns A, Denton CP. UK Scleroderma Study Group (UKSSG) guidelines on the diagnosis and management of scleroderma renal crisis. Clin Exp Rheumatol. 2016;34(5 Suppl 100):106–9.

54. Fenves AZ, Murphy JS, Emmett M. Scleroderma renal crisis and recovery from end-stage renal disease. Semin Dial. 1998;11(3):189–91.

55. Gibney EM, Parikh CR, Jani A, Fischer MJ, Collier D, Wiseman AC. Kidney transplantation for systemic sclerosis improves survival and may modulate disease activity. Am J Transplant. 2004;4(12):2027–31.

56. Cozzi F, Marson P, Cardarelli S, Favaro M, Tison T, Tonello M, et al. Prognosis of scleroderma renal crisis: A long-term observational study. Nephrol Dial Transplant. 2012;27(12):4398–403.

57. Nagamura N, Kin S. Scleroderma renal crisis during intravenous cyclophosphamide pulse therapy for complicated interstitial lung disease was successfully treated with angiotensin converting enzyme inhibitor and plasma exchange. Nagoya J Med Sci. 2016;78(3):329–34.

58. Kambham, N. et al. Scleroderma. In: Colvin R, Chang A, Cornell L, editors. *Diagnostic Pathology: Kidney Diseases*. 4th ed. Copyright Elsevier; 2023.

10 Renal Manifestations of Rheumatoid Arthritis, Spondyloarthropathies, Inflammatory Myopathies and MCTD

Suguni Loku Galappaththy, Jemima Albayda and Didem Saygin

10.1 INTRODUCTION

In this chapter, we will focus on systemic autoimmune conditions that are infrequently associated with renal involvement. These conditions include rheumatoid arthritis, spondyloarthropathies, idiopathic inflammatory myopathies and mixed connective tissue disease. Renal involvement in these autoimmune diseases includes vascular complications, glomerular disease and tubulointerstitial changes. The presentation of renal involvement in these conditions can be subclinical or overt but usually has prognostic and treatment implications. Importantly, the differential diagnosis of renal dysfunction in a patient with these conditions should include renal toxicity from the drugs used in the management of these conditions.

Here, we first provide a brief overview of rheumatoid arthritis, spondyloarthropathies, idiopathic inflammatory myopathies and mixed connective tissue disease, followed by the epidemiology, prognosis and management of renal manifestations associated with each of these conditions (Table 10.1).

Table 10.1: Summary of Renal Manifestations in Rheumatoid Arthritis, Spondyloarthropathies, Idiopathic Inflammatory Myopathies and Mixed Connective Tissue Disease

Autoimmune Condition	Frequency of Renal Disease	Renal Manifestations
Rheumatoid arthritis	5–50%	**Due to disease process** Glomerulonephritis (GN) • Mesangial GN • Membranous GN • IgA nephropathy • Minimal change disease • Focal segmental glomerulosclerosis Rheumatoid vasculitis Secondary AA amyloidosis **Medication-induced toxicity** GN • Membranous GN (gold, penicillamine) • Minimal change disease (gold) Interstitial nephritis (NSAIDs) Papillary necrosis (NSAIDs) Acute tubular necrosis (NSAIDs)
Spondyloarthropathy	8–35%	**Due to disease process** GN • IgA nephropathy (most common) • Membranoproliferative GN • Membranous GN • Focal segmental glomerulosclerosis Secondary AA amyloidosis **Medication-induced toxicity** Acute tubular necrosis Interstitial nephritis

(Continued)

Table 10.1: (Continued)

Autoimmune Condition	Frequency of Renal Disease	Renal Manifestations
Idiopathic inflammatory myopathies (IIM)	21–50%	**Rhabdomyolysis-related kidney injury** **Renal impairment due to autoimmune process** GN • Mesangial proliferative GN • Membranous nephropathy • Minimal change disease • Crescentic GN • IgA nephropathy • Focal segmental glomerulosclerosis Tubulointerstitial nephritis (rare)
Mixed connective tissue disease	4–64%	GN • Membranous GN (most common) • Membranoproliferative GN Tubulointerstitial nephritis Disease specific to phenotype • Scleroderma renal crisis • Lupus nephritis • ANCA-associated vasculitis

Abbreviations: GN, glomerulonephritis; NSAIDs, nonsteroidal anti-inflammatory drugs

10.2 RENAL MANIFESTATIONS OF RHEUMATOID ARTHRITIS

Rheumatoid arthritis (RA) is a systemic autoimmune condition that causes chronic inflammation in the synovial joints but also has several extra-articular manifestations. The worldwide prevalence is estimated to be around 1%, predominantly affecting women (1). Despite cardiovascular disease taking the center stage in terms of causing morbidity and mortality in patients with RA, renal dysfunction also carries a significant importance due to its effect on prognosis and implications for treatment. Furthermore, subclinical renal dysfunction is also an independent risk factor for cardiovascular events in patients with RA (2).

The prevalence of kidney disease in RA varies from 5 to 50%, depending on the study design and the study population (3, 4). In the MATRIX study, the prevalence of elevated creatinine was reported in 19% of patients with RA (5). Of this subset of patients, 20% were in stage 2 and 15% were in stage 3 of chronic kidney disease (CKD) (5). Proteinuria, hematuria and pyuria were observed in 16%, 17% and 20% of the patients, respectively (5).

In RA, renal disease could result from the medications used in the treatment of RA and/or the effects of the primary disease process. Direct effects on the kidney can result in focal glomerulonephritis, which is typically not rapidly progressive or can manifest as rheumatoid vasculitis. Chronic inflammation resulting in amyloidosis can affect multiple segments of the kidney, including the glomeruli, renal tubules, vasculature and interstitium. The landscape of kidney disease in RA has evolved with the advent of targeted biologics, moving away from older disease-modifying anti-rheumatic drugs (DMARDs) such as penicillamine, gold and cyclosporine, which were more nephrotoxic. A more aggressive treat-to-target therapeutic approach has led to reduced medication toxicity and improved disease control with less secondary amyloidosis.

Regardless of the etiology, renal involvement is an independent predictor of mortality in RA patients and can present as hematuria and/or proteinuria, CKD, microalbuminuria or histologically confirmed amyloidosis (6). It is difficult to accurately predict the renal morphologic lesions in RA patients based solely on abnormalities in urinalysis, impaired creatinine clearance or clinical features (7). Therefore, a renal biopsy should be considered in determining the diagnosis, assessment of prognosis and therapeutic decisions (7).

10.2.1 Glomerulonephritis in RA

Glomerulonephritis (GN) has a prevalence of 60–65% on histological evaluation in patients with RA who have kidney dysfunction (8). Studies have reported a variety of histologic findings, including mesangial GN, membranous GN, IgA nephropathy, minimal change disease and focal segmental glomerulosclerosis (FSGS). In general, GN in RA has a good prognosis and is rarely associated with renal impairment.

Mesangial GN is the most common histologic finding, with a prevalence of around 35–78% among patients with RA-related nephropathy (7, 9). It is commonly associated with long-standing RA with an average disease duration of 13 years and has a mild course, with only the rare occurrence of nephrotic syndrome and renal dysfunction (10). It is much more likely to present with isolated hematuria, proteinuria or a combination of the two.

While mesangial GN is thought to be due to RA itself, membranous GN is rarely due to RA and is often the result of medications, including older DMARDs such as gold and penicillamine (7, 9, 10). It is typically self-limited with improvement after the discontinuation of the offending agent. On rare instances when membranous GN is associated with RA itself, it is seen within approximately 4 years of disease onset and commonly presents with nephrotic syndrome (7).

The prevalence of IgA nephropathy is similar among patients with RA and the general population and is histologically indistinguishable (11, 12). Therefore, when an RA patient presents with IgA nephropathy, a presumptive diagnosis of a secondary IgA nephropathy is made. Treatment and prognosis are similar to those for primary IgA nephropathy (13). There have been reports of rare cases of IgA nephropathy from tumor necrosis factor inhibitors (TNFis) (14) (Table 10.2).

FSGS is the most common primary glomerular pathology leading to end-stage renal disease in the United States; however, the co-existence of FSGS and RA is limited to a few case reports

Table 10.2: Medication-Induced Nephrotoxicity and Dose Adjustments

Medication	Renal Manifestations	Dosage Adjustments in Renal Impairment
Methotrexate	Crystal-induced AKI (uncommon in doses used in RA)	CrCl >50 mL/minute: No adjustments CrCl 31–50 mL/minute: Reduce dose by 50% CrCl <30 mL/minute or renal replacement therapy (RRT): Contraindicated
Leflunomide	Interstitial nephritis (rare) IgA nephropathy (rare)	No adjustment is needed in renal impairment or in RRT.
Sulfasalazine	Interstitial nephritis (rare) Nephrotic syndrome (rare)	No adjustment is needed in renal impairment or in RRT.
Hydroxychloroquine	No renal involvement reported	Dosing should be guided by plasma hydroxychloroquine levels. If therapeutic drug monitoring unavailable: *CrCl >50 mL/minute:* No dosage adjustment *CrCl 30–50 mL/minute:* Maximum 75% of the dose *CrCl <30 mL/minute:* Maximum 25–50% of dose Consider reducing the dose to three times a week after hemodialysis if on hemodialysis.
NSAIDs	Acute kidney injury Acute tubular nephritis Papillary necrosis and chronic interstitial nephritis Glomerulonephritis: Minimal change/membranous Type 4 renal tubular acidosis (hyperkalemia)	*CrCl 30–59 mL/minute:* Use with caution with close monitoring *CrCl <30 mL/minute and RRT:* Contraindicated

(Continued)

Table 10.2: (Continued)

Medication	Renal Manifestations	Dosage Adjustments in Renal Impairment
TNF inhibitors	Lupus-like events with new ANA, dsDNA positivity and biopsy-proven GN (rare) ANCA-associated vasculitis with pauci-immune glomerulonephritis (rare) IgA nephropathy (rare)	No adjustment is needed in renal impairment or in RRT
Tofacitinib	Mild renal impairment (rare)	*CrCl >50 mL/minute:* No adjustments in dosing needed *CrCl <50 mL/minute and in RRT:* Decrease dose to 5 mg once a day
Abatacept	No renal involvement reported	No adjustment is needed in renal impairment or in RRT.
Tocilizumab	No renal involvement reported	No adjustment is needed in renal impairment or in RRT.
Rituximab	No renal involvement reported	No adjustment is needed in renal impairment or in RRT.
Immunoglobulins	Acute kidney injury Osmotic nephrosis (due to stabilizers)	No dosage adjustment needed for renal impairment or in RRT, but rate of infusion or concentration of solution should be minimized with attention to volume status. A lower, more frequent dosing should be attempted.
IL-17 inhibitors	No renal involvement reported	No adjustment is needed in renal impairment or in RRT.
Mycophenolate mofetil Mycophenolate sodium	No renal involvement reported	*CrCl >25 mL/minute:* No dose adjustment necessary *CrCl <25 mL/minute:* Limit dose to mycophenolate mofetil 1 g twice daily or mycophenolate sodium delayed release 720 mg twice daily or closely monitor for adverse effects of increased drug exposure (e.g., leukopenia, anemia, GI symptoms)
Calcineurin inhibitors	Drug-induced thrombotic microangiopathy Acute calcineurin inhibitor toxicity (vasoconstriction of the glomerular arterioles) *Chronic calcineurin inhibitor toxicity:* Nodular arteriolar hyalinosis, interstitial fibrosis, tubular atrophy and glomerular sclerosis (focal or global)	*Tacrolimus:* Dose adjustments should be based on therapeutic drug monitoring. No initial dose adjustments needed for any degree of kidney dysfunction/RRT. *Cyclosporine:* Dose adjustments should be based on therapeutic drug monitoring. No initial dose adjustments needed for any degree of kidney dysfunction/RRT.

Abbreviations: RRT, renal replacement therapy; CrCl, creatinine clearance; AKI, acute kidney injury; RA, rheumatoid arthritis; GI, gastrointestinal; NSAIDs, nonsteroidal anti-inflammatory drugs

(15, 16). The two diseases have some overlap in pathogenesis with immune complex deposition, T-cell mediated damage and cytokine production, but there is typically no correlation between RA disease activity and FSGS risk (15). The initial treatment of FSGS associated with RA is conservative management that involves blood pressure control and RA-targeted therapy (15, 16).

10.2.2 Renal Involvement in Rheumatoid Vasculitis

Renal dysfunction with rheumatoid vasculitis is rare and limited to case reports (17–19). Renal artery involvement similar to polyarteritis nodosa and pauci-immune GN comparable to anti-neutrophil cytoplasmic antibody (ANCA)-associated vasculitis are reported and are often associated with necrotizing cutaneous ulcerations (17–20). This is sometimes associated with crescent formation on renal biopsy and the presence of antineutrophilic antibodies (18, 19). Management is similar to that for primary systemic vasculitides involving high-dose glucocorticoids, rituximab and cyclophosphamide (18, 19).

10.2.3 Secondary Amyloidosis Due to RA

Secondary amyloidosis is a sequela of chronic inflammatory disorders that leads to the overproduction of the acute phase reactant serum amyloid A protein (SAA). Secondary amyloidosis used to be a common cause of nephrotic syndrome in RA before the use of methotrexate and biologics in the 1970s (21). Patients with long-standing, poorly controlled, seropositive RA and those with extra-articular manifestations are reported to be at a higher risk of developing AA amyloidosis (22, 23). The primary principle of the management of AA amyloidosis is controlling the activity of the underlying RA. There have been reports of the successful treatment of secondary amyloidosis due to RA with TNFis, interleukin-6 (IL-6) inhibitors and rituximab (24–26).

10.3 RENAL MANIFESTATION OF SPONDYLOARTHROPATHIES

Spondyloarthropathies (SpAs) are a group of chronic inflammatory diseases that primarily involve the spine and sacroiliac joints (27). The most common extra-articular manifestations of SpA include uveitis, psoriasis (in case of psoriatic arthritis) and inflammatory bowel disease (in case of enteropathic arthritis) (28). Renal manifestations of SpA have a reported prevalence ranging between 8 and 35%, depending on the definition used for renal involvement, including urinary abnormalities, renal dysfunction or histopathological findings (29–31). Risk factors for renal involvement include advanced age, human leukocyte antigen B27 (HLA-B27) positivity, cardiovascular risk factors (hypertension, diabetes mellitus, high Framingham score), high disease activity scores (such a Bath Ankylosing Spondylitis Activity Index [BASDAI], Ankylosing Spondylitis Disease Activity Score c-reactive protein [ASDAS-CRP]), elevated inflammatory markers and nonsteroidal anti-inflammatory drug (NSAID) use (31). Renal involvement in SpA includes secondary AA amyloidosis, NSAID-induced nephropathy and GN, particularly IgA nephropathy and less commonly membranoproliferative GN, membranous GN, FSGS and unspecified proliferative GN.

10.3.1 Secondary Amyloidosis Due to SpA

Clinically apparent secondary amyloidosis is reported in approximately 1% of patients with SpA, but subclinical secondary amyloidosis can be as high as 7% (32, 33). It is seen more commonly in older patients and those with long-standing disease with an average disease duration of 14 years (32, 34). Elevated inflammatory markers, high disease activity levels and peripheral arthritis are independent risk factors for amyloidosis (32, 34). The mortality rate of patients with SpA is 1.5 times higher than that the general population, which is primarily attributed to AA amyloidosis (35). Presentation can vary from mild proteinuria to nephrotic syndrome and renal dysfunction. Renal biopsy is needed for a definitive diagnosis and shows amorphous deposition in the mesangium that is Congo red positive with an apple-green birefringence under polarized light. Several studies have reported an improvement in proteinuria and renal function with TNFi therapy (32, 36)

10.3.2 NSAID-Induced Renal Injury

NSAIDs are the mainstay of treatment in SpA, and their pervasive use can lead to kidney injury (Table 10.2). NSAIDs can have a particularly negative impact on patients with preexisting risk factors such as older age, decreased renal function and comorbidities (37).

Kidney injury can occur due to several mechanisms, which include acute tubular necrosis secondary to hemodynamic alterations and a reduction in kidney perfusion and NSAID-induced acute interstitial nephritis. The exact mechanism of interstitial nephritis is unknown, but it is thought to be a hypersensitivity reaction (38). With prolonged uncontrolled NSAID use, acute interstitial nephritis can progress to chronic interstitial nephritis and CKD. The definitive treatment of NSAID-induced kidney injury is the discontinuation of NSAIDs and supportive therapy.

10.3.3 IgA Nephropathy

IgA nephropathy is commonly associated with SpA. However, given that IgA nephropathy is the most prevalent GN worldwide, this association may be incidental rather than causal (39). On the other hand, it has been suggested that ankylosing spondylitis and IgA nephropathy share some immunological features (40). In both disease conditions, there is impaired expression of IgA Fc receptors that are involved in the clearance of IgA complexes, which in turn causes elevated serum IgA levels and IgA immune complexes (40). IgA nephropathy secondary to ankylosing spondylitis generally has worse renal outcomes than primary IgA nephropathy, along with a greater prevalence of crescents on biopsy and similar prognostic factors (41). These poor prognostic factors include the presence of hypertension, high-grade proteinuria (>1 g/day) and the presence of segmental sclerosis and tubular atrophy/interstitial fibrosis (S and T score) on biopsy (41). Patients are treated with supportive therapy, including angiotensin-converting enzyme (ACE) inhibitors for proteinuria as well as glucocorticoids in those with renal impairment and nephrotic-range proteinuria. TNFis usually do not have an impact on the rate of decline in renal function (41)

10.4 RENAL MANIFESTATIONS OF IDIOPATHIC INFLAMMATORY MYOPATHIES

Idiopathic inflammatory myopathies (IIMs) are a heterogenous group of autoimmune conditions that cause muscle inflammation as their predominant feature. The worldwide prevalence is approximately seven cases per 100,000 persons (42). IIMs encompass dermatomyositis, polymyositis, immune-mediated necrotizing myopathy, anti-synthetase syndrome and inclusion body myositis. IIMs frequently cause extra-muscular complications, including interstitial lung disease in 25–45% of cases (43). Renal involvement, which was previously thought to be a rare occurrence, has a reported prevalence as high as 21–23% in patients with IIM (44, 45). AKI occurs in the first 6 months after the diagnosis in about 50% of patients with IIM (45). Male sex, cardiovascular risk factors and initial proteinuria >0.3 g/day are associated with an increased risk of AKI (45). The outcomes in patients with AKI are generally poor, with the majority progressing into CKD (45).

There are two main types of renal disease described in patients with IIM, which include acute tubular injury resulting in acute renal failure secondary to rhabdomyolysis and chronic glomerulonephritis related to the primary disease process.

10.4.1 Rhabdomyolysis-Induced AKI

IIM typically causes a subacute to chronic progressive muscle injury, which develops over weeks to months. Therefore, AKI from rhabdomyolysis is rarely seen in patients with IIM and generally should point towards a toxic myopathic process rather than IIM. The AKI in rhabdomyolysis is seen as a result of the direct toxic effects of myoglobin on renal tubules with the formation of pigmented granular casts and iron-induced oxidative stress (46). Third spacing into edematous damaged muscle results in the activation of the sympathetic system, which in return causes renal vasoconstriction, which also contributes to AKI (46).

Prompt diagnosis and treatment are imperative in rhabdomyolysis, as this can cause life-threatening electrolyte and acid–base imbalances due to the release of intracellular components during muscle inflammation. This includes metabolic acidosis (due to the release of organic acids), hyperkalemia and hyperphosphatemia (47). The calcium levels have a biphasic behavior, with significant hypocalcemia due to the sequestration of calcium in damaged muscle due to the failure of the dependent calcium channel that actively pumps calcium out of the cell (46). Later in the disease, there can be a slow release of this deposited calcium to cause severe hypercalcemia (46). All these electrolyte abnormalities, especially hyperkalemia and hypocalcemia, can cause life-threatening cardiac arrythmias.

For the diagnosis of rhabdomyolysis, the urine dipstick test is not generally helpful, as this cannot distinguish between hematuria (seen in glomerular disease) and myoglobin. Testing for urinary sediment is necessary to differentiate red blood cells/red cell casts from pigmented granular casts.

Aggressive fluid resuscitation and alkalization are the mainstays of the treatment of rhabdomyolysis, along with the treatment of underlying IIM. Fluids ensure the forced diuresis of myoglobin and potassium, while alkalinization of the serum with sodium bicarbonate addresses metabolic acidosis and hyperkalemia and prevents the precipitation of myoglobin in renal tubules (47). If oliguria, hyperkalemia and metabolic acidosis are not responsive to these measures, renal replacement therapy should be considered.

10.4.2 Glomerulonephritis and Other Renal Pathologies Related to IIM

The spectrum of renal involvement in IIM includes GN and, less commonly, amyloidosis, tubulointerstitial nephritis and vascular involvement with edematous thickening of the intima of the arterioles resembling malignant hypertension/scleroderma renal crisis (45). These renal diseases can occur before or after the onset of IIM, and the overall outcome is favorable, with approximately 70% of patients showing improvement and the rest of the patients showing progression into CKD or end-stage renal disease (46).

Immune complex-mediated GN, including mesangial proliferative and membranous nephropathy, remains as the most common form of GN in IIM (46). Other types of GN include minimal change disease, crescentic GN, IgA nephropathy and FSGS (46). Given that a variety of GN types have been reported, it is difficult to delineate whether it is the same autoimmune mechanism affecting both the kidney and the muscle.

The presentation of GN in IIM is variable, ranging from minor urinary abnormalities, including a combination of proteinuria and hematuria, to rapidly progressive renal impairment (46). However, rapidly progressive crescentic GN is a rare event, with only a few cases reported to date (48, 49). In the situation of a rapidly worsening renal function with oliguria, it is important to consider IIM-induced rhabdomyolysis in the differential diagnosis and investigate accordingly, as the management will be drastically different from that for GN. Fluid resuscitation will help rhabdomyolysis, while this can precipitate pulmonary edema in GN. High blood pressure with peripheral edema, urinary sediment with dysmorphic red blood cells and casts suggests glomerular involvement, while high creatine kinase levels, hypotension and pigmented casts may be seen in rhabdomyolysis. For the treatment of GN with mild degrees of proteinuria and/or hematuria with normal renal function, steroid dosages used for IIM can be used (1 mg/kg for 4–6 weeks). For more symptomatic GN, including patients with nephrotic syndrome and/or worsening renal function, there have been reports of using cyclophosphamide, azathioprine, rituximab, intravenous immunoglobulin, cyclosporine and mycophenolate mofetil (45, 46, 50).

10.5 RENAL MANIFESTATIONS OF MIXED CONNECTIVE TISSUE DISEASE

Mixed connective tissue disease (MCTD) is a systemic rheumatic disease characterized by high-titer anti-U1 ribonucleoprotein (RNP) antibodies in combination with overlapping clinical features of systemic lupus erythematosus, systemic sclerosis, inflammatory arthritis/RA and inflammatory myopathy. In the initial description of MCTD, the absence of severe renal disease was reported as a characteristic feature of this condition (51, 52). The anti-U1 ribonucleoprotein (RNP) antibodies are thought to be protective against diffuse proliferative GN (51, 52). The frequency of renal disease ranges between 4 and 64% depending on the definition used for renal disease, including renal biopsy findings, urinary abnormalities or decreased renal function (53, 54). Renal biopsy is required to make a definitive diagnosis. Membranous nephropathy is the most common renal disease in MCTD, but there have been a few cases of tubular interstitial nephritis and membranoproliferative GN (51, 54). Kidney involvement is mostly subclinical, with an overall favorable prognosis and with good response to glucocorticoids.

Renal complications of other associated autoimmune conditions can also be seen in MCTD. These complications include hypertensive crisis similar to scleroderma renal crisis and GN similar to ANCA-associated vasculitis and systemic lupus erythematosus (55–59). The treatment of these conditions is similar to that of their original counterparts (e.g., ACE inhibitors in scleroderma renal crisis and glucocorticoids with cyclophosphamide or rituximab in ANCA-associated vasculitis).

Urinary abnormalities such as proteinuria and/or hematuria on urinalysis during the clinical course of MCTD may indicate a higher risk of developing other associated autoimmune conditions and an overall poor prognosis (60). Therefore, we recommend monitoring urinalysis in patients with MCTD, even if their baseline urinalysis is normal.

REFERENCES

1. Mutru O, et al. Ten year mortality and causes of death in patients with rheumatoid arthritis. Br Med J (Clin Res Ed). 1985;290(6484):1797–9.
2. Chiu HY, et al. Increased risk of chronic kidney disease in rheumatoid arthritis associated with cardiovascular complications—A national population-based cohort study. PLoS ONE. 2015;10(9):e0136508.

3. Koseki Y, et al. A prospective study of renal disease in patients with early rheumatoid arthritis. Ann Rheum Dis. 2001;60(4):327–31.
4. Hickson LJ, et al. Development of reduced kidney function in rheumatoid arthritis. Am J Kidney Dis. 2014;63(2):206–13.
5. Karie S, et al. Kidney disease in RA patients: Prevalence and implication on RA-related drugs management: The MATRIX study. Rheumatology (Oxford). 2008;47(3):350–4.
6. Sihvonen S, et al. Renal disease as a predictor of increased mortality among patients with rheumatoid arthritis. Nephron Clin Pract. 2004;96(4):c107–14.
7. Helin HJ, et al. Renal biopsy findings and clinicopathologic correlations in rheumatoid arthritis. Arthritis Rheum. 1995;38(2):242–7.
8. Icardi A, et al. [Kidney involvement in rheumatoid arthritis]. Reumatismo. 2003;55(2):76–85.
9. Kapoor T, et al. Renal manifestations of rheumatoid arthritis. Rheum Dis Clin North Am. 2018;44(4):571–84.
10. Makino H, et al. Renal involvement in rheumatoid arthritis: Analysis of renal biopsy specimens from 100 patients. Mod Rheumatol. 2002;12(2):148–54.
11. Nakano M, et al. Determination of IgA- and IgM-rheumatoid factors in patients with rheumatoid arthritis with and without nephropathy. Ann Rheum Dis. 1996;55(8):520–4.
12. Korpela M, et al. Immunological comparison of patients with rheumatoid arthritis with and without nephropathy. Ann Rheum Dis. 1990;49(4):214–18.
13. Lv J, et al. Corticosteroid therapy in IgA nephropathy. J Am Soc Nephrol. 2012;23(6):1108–16.
14. Premužić V, et al. The association of TNF-alpha inhibitors and development of IgA nephropathy in patients with rheumatoid arthritis and diabetes. Case Rep Nephrol. 2020;2020:9480860.
15. Liu Y, et al. Focal segmental glomerulosclerosis lagged behind the onset of rheumatoid arthritis by 7 years: A case report and literature review. Medicine (Baltimore). 2017;96(1):e5789.
16. Albandak M, et al. Rheumatoid arthritis with focal segmental glomerulosclerosis: A case report and literature review. Cureus. 2023;15(4):e37161.
17. Boers M, et al. Renal findings in rheumatoid arthritis: Clinical aspects of 132 necropsies. Ann Rheum Dis. 1987;46(9):658–63.
18. Harper L, et al. Focal segmental necrotizing glomerulonephritis in rheumatoid arthritis. QJM. 1997;90(2):125–32.
19. Qarni MU, et al. Pauci-immune necrotizing glomerulonephritis complicating rheumatoid arthritis. Clin Nephrol. 2000;54(1):54–8.
20. Scott DG, et al. Systemic rheumatoid vasculitis: A clinical and laboratory study of 50 cases. Medicine (Baltimore). 1981;60(4):288–97.
21. Lawson AA, et al. Renal disease and drug therapy in rheumatoid arthritis. Ann Rheum Dis. 1966;25(5):441–9.
22. Nakamura T. Clinical strategies for amyloid A amyloidosis secondary to rheumatoid arthritis. Mod Rheumatol. 2008;18(2):109–18.
23. Prete M, et al. Extra-articular manifestations of rheumatoid arthritis: An update. Autoimmun Rev. 2011;11(2):123–31.
24. Courties A, et al. AA amyloidosis treated with tocilizumab: Case series and updated literature review. Amyloid. 2015;22(2):84–92.
25. Pamuk ON, et al. Turkish experience in rheumatoid arthritis patients with clinical apparent amyloid deposition. Amyloid. 2013;20(4):245–50.
26. Kilic L, et al. Rituximab therapy in renal amyloidosis secondary to rheumatoid arthritis. Biomolecules. 2018;8(4).
27. Rodrigues AC, et al. Kidney disease in ankylosing spondylitis: A case series and review of the literature. J Bras Nefrol. 2023;45(1):36–44.
28. Stolwijk C, et al. Prevalence of extra-articular manifestations in patients with ankylosing spondylitis: A systematic review and meta-analysis. Ann Rheum Dis. 2015;74(1):65–73.
29. Samia B, et al. [Renal abnormalities in ankylosing spondylitis]. Nephrol Ther. 2012;8(4):220–5.
30. Vilar MJ, Cury SE, Ferraz MB, Sesso R, Atra E. Renal abnormalities in ankylosing spondylitis. Scand J Rheumatol. 1997;26(1):19–23.
31. Couderc M, et al. Prevalence of renal impairment in patients with rheumatoid arthritis: Results from a cross-sectional multicenter study. Arthritis Care Res (Hoboken). 2016;68(5):638–44.
32. Dönmez S, et al. Secondary amyloidosis in ankylosing spondylitis. Rheumatol Int. 2013;33(7):1725–9.

33. Gratacos J, et al. Secondary amyloidosis in ankylosing spondylitis. A systematic survey of 137 patients using abdominal fat aspiration. J Rheumatol. 1997;24(5):912–15.
34. Barbouch S, et al. Renal amyloidosis in ankylosing spondylitis: A monocentric study and review of literature. Saudi J Kidney Dis Transpl. 2018;29(2):386–91.
35. Lehtinen K. Mortality and causes of death in 398 patients admitted to hospital with ankylosing spondylitis. Ann Rheum Dis. 1993;52(3):174–6.
36. Lee SH, et al. Renal involvement in ankylosing spondylitis: Prevalence, pathology, response to TNF-a blocker. Rheumatol Int. 2013;33(7):1689–92.
37. Kim JW. Are nonsteroidal anti-inflammatory drugs safe for the kidney in ankylosing spondylitis? J Rheum Dis. 2023;30(3):139–45.
38. Lucas GNC, et al. Pathophysiological aspects of nephropathy caused by non-steroidal anti-inflammatory drugs. J Bras Nefrol. 2019;41(1):124–30.
39. D'Amico G. The commonest glomerulonephritis in the world: IgA nephropathy. Q J Med. 1987;64(245):709–27.
40. Montenegro V, et al. Elevation of serum IgA in spondyloarthropathies and IgA nephropathy and its pathogenic role. Curr Opin Rheumatol. 1999;11(4):265–72.
41. Champtiaux N, et al. Spondyloarthritis-associated IgA nephropathy. Kidney Int Rep. 2020;5(6):813–20.
42. Mammen AL. Dermatomyositis and polymyositis: Clinical presentation, autoantibodies, and pathogenesis. Ann N Y Acad Sci. 2010;1184:134–53.
43. Fathi M, et al. Pulmonary complications of polymyositis and dermatomyositis. Semin Respir Crit Care Med. 2007;28(4):451–8.
44. Yen TH, et al. Renal involvement in patients with polymyositis and dermatomyositis. Int J Clin Pract. 2005;59(2):188–93.
45. Couvrat-Desvergnes G, et al. The spectrum of renal involvement in patients with inflammatory myopathies. Medicine (Baltimore). 2014;93(1):33–41.
46. Cucchiari D, et al. Renal involvement in idiopathic inflammatory myopathies. Clin Rev Allergy Immunol. 2017;52(1):99–107.
47. Bosch X, et al. Rhabdomyolysis and acute kidney injury. N Engl J Med. 2009;361(1):62–72.
48. Tsunemi M, et al. A case of crescentic glomerulonephritis associated with polymyositis. Nephron. 1993;64(3):488–9.
49. Yuste C, et al. Overlap between dermatomyositis and ANCA vasculitides. Clin Kidney J. 2014;7(1):59–61.
50. Dyck RF, et al. Glomerulonephritis associated with polymyositis. J Rheumatol. 1979;6(3):336–44.
51. Kitridou RC, et al. Renal involvement in mixed connective tissue disease: A longitudinal clinicopathologic study. Semin Arthritis Rheum. 1986;16(2):135–45.
52. Lundberg IE. The prognosis of mixed connective tissue disease. Rheum Dis Clin North Am. 2005;31(3):535–47, vii–viii.
53. Sawai T, et al. Morphometric analysis of the kidney lesions in mixed connective tissue disease (MCTD). Tohoku J Exp Med. 1994;174(2):141–54.
54. Yoshida A, et al. [Nephropathy in patients with mixed connective tissue disease]. Ryumachi. 1994;34(6):976–80.
55. Germain MJ, et al. Pulmonary hemorrhage and acute renal failure in a patient with mixed connective tissue disease. Am J Kidney Dis. 1984;3(6):420–4.
56. Hernández-Molina G, et al. ANCA associated glomerulonephritis in a patient with mixed connective tissue disease. Ann Rheum Dis. 2006;65(3):410–11.
57. Abdul Mabood Khalil M, et al. Scleroderma renal crisis in a newly diagnosed mixed connective tissue disease resulting in dialysis-dependent chronic kidney disease despite angiotensin-converting enzyme inhibition. CEN Case Rep. 2013;2(1):41–5.
58. Madieh J, et al. Scleroderma renal crisis in a case of mixed connective tissue disease treated successfully with angiotensin-converting enzyme inhibitors. Case Rep Nephrol. 2021;2021:8862405.
59. Ali S, et al. A novel case of lupus nephritis and mixed connective tissue disorder in a COVID-19 patient. Ann Med Surg (Lond). 2022;78:103653.
60. Nishioka R, et al. Urinary abnormality in mixed connective tissue disease predicts development of other connective tissue diseases and decrease in renal function. Mod Rheumatol. 2022;32(1):155–62.

11 Kidney Disease in Sarcoidosis, Sjögren's Disease, and IgG4-Related Disease

Ellen Romich[†], Maria Jose Zabala Ramirez[†], Vanessa Romero, Dana Direnzo[‡], and Koyal Jain[‡]
[†]These are co-first authors.
[‡]These are co-senior authors.

11.1 INTRODUCTION

Sarcoidosis, Sjögren's disease, and IgG4-related disease are a grouping of inflammatory disorders that can have variable clinical presentations affecting multiple organ systems. The goals of this chapter are to discuss the diagnostic and clinical characteristics of sarcoidosis, Sjögren's disease, and IgG4-related disease and define renal manifestations associated with each entity.

11.2 SARCOIDOSIS

Sarcoidosis is a multisystem disease, originally described in 1899 by Ceasar Boeck, with granulomatous inflammation of tissues (1).

11.2.1 General Diagnostic/Classification Criteria

No standardized diagnostic or classification criteria exist for the diagnosis of sarcoidosis. However, the American Thoracic Society clinical practice guidelines recommend that the diagnosis be based on a compatible clinical presentation, the finding of non-necrotizing granulomatous inflammation in one or more tissue samples, and the exclusion of alternative causes of granulomatous disease (2). In certain scenarios with well-defined presentations such as Lofgren's syndrome (bilateral hilar adenopathy with erythema nodosum and periarticular arthritis), biopsy may not be required (2).

11.2.2 Renal Diagnostic Criteria

The reported frequency of kidney involvement in sarcoidosis is widely variable and believed to be underreported (3–6). It is more prevalent in men compared to women 1.7:1 and in the Black/African American population. Mean age at presentation is 55 years (6, 7). Presentation may include interstitial nephritis, glomerulonephritis, nephrolithiasis, nephrocalcinosis, renal masses, and AA amyloidosis (3, 5). Severity can vary widely from asymptomatic, to acute kidney injury (AKI), to end-stage kidney disease (ESKD); however, the latter is rare (6). Isolated renal sarcoidosis is rare (5, 6). Hypercalcemia can cause AKI through different mechanisms, including obstructing tubules with calcium precipitates, renal vasoconstriction, dehydration due to sodium losses in urine, and increasing resistance to vasopressin (4, 5).

The presence of hematuria, aseptic pyuria, proteinuria, elevated creatinine, and hypercalcemia suggests the presence of kidney involvement. Urine sediment can reveal microscopic hematuria and aseptic pyuria, and the presence of cellular casts is often not observed (4–6). Renal biopsy remains the gold standard for diagnosis and should be done whenever kidney involvement is suspected (Figure 11.1). Renal ultrasound should be performed in all patients to evaluate for evidence of chronic kidney disease (CKD), nephrolithiasis, and nephrocalcinosis. For all patients

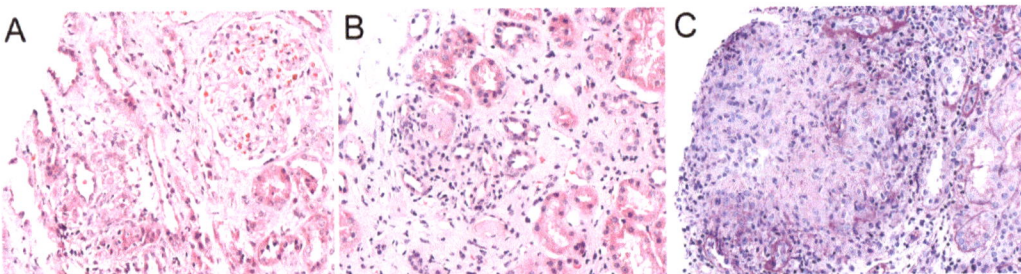

Figure 11.1 Renal sarcoidosis often shows granulomatous inflammation. (A) Some cases can present with ill-defined granulomas with epithelioid histiocytes (H&E stain; 10×). (B) Scattered and rare giant cells can be seen (H&E stain; 20×). (C) The hallmark of sarcoidosis is the presence of non-necrotizing, well-formed sharply defined granulomas (PAS stain; 20×).

DOI: 10.1201/9781003438373-13

presenting with isolated renal involvement, screening for extrarenal involvement should be pursued, and other forms of granulomatous disease should be excluded, including Mycobacterial infections (5, 6).

11.2.3 General Treatment Approach

The European Respiratory Society (ERS) has published clinical practice guidelines for treatment that vary based on clinical presentation. Observation may be appropriate in mild cases, while treatment is indicated for life- or organ-threatening disease or symptoms negatively impacting quality of life. The ERS guidelines provide recommendations for the treatment of pulmonary, cutaneous, cardiac, and neurologic disease, while recommendations for other manifestations, including renal disease, are limited (8).

In general, glucocorticoids are the first-line treatment for most forms of symptomatic disease. Second- and third-line treatments beyond glucocorticoids are highly variable. Methotrexate (or another disease-modifying anti-rheumatic drug [DMARD]—azathioprine, leflunomide, mycophenolate mofetil, hydroxychloroquine) is commonly used as a second-line treatment for active disease despite glucocorticoids, unacceptable glucocorticoid side-effects, or relapse. Third-line treatments include infliximab, adalimumab, and rituximab (8).Treatment is typically continued once disease manifestations have been controlled, as relapse is common within 2 years after withdrawing therapy in 20–80% of individuals (8).

11.2.4 Renal Treatment Approach

Recommendations for renal sarcoidosis management are limited. Similar to extrarenal manifestations, glucocorticoids remain the mainstay of treatment (5, 6). Treatment goals are to preserve and improve kidney function, and response to treatment after the first 4 weeks of therapy remains an important prognostic factor (6, 9). Complete response to treatment occurs in around 31% of cases (6, 9). No racial difference was noted in the response to treatment (10).

The need for dialysis is rare, associated mainly with granulomatous interstitial nephritis, hypercalcemia, nephrocalcinosis, and hypergammaglobulinemia (4).

Limited data exists regarding kidney transplantation in patients with sarcoidosis. Small studies suggest that patient/graft survival (94.4% at 42-month follow-up) and complication rates in kidney transplants are similar to those in other patient populations (4, 5). Recurrence has been reported in up to 17% of patients (5). Lower amounts of interstitial fibrosis on biopsy and initial response to treatment indicate a favorable prognosis (6, 9).

11.3 SJÖGREN'S DISEASE

Sjögren's disease (SD) is also a multi-organ system disease defined by hallmark sicca symptoms and glandular inflammation (11). SD can be associated with hematologic, pulmonary, nervous system, skin, and renal manifestations (12). SD is also referred to as sicca syndrome or Mikulicz's disease and was first described in the late 1800s (13).

11.3.1 Classification Criteria

The 2016 American College of Rheumatology (ACR)/European League Against Rheumatism (EULAR) Classification Criteria for primary SD are used in patients with signs and symptoms suggestive of SD (14). The criteria consist of a weighted sum of five items (Table 11.1), where individuals with ≥4 points meet criteria for primary SD with 96% sensitivity and 95% specificity (14).

Table 11.1: 2016 ACR Classification Criteria for Sjögren's Disease

Feature	Points
Anti-SSA/Ro positivity	3 points
Minor salivary gland lip biopsy demonstrating focal lymphocytic sialadenitis with focus score of ≥1 foci/4 mm2	3 points
Abnormal ocular staining score ≥5	1 point
Schirmer's test ≤5 mm/5 minutes	1 point
Unstimulated salivary flow rate ≤0.1 mL/minute	1 point

Note: Score of ≥4 for classification of Sjögren's Disease

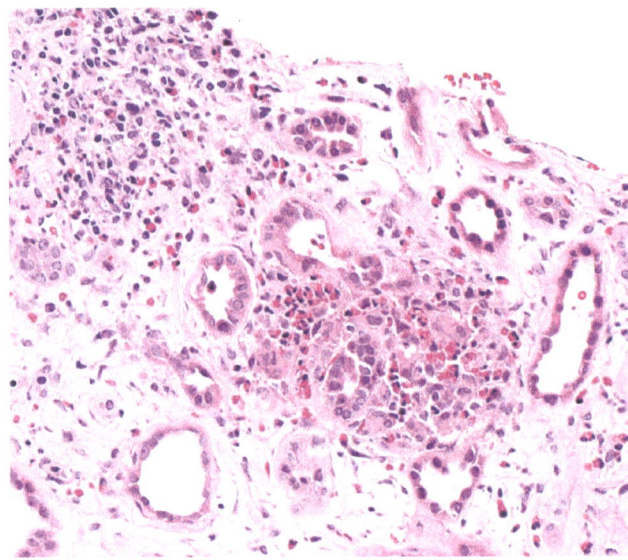

Figure 11.2 Acute interstitial nephritis characterized by interstitial edema accompanied by mononuclear leukocytes infiltrates with increased number of eosinophils (H&E stain; 20×).

11.3.2 Renal Diagnostic Criteria

Clinical manifestations from kidney involvement occur in 5% of patients with primary SD, most commonly affecting women (15, 16) (Figure 11.2). They can present as interstitial nephritis (IN) with or without tubular dysfunction or more rarely as glomerulonephritis (GN). IN is the most common presentation, and it accounts for 40–85% of renal lesions in this patient population (15, 16). IN usually presents early in the disease, and its progression is generally slow, whereas with GN, prognosis is less favorable (15). GN usually presents as membranoproliferative GN due to type II cryoglobulins with immune complex deposition and C4 consumption.

Lymphocytic infiltration of the interstitium can cause tubular dysfunction and can present as distal RTA (occurring in 5–70% of cases) with hypokalemia, normal anion gap metabolic acidosis (NAGMA), and urine pH >5.5. Hypercalciuria and hypocitraturia in the setting of distal RTA can result in nephrolithiasis, and in these cases, renal ultrasound should be considered. In around 3% of cases, it presents as Fanconi syndrome with NAGMA, phosphaturia, glycosuria, and aminoaciduria. It can rarely present as Gitelman or Bartter syndrome (15). Concentrating defects (nephrogenic DI) have been reported in association with SD, presenting with polydipsia, polyuria, and nocturia. Tubulo-interstitial nephritis (TIN) has an indolent course. GN usually presents as AKI with nephritic or nephrotic syndromes and CKD.

Diagnostic approach should include the assessment of kidney function (serum, complete urine studies), complements, cryoglobulins, rheumatoid factor, immunoglobulins, and paraproteins. Kidney biopsy remains the gold standard for diagnosis of IN and GN (15, 16).

11.3.3 General Treatment Approaches

Treatment of SD is centered on the management of sicca symptoms (i.e., dry eye, dry mouth). Immunosuppression is added for systemic disease and tailored to specific organ involvement. The 2019 EULAR recommendations for the management of SD provide recommendations for symptomatic and organ-specific treatment (17). Ocular dryness is frequently managed with artificial tears and ointments or topical immunosuppressants (i.e., cyclosporine A), while oral dryness is managed with non-pharmacologic stimulation (sugar-free lozenges/gum) or pharmacologic stimulation (muscarinic agonists—pilocarpine and cevimeline). Systemic immunosuppressive treatments have shown little benefit for sicca symptoms.

The selection of an immunosuppressive agent depends on the severity of systemic disease (17). DMARDs may include hydroxychloroquine, methotrexate, leflunomide, azathioprine, mycophenolate mofetil (MMF), rituximab, cyclophosphamide, or IVIG, depending on the type and severity of disease manifestation (17).

11.3.4 Renal Treatment Approach

No specified guidelines for management of Sjögren's-related kidney disease exist, and management depends on disease presentation. TIN management is largely supportive, with conflicting data for immunosuppression. Some studies have shown a possible role of corticosteroids and other immunosuppressive therapy, but this is not supported in other studies (15, 18, 19). The use of immunosuppression for TIN remains controversial but can be considered, especially if no significant chronic changes (interstitial fibrosis and tubular atrophy) are noted on kidney biopsy. MMF and rituximab have been used, but data from randomized controlled trials are lacking (16). Immunosuppression is required for the management of GN to avoid progression to ESKD. MMF, rituximab, or cyclophosphamide (severe cases) along with corticosteroids is usually used. Rituximab and corticosteroids are the preferred agents in cryoglobulinemia (16).

11.4 IGG4-RELATED DISEASE

IgG4-related disease (IgG4-RD) also can be challenging to diagnose and is a relatively newly recognized fibroinflammatory disease. IgG4-RD was first described as an entity after noticing lymphoplasmacytic infiltrates depositing outside of the pancreas in individuals with autoimmune pancreatitis (20).

11.4.1 General Diagnostic/Classification Criteria

The IgG4-RD classification criteria, published jointly in 2019 by the ACR and EULAR, incorporate several histological, serological, and clinical features (21). Inclusion criteria consist of characteristic clinical or radiological involvement of a typical organ (such as the pancreas, salivary glands, bile ducts, orbits, kidney, lung, aorta, retroperitoneum, pachymeninges, or thyroid) or pathological evidence of an inflammatory process with lymphoplasmacytic infiltrate in one of these same organs. Exclusion criteria consist of features that would suggest an alternative diagnosis, including autoantibodies (e.g., ANCA, SSA/B, dsDNA, Smith/RNP), peripheral eosinophilia >300 mm^3, radiological findings suggestive of infection or malignancy, and prominent neutrophilic inflammation on biopsy, among others (21).

Key histopathological features include dense lymphocytic infiltrate, storiform fibrosis, and obliterative phlebitis (22). Immunostaining is significant if the ratio of IgG4 to total IgG staining is >40% or there are at least 10 IgG4+ cells per high-power field. Serologically, elevated serum IgG4 levels are characteristic. Clinical features may include the involvement of bilateral lacrimal, parotid, sublingual, and submandibular glands; peribronchovascular and septal thickening in the lungs; pancreatic or biliary tree involvement; and soft tissue thickening in the retroperitoneum or around the infrarenal aorta or iliac arteries. From a renal perspective, classification points are assigned for hypocomplementemia, renal pelvis thickening, or bilateral renal cortex low-density areas on imaging (21).

11.4.2 Renal Diagnostic Criteria

Kidney involvement in IgG4 RD is relatively common (23, 24). Middle-aged men are most commonly affected (23). Patients usually present with kidney impairment or an incidental finding of renal lesions on imaging (25). TIN is the most common presentation, but IgG4-RD can also present as GN (commonly membranous nephropathy), renal pelvic lesions, and hydronephrosis due to ureteral lesions or retroperitoneal fibrosis (23–26).

Urine sediment is frequently bland, but hematuria and proteinuria have been reported. Proteinuria is usually non-nephrotic (<3.5 g/day) unless there is glomerular involvement. Renal imaging should be considered to assess for other renal lesions. Contrast-enhanced CT is preferred, but MRI should be considered when there is renal impairment (24, 25). Kidney biopsy should be pursued, if possible, for definitive diagnosis. The presence of IgG4+ and plasma-infiltrating cells is necessary for a diagnosis of IgG4-TIN, but it is not specific for this disease. Eosinophilic infiltration can also be found (24, 27, 28). Storiform fibrosis is common, as well as varying stages of fibrosis. Other prominent findings on biopsy are tubular atrophy with thickened tubular basement membrane and the disappearance of tubules. Lymphoplasmacytic infiltration of the renal capsule is another distinctive feature of IgG4-RD. Immune complex deposition composed of IgG and C3 in the tubular basement membrane are typically found, reported in at least 80% of patients with IgG4-TIN (24, 27, 29). Secondary membranous nephropathy has been reported in 7–10% of patients (28). Pathologic findings are characterized by granular deposits of IgG and C3 along the glomerular capillary walls. GBM deposits are predominantly IgG4, and in some cases C1q deposits can be found (24, 27, 28).

11.4.3 General Treatment Approaches

According to the 2015 international consensus guidance statement for the management and treatment of IgG4-RD, first-line treatment typically includes glucocorticoids with the goal of minimizing symptoms and improving biochemical and radiological findings (27). The earlier inflammatory phase of the disease, which is characterized by prominent lymphoplasmacytic infiltrate, is more likely to respond to immunosuppression than later fibrotic stages of the disease (30). The optimal doses and duration of steroid treatment have not been defined but typically start at 30–40 mg/day of prednisone or equivalent with a gradual taper over 4–6 months. Higher glucocorticoid doses may be considered for severe disease (27).

Beyond glucocorticoids, there are no established guidelines on the use of immunomodulatory agents for inducing or maintaining remission, but relapse after glucocorticoid taper is common. Medications including azathioprine, mycophenolate mofetil, methotrexate, leflunomide, tacrolimus, and cyclophosphamide have been used, but data on efficacy is limited. There is increasing interest in the use of rituximab for B-cell depletion in the treatment of IgG4-RD (31, 32).

11.4.4 Renal Treatment Approach

Early diagnosis and treatment are imperative to preserve kidney function. A characteristic feature of IgG4-RD disease is the rapid response to corticosteroids (24, 26, 27), which are first-line treatment. Rituximab has been associated with a lower risk for relapse (23), and there is also evidence for the use of azathioprine (27).

There are no established biomarkers that can be followed to monitor for relapse. Complements (both C3 and C4) have been noted to be extremely low at diagnosis and during relapse and may be useful to monitor for relapse (24, 27). On the contrary, IgG4 level is elevated at diagnosis in more than 90% of patients, and levels can decrease with treatment, although the prognostic value of IgG4 levels is not established (25, 26).

In a study by Chaba et al., 71% of patients had CKD, of which 30% had an eGFR < 30 mL/minute per 1.73 m^2, and 12% of patients progressed to ESKD (23).

11.5 OUTCOMES

In general, disease outcomes can vary widely in sarcoidosis, SD, and IgG4-RD. Residual or prior tissue damage stemming from inflammation can significantly impact health-related quality of life (HRQoL). In sarcoidosis, pulmonary fibrosis/scarring and resultant lung dysfunction greatly contribute to a patient's overall health status (33). The health impacts and burden of long-term corticosteroid use also can be detrimental, where higher doses of steroids have been associated with worse a HRQoL compared to lower doses of steroids (<500 mg of prednisone/year) (34). Healthcare utilization is also significantly impacted by psychosocial factors and patient comorbid conditions in sarcoidosis (35). Older adults and African Americans tend to have worse disease outcomes and HRQoL.

Similar findings may be found in SD. Based on a cluster analysis of a large Asian Indian cohort, patients tend to subset into mild and severe disease. Mild SD, or SD with negative antibodies, has a good prognosis but poses a major detriment to HRQoL due to intractable sicca (36). Severe SD represents patients with major organ manifestations and high titer antibodies with an increased risk for lymphoma. SSA antibodies can also contribute to pregnancy complications, with increased risks for spontaneous abortions and neonatal lupus (37). However, overall, the prognosis of SD is favorable and similar to the general population (38).

IgG4-RD also has a favorable prognosis if diagnosed and treated promptly. IgG4-RD responds well to glucocorticoids as well as targeted biologic therapy (39). However, disease severity varies widely (40). Table 11.2 summarizes the manifestations and evaluation of kidney disease in sarcoidosis, SD, and IgG4-RD.

11.6 CONCLUSION

Sarcoidosis, Sjögren's disease, and IgG4-related disease are a grouping of inflammatory disorders that can have a variety of clinical presentations affecting multiple organ systems. Kidney involvement is variable both in terms of frequency and presentation. Glucocorticoids are generally the first-line treatment, with systemic immunosuppressive medications as additional options for severe or refractory disease. Prognosis also varies widely depending on disease and severity but is generally favorable.

Table 11.2: Predicted dose of Allopurinol (mg/day) based (adapted from Wright 2024)

Descriptor	Sarcoidosis	Sjögren's Disease	IgG4-Related Disease
Kidney involvement	Varies widely (believed to be underreported)	Rare (5% of cases)	Common (around 30% of cases)[++]
Common presentations	Interstitial nephritis (granulomatous and non-granulomatous) Glomerulonephritis (IgA) Nephrolithiasis Nephrocalcinosis AA amyloidosis	Tubulo-interstitial nephritis (TIN)[*] Distal RTA Fanconi syndrome Nephrogenic diabetes insipidus Glomerulonephritis (membranoproliferative GN[**])	TIN GN (membranous nephropathy) Renal pelvic lesions Hydronephrosis[&]
Urine sediment	Microscopic hematuria Aseptic pyuria +/− Proteinuria	Bland +/− Hematuria and proteinuria	Bland +/− Hematuria and proteinuria
Imaging findings	Nephrolithiasis Nephrocalcinosis	Nephrolithiasis[+]	Multiple parenchymal low-density lesions Mass-like lesions Rim-like lesion along the renal capsule
Required workup	Basic metabolic panel Urine analysis Urine protein–creatinine ratio Kidney biopsy	Basic metabolic panel Complements Cryoglobulins Rheumatoid factor Immunoglobulins Paraproteins Urine analysis Urine protein–creatinine ratio Kidney biopsy	Basic metabolic panel IgG4 serum level Complements Urine protein–creatinine ratio Kidney biopsy
Histological features	Numerous interstitial non-caseating granulomas Interstitial fibrosis and tubular atrophy +/− Calcifications [***]	TIN with lymphocytic infiltration (CD4+ T lymphocytes) Membranoproliferative glomerulonephritis with intracapillary hypercellularity Several hyaline thrombi in capillaries in cryoglobulinemia	Plasma-cell-rich TIN (IgG4+) Different stages of fibrosis Storiform fibrosis Tubular atrophy with thickened TBM Patchy lesions
First-line treatment	Glucocorticoids	*TIN*: Largely supportive *GN*: Immunosuppression (MMF, rituximab, cyclophosphamide)	Glucocorticoids

[*]Most common 40–85% of cases (15, 16)
[**]Due to type II cryoglobulinemia (15, 16)
[+]In patients presenting with RTA (15)
[++] Has been reported in 7–24.6% of patients in a Japanese study and up to 30% in a European study (23, 24)
[&] Due to ureteral lesions or retroperitoneal fibrosis (23, 24, 27)
[***]Only in cases where membranous nephropathy granular glomerular capillary loop deposits on immunofluorescence and subepithelial glomerular capillary loop deposits on electron microscopy are present (7)
Abbreviations: GN, glomerulonephritis; MMF, mycophenolate mofetil; RTA, renal tubular acidosis; TBM, tubular basement membrane; TIN, tubule-interstitial nephritis

REFERENCES

1. Iannuzzi MC, et al. Sarcoidosis. N Engl J Med. 2007;357(21):2153–65.
2. Crouser ED, et al. Diagnosis and detection of sarcoidosis. An official American thoracic society clinical practice guideline. Am J Respir Crit Care Med. 2020;201(8):E26–51.
3. Bergner R, et al. Renal sarcoidosis: Approach to diagnosis and management. Curr Opin Pulm Med. 2018;24(5):513–20.

4. Calatroni M, et al. Renal sarcoidosis. J Nephrol. 2023;36(1):5–15.
5. Hilderson I, et al. Treatment of renal sarcoidosis: Is there a guideline? Overview of the different treatment options. Nephrol Dial Transplant 2014;29(10):1841–7.
6. Löffler C, et al. Renal sarcoidosis: Epidemiological and follow-up data in a cohort of 27 patients. Sarcoidosis Vasc Diffus Lung Dis. 2015;31(4):306–15.
7. Fogo AB, et al. AJKD Atlas of Renal Pathology: Sarcoidosis. Am J Kidney Dis. 2016;68(1):e5–6.
8. Baughman RP, et al. ERS clinical practice guidelines on treatment of sarcoidosis. Eur Respir J. 2021;58(6):2004079.
9. Mahévas M, et al. Renal sarcoidosis: Clinical, laboratory, and histologic presentation and outcome in 47 patients. Medicine (Baltimore). 2009;88(2):98–106.
10. Rajakariar R, et al. Sarcoid tubulo-interstitial nephritis: Long-term outcome and response to corticosteroid therapy. Kidney Int. 2006;70(1):165–9.
11. Mariette X, et al. Primary Sjögren's syndrome. N Engl J Med. 2018;378(10):931–9.
12. Negrini S, et al. Sjögren's syndrome: A systemic autoimmune disease. Clin Exp Med. 2022;22(1):9–25.
13. Ghafoor M. Sjögren's before Sjögren: Did henrik Sjögren (1899–1986) really discover Sjögren's disease? Maxillofac Oral Surg. 2012;11(3):373–4.
14. Shiboski CH, et al. 2016 ACR-EULAR classification criteria for primary Sjögren's syndrome: A consensus and data-driven methodology involving three international patient cohorts. Arthritis Rheumatol. 2017;69(1):35–45.
15. Goules A, et al. Renal involvement in primary Sjögren's syndrome: Natural history and treatment outcome. Clin Exp Rheumatol. 2019;37(3 Suppl 1):123–32.
16. Aiyegbusi O, et al. Renal disease in primary Sjögren's syndrome. Rheumatol Ther. 2021;8(1):63–80.
17. Ramos-Casals M, et al. EULAR recommendations for the management of Sjögren's syndrome with topical and systemic therapies. Ann Rheum Dis. 2020;79(1):3–18.
18. Maripuri S, et al. Renal involvement in primary Sjögren's syndrome: A clinicopathologic study. Clin J Am Soc Nephrol. 2009;4(9):1423–31.
19. Kidder D, et al. Kidney biopsy findings in primary Sjögren syndrome. Nephrol Dial Transplant. 2015;30(8):1363–9.
20. Stone JH, et al. IgG4-related disease. N Engl J Med. 2012;366(6):539–51.
21. Wallace ZS, et al. The 2019 American college of rheumatology/European league against Rheumatism classification criteria for IgG4-related disease. Ann Rheum Dis. 2020;79(1):77–87.
22. Kamisawa T, et al. IgG4-related disease. Lancet. 2015;385(9976):1460–71.
23. Chaba A, et al. Clinical and prognostic factors in patients with IgG4-Related kidney disease. Clin J Am Soc Nephrol. 2023;18(8):1031–40.
24. Kawano M, et al. IgG4-related kidney disease and retroperitoneal fibrosis: An update. Mod Rheumatol. 2019;29(2):231–9.
25. Kawano M, et al. IgG4-related kidney disease—an update. Curr Opin Nephrol Hypertens. 2015;24(2):193–201.
26. Kawano M, et al. Recent advances in IgG4-related kidney disease. Mod Rheumatol. 2023;33(2):242–51.
27. Khosroshahi A, et al. International consensus guidance statement on the management and treatment of IgG4-related disease. Arthritis Rheumatol. 2015;67(7):1688–99.
28. Quattrocchio G, et al. IgG4-related nephropathy. J Nephrol. 2016;29(4):487–93.
29. Raissian Y, et al. Diagnosis of IgG4-related tubulointerstitial nephritis. J Am Soc Nephrol. 2011;22(7):1343–52.
30. Lanzillotta M, et al. Emerging therapy options for IgG4-related disease. Expert Rev Clin Immunol. 2021;17(5):471–83.
31. Carruthers MN, et al. Rituximab for IgG4-related disease: A prospective, open-label trial. Ann Rheum Dis. 2015;74(6):1171–7.
32. Della-Torre E, et al. Efficacy and safety of rituximab biosimilar (CT-P10) in IgG4-related disease: An observational prospective open-label cohort study. Eur J Intern Med. 2021;84:63–7.
33. Nagai S, et al. Outcome of sarcoidosis. Clin Chest Med. 2008;29(3):565–74,
34. Judson MA, et al. The effect of corticosteroids on quality of life in a sarcoidosis clinic: The results of a propensity analysis. Respir Med. 2015;109(4):526–31.
35. Gerke AK, et al. Disease burden and variability in sarcoidosis. Ann Am Thorac Soc. 2017;14(Suppl 6):S421–8.

36. Sandhya P, et al. Clinical characteristics and outcome of primary Sjogren's syndrome: A large Asian Indian cohort. Open Rheumatol J. 2015;9:36–45.
37. Gupta S, et al. Sjögren syndrome and pregnancy: A literature review. Perm J. 2017;21:16–47.
38. Stefanski AL, et al. The diagnosis and treatment of Sjögren's syndrome. Dtsch Arztebl Int. 2017;114(20):354–61.
39. Lanzillotta M, et al. Advances in the diagnosis and management of IgG4 related disease. BMJ. 2020;369:m1067.
40. Floreani A, et al. IgG4-related disease: Changing epidemiology and new thoughts on a multisystem disease. J Transl Autoimmun. 2020;4:100074.

12 Renal Disease in Gout

Chen Xie and John FitzGerald

12.1 PREVALENCE OF RENAL FAILURE IN PATIENTS WITH GOUT

The prevalence of gout in the United States of America (USA) is estimated to be about 3.9%. The US prevalence doubled between the 1960s and the 1980s (1) but stabilized between 2007–08 and 2015–16 based on recent National Health and Nutrition Examination Survey (NHANES) data (2, 3). The prevalence of patients with chronic kidney disease (CKD), defined as low estimated glomerular filtration rate (eGFR), albuminuria, or both, is 14%, also based on recent NHANES data. The prevalence of CKD is recognized to be higher in older patients (33% for ≥ 65 years) and in patients with diabetes (34%) (4). The prevalence of CKD stage 3 is 5.1% (20% for ≥ 65 years). The age-standardized prevalence of CKD globally has remained relatively stable throughout the last several decades, with approximately 9.5% of females and 7.3% of males affected in 2017 (5). The recent stabilization of gout prevalence in the US mirrors similar trends for CKD and hypertension (6, 7).

Gout and CKD are both common and frequently coexist due to shared risk factors and interactions between the diseases. It is estimated that 71% of adults with gout (vs. 42% of adults without gout) have CKD stage ≥ 2, and 24% of adults with gout (vs. 5.2% of adults without gout) have CKD stage ≥ 3 (8, 9). The prevalence of CKD among adults with gout is similar in magnitude to the prevalence of CKD among adults with hypertension or diabetes (4). While both gout and CKD have been observed to be independent risk factors for each other, and cohort and cross-sectional studies have demonstrated that the incidence and prevalence of CKD increases with higher serum urate levels, the role of hyperuricemia as a causative factor in CKD remains controversial (8–12). Numerous potential mechanisms have been postulated invoking the effects of urate on glomerular hydrostatic pressure, inflammation, vasoconstriction/vasodilation, endothelial cell function, and cellular metabolism (13). In addition, in a study of US veterans with gout (at least two ICD-9 diagnoses of gout) and hyperuricemia (defined as two values > 7 mg/dL) predicted incident diagnosis of CKD with a hazard ratio (HR) of 1.43 (95% CI 1.20–1.70) compared to veterans with gout but without hyperuricemia (14). This study controlled for age, race, region, study year, BMI, other metabolic disease, and tobacco use. Finally, hyperuricemia may also interact with microalbuminuria for poorer renal function in patients with diabetes (15).

Given the potential significant causative role of hyperuricemia in the development of CKD, one might expect that lowering urate levels would have a protective effect; however, this has not been consistently demonstrated. In a retrospective cohort study of Medicare recipients, a higher dose and longer use of allopurinol was associated with a decreased incidence of renal disease (16). However, in two recent randomized controlled trials, urate-lowering therapy did not have a significant impact on reducing the rate of renal function decline (17, 18).

Racial disparities have been identified in the prevalence of both gout and CKD in the USA. There is a higher prevalence of both conditions among Black adults compared to White adults. The prevalence of gout in Asian adults exceeds that of all other racial and ethnic groups (19–21).

12.2 URATE TRANSPORT IN THE KIDNEY AND GUT

Urate is produced by the liver during the metabolism of endogenous and dietary purines. Human tissues have almost no ability to metabolize urate. Therefore, kidney and gut excretion are essential in maintaining urate homeostasis. Under normal circumstances, renal excretion accounts for about two-thirds of urate disposal, while the gastrointestinal tract accounts for the remaining one-third (22, 23).

In healthy nephrons, nearly all urate undergoes filtration at the glomerulus. Roughly 90% of the filtered urate is reabsorbed and then excreted in the proximal tubule (24). The key transporters involved in reabsorption and excretion are shown in Figure 12.1. The apical membrane urate-anion exchangers URAT1 and OAT4 absorb the filtered urate. Urate exits proximal tubular cells at the basolateral membrane via the GLUT9 transporter. Urate secretion involves the anion exchangers OAT1, OAT2, and OAT3, which transport urate across the basolateral membrane into the proximal tubule cells. This is followed by transport out to the tubule lumen via different transporters in the apical membrane, including ABCG2 (23). The high-capacity urate transporter ABCG2 is also expressed on intestinal epithelium cells and is responsible for the majority of gut urate excretion (25–27). Defects in ABCG2 are a significant risk factor for hyperuricemia and gout (26, 27). As renal function fails, the role of the gut as a primary urate secretory organ grows in importance,

DOI: 10.1201/9781003438373-14

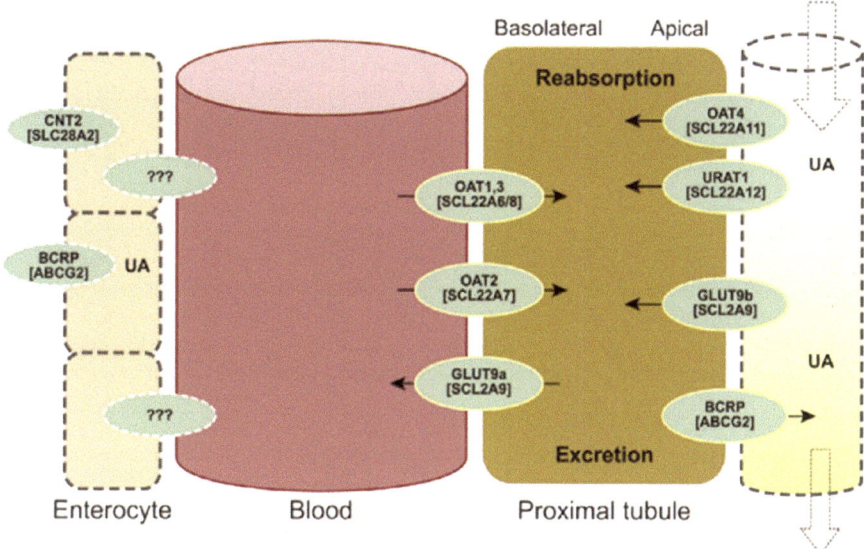

GLUT = glucose transporter; OAT = organic anion transporter; BCRP = breast cancer resistance protein.
Adapted from: George RL, Keenan RT. *Current Rheum Reports*. 2013;15(2):309.(16)

Figure 12.1   Urate transporters.

expanding to excrete up to 60% of daily urate production (25). Therefore, the impact of defects in ABCG2 has greater potential consequences in patients with CKD (25, 28).

The protein uromodulin, which is produced exclusively by renal epithelial cells and is the most abundant urinary protein, may also play a significant role in urate excretion. Mutations in the *UMOD* gene encoding uromodulin give rise to autosomal dominant tubulointerstitial kidney disease (ADTKD-*UMOD*) characterized by the decreased fractional excretion of urate. In fact, hyperuricemia is often the first symptom, preceding the development of CKD, and may cause early onset gout (29).

12.3 DIALYSIS AND URATE EXCRETION

Despite enhanced gastrointestinal urate excretion in CKD, urate excretion remains insufficient in CKD and end-stage renal disease (ESRD). Patients with ESRD rely on renal replacement therapy for urate excretion. Urate has a molecular weight of 168 Daltons and circulates unbound to proteins, translating into easy clearance by hemodialysis (HD), with filtration rates from 70 to 150 mL/minute (80% reduction) (30, 31). Though peritoneal dialysis (PD) is less efficient than HD, with a filtration rate ranging from 10 to 20 mL/minute (31), the total urate clearance over a 1-week period is similar on average between thrice-weekly HD and daily PD when PD is performed with daily dialysis and an increased duration (32, 33).

Despite the ability of HD and PD to clear urate from circulation, a wide range of mean serum urate levels has been reported in patients receiving renal replacement therapy, with several studies demonstrating persistently high rates of hyperuricemia. In a single-site retrospective cross-sectional study of 61 patients with gout undergoing dialysis (33 HD, 28 PD, 42 prescribed allopurinol), serum urate levels were below the target of 6 mg/dL only 41% of the time, with no statistically significant difference between those on HD or PD (34). In a population study of 146 Chinese patients on at least 1 year of HD, 60% of patients had hyperuricemia, as measured by a pre-HD urate value > 7.2 mg/dL (35). Beyond the impact of persistent hyperuricemia on gout, these authors reported increased mortality rates, with a three-fold increase for the highest urate pentile, in patients on HD with hyperuricemia. In this observational study, increased mortality was also reported for the lowest and highest pentiles of urate. This U-shaped all-cause mortality was also observed in a large retrospective cohort of 16,057 patients on HD (49% with pre-HD urate levels > 6.0 mg/dL, 24% with pre-HD urate > 7.1 mg/dL) (36). An association between urate and mortality was not seen in a smaller (n = 601) cohort (37).

Serum urate levels can fluctuate dramatically before and after dialysis. In a study of 123 anuric patients on HD, those with normal ABCG2 function had a mean pre-HD urate level of 7.1 mg/dL, which fell to 2.0 mg/dL post-HD and then built back to a range of 6.3–7.1 mg/dL after a 2- or 3-day interval prior to the next HD session (25). However, with a 50% reduction in ABCG2 function, urate levels can rise to a mean level of 8.4 mg/dL pre-HD. Other authors note mean urate levels post-HD of around 1 mg/dL, depending on settings and the type of dialyzer (30).

HD is an effective albeit intermittent form of urate-lowering therapy. These sharp changes likely explain the observed increase in gout flare rates around HD initiation (38). It is common for patients undergoing dialysis to frequently experience gout attacks. Based on Medicare claims analysis of 231,841 ESRD patients (on HD or PD without description of a prior history of gout), 13.5% of patients had a claim supportive of an inflammatory attack (39). The risk of a gout flare falls with a longer duration (in years) of dialysis. Compared to patients with fewer than 2 years of dialysis, those with 2 to 4 years of dialysis had a 20% lower risk of gout attack, and those with ≥ 5 years of dialysis had a 50% lower risk. Additionally, patients undergoing PD had a 10% higher rate of gout flares than those with HD (39).

12.4 URATE MANAGEMENT IN CKD

The 1984 Hande article effectively documented oxypurinol levels in relation to creatinine clearance and described the risk of allopurinol hypersensitivity syndrome (AHS) (40). However, it also provided allopurinol maintenance dosing recommendations that became the basis for renally adjusted allopurinol dosing for decades. Subsequent studies documented that only 19% of patients treated with allopurinol dosing based on Hande's recommendations achieve target serum urate levels (< 6 mg/dL) (41). From a population dose-escalation study, it was found that most patients required doses of allopurinol 100–200 mg above the Hande recommendations (42).

Fortunately, the literature has progressed since the original Hande recommendations. With respect to allopurinol, there are two main considerations: initial dosing and the final titration dose required to achieve serum urate target < 6 mg/dL. With poorer renal function, there is greater concern about high opxypurinol levels and AHS. Starting dose, renal function, and HLA-B* 5801 presence are major risk factors for AHS (43). These authors recommend a starting dose of 1.5 mg per unit of estimated GFR with slow (monthly) uptitration. This is detailed in Table 12.1 and summarized by 100 mg per day for no or mild CKD, 50 mg per day for CKD stage 3 (eGFR 31–45 mL/minute/1.73 m^2), and intermittent dosing for CKD ≥ 4. The greatest risk of AHS is in the first 30 days of starting allopurinol; however, half of cases can present later, but rarely (10% of cases) after 180 days.

Hyperuricemia is postulated to cause worsening CKD through the exacerbation of glomerular hypertension, oxidative stress, endothelial dysfunction, or urate deposition in the medulla (44–46). More increased use of and higher doses of urate-lowering therapy in CKD has been driven by observational studies that have described the delayed progression of CKD in patients with either lower urate levels or the use of urate-lowering therapy (47). In a 2017 meta-analysis of 16 articles (1211 patients with CKD), the use of ULT was associated with a 41% reduction in the risk of ESRD, slowing the rate of eGFR decline by 4.10 mL/minute/1.73 m^2 per year and decreasing the severity of albuminuria or proteinuria (48). These and other observations led to two randomized control trials evaluating the impact of allopurinol on CKD separately for patients with diabetes and gout. The Preventing Early Renal Loss in Diabetes (PERL) trial looked at 267 patients with type 1 diabetes, early-to-moderate diabetic kidney disease, and a serum urate level of at least 4.5 mg/dL (but not necessarily gout) (18). Patients were randomized to receive either an oral placebo or allopurinol (100

Table 12.1: Proposed Starting Dosage of Allopurinol Based on 1.5 mg per Estimated GFR

Estimated GFR, mL/minute/1.73 m^2	Allopurinol Starting Dosage
<5	50 mg/week
5–15	50 mg twice weekly
16–30 (CKD 4)	50 mg every 2 days
31–45 (CKD 3b)	50 mg/day
46–60 (CKD 3a)	50 mg and 100 mg on alternate days
61–90 (CKD 2)	100 mg/day
> 90	≥ 100 mg/day

Source: Adapted from Stamp et al., 2012

mg per day for 4 weeks, with titration to 200–400 mg daily based on baseline eGFR). There was a significant serum urate response in the allopurinol group, but despite 3 years of urate reduction (6.1 mg/dL to 3.9 mg/dL), no difference in eGFR, creatinine, or albumin excretion was observed.

A second RCT, the Controlled Trial of Slowing of Kidney Disease Progression from the Inhibition of Xanthine Oxidase (CKD-FIX), involved 369 patients (mean age, 62) with stage 3 or 4 CKD (17). These patients had either proteinuria or a reduction in eGFR of ≥3 mL/minute during the previous year. About half the patients had diabetic nephropathy, but patients with gout were excluded. Patients were randomly assigned, using block allocation, to either placebo or allopurinol, starting at 100 mg daily and titrated up to 300 mg over 12 weeks, regardless of serum urate levels, for 2 years. Again, there was significant reduction in urate levels (from 8.2 mg/dL to 5.3 mg/dL), but allopurinol did not slow the decline in eGFR or affect albuminuria compared to the placebo.

In a third study, the Febuxostat Versus Placebo Randomized Controlled Trial Regarding Reduced Renal Function in Patients with Hyperuricemia Complicated by Chronic Kidney Disease Stage 3 (FEATHER), febuxostat (40 mg) was evaluated against a placebo among 443 patients with stage 3 CKD and asymptomatic hyperuricemia. The study found no difference in the mean eGFR slope between the treatment groups (49).

On a brighter note, the introduction of sodium-glucose cotransporter type 2 inhibitors (SGLT2is) has s clear renal benefit, as shown in studies like CREDENCE and DAPA-CKD (50–55). Additionally, SGLT2is have the added benefit of urate lowering (through GLUT9 and URAT1 inhibition) (56–58), leading to reduced incident gout (59–62) and gout flare rates (56). The magnitude of urate reduction is dependent on the presence of baseline hyperuricemia; a higher baseline permits a greater reduction in urate with an SGLT2i, an outcome that appears to be independent of the severity of renal disease (57).

12.4.1 Dose Escalation in Patients with CKD

As noted, most patients require doses above the Hande-recommended dosing to achieve serum urate targets (42). In a detailed pharmacokinetics/pharmacodynamics study, researchers identified that body weight was the primary predictor of the final allopurinol dose required to achieve serum urate targets (63). As weight increased from <90 kg to >130 kg, the predicted mean allopurinol dose increased from 200 mg/ day to 400 mg/day. With CKD4, the expected mean dose of allopurinol rises by 100 mg/day (for peoples of non-Pacific Island descent) (Table 12.2). A more detailed target titration schedule is provided in the article if the pre-ULT SU value is known.

These PK/PD results were corroborated in an RCT evaluating allopurinol dose escalation (64). A post-hoc analysis evaluated the mean allopurinol dose to achieve the serum urate target (< 6 mg/dL). For patients with creatine clearance (CrCl) < 30 mL/minute, the geometric mean allopurinol dose was 285 mg/day. This dose rose to 320 mg/day for patients with CrCl 30–60 mL/minute and to 440 mg/day for those with CrCl > 60 mL/minute. No statistically significant increase in adverse events was noted.

12.5 ANTI-INFLAMMATORY MANAGEMENT IN CKD

Anti-inflammatory medications for the treatment or prophylaxis of gout attacks include non-steroidal anti-inflammatory drugs (NSAIDs), colchicine, glucocorticoids, and the interleukin-1 (IL-1) inhibitors anakinra and canakinumab (65). There is a general absence of conclusive data on the safety and efficacy of these medications in patients with gout and CKD. The efficacy of these drugs is primarily inferred from studies with outcomes not specifically stratified by renal function. Therefore, most of the recommendations surrounding the selection and dosage of these medications are empiric, guided heavily by the potential for increased side effects in patients with CKD.

12.6 NSAIDS

NSAIDs are generally contraindicated in patients with CKD and residual kidney function due to their association with worsening kidney function (66–69). The safety and efficacy of NSAID use in patients with ESRD and those who are dialysis dependent with gout remains unknown. Some experts advocate for the cautious use of NSAIDs in these patients (70, 71).

12.7 COLCHICINE

Colchicine has been used for centuries to treat gout attacks, but there is a lack of formal data addressing its safety and efficacy specifically in patients with both gout and CKD (72). Colchicine's narrow therapeutic margin may pose an even greater challenge in the presence of CKD. While the kidney only accounts for 10 to 20% of colchicine clearance, kidney impairment is a significant risk factor for colchicine toxicity, particularly neuromyopathy (73–75). Drugs that inhibit CYP3A4 and the P-glycoprotein efflux pump further reduce the clearance of colchicine and enhance its toxicity; such

Table 12.2: Predicted dose of Allopurinol (mg/day) based (adapted from Wright 2024)

Allopurinol daily maintenance dose (mg/day)				
	CrCL (mL/min)	Body weight		
		<90 kg	90–129.9 kg	>130 kg
Any ethnicity (not Pacific Peoples)	<30	200	300	400
	≥30	300	400	500
Pacific Peoples	<30	300	400	500
	≥30	400	500	600

Note: The doses are expected to achieve target serum urate concentrations < 6 mg/dL in >80% of people with gout.
Abbreviation: CrCL, creatinine clearance using the Cockcroft-Gault equation.

drugs include commonly used antibiotics, antiretrovirals, and antihypertensive medications (76). These safety concerns limit the use of colchicine in patients with CKD and especially in those with dialysis-dependent ESRD, as there is minimal clearance of colchicine by hemodialysis (77). Some experts recommend avoiding the drug entirely in patients with severe kidney impairment (70, 78, 79).

12.8 GLUCOCORTICOIDS

Systemic and intra-articular glucocorticoids are generally regarded as the safest anti-inflammatory medications in patients with CKD and gout, although, once again, there is an absence of high-quality data (72, 80). The detrimental impact of glucocorticoids on common comorbidities associated with gout and CKD, including hypertension, diabetes, obesity, and increased infection, may limit their use.

12.9 IL-1 INHIBITORS

The IL-1 inhibitors anakinra and canakinumab are the newest gout anti-inflammatory therapies. Guidelines recommend their use when NSAIDs, colchicine, and glucocorticoids are ineffective or cannot be used (65, 78). Major clinical trials of these IL-1 inhibitors in gout did not stratify outcome data by CKD severity and entirely excluded patients with CKD stage ≥ 4 (81–83). Case series and reports that include the use of anakinra in patients with CKD and gout are mostly reassuring in terms of safety (72, 80). However, the clearance of anakinra is directly related to kidney function, and the drug is not cleared by dialysis. As a result, some experts recommend dosing anakinra every other day, rather than daily, in patients with an eGFR of < 30 mL/minute/1.73 m^2 (80, 84, 85). By comparison, canakinumab, with its large molecular size (approximately nine times that of anakinra), is unlikely to have its clearance influenced by kidney function or renal replacement (86).

12.10 CONCLUSION

Gout and CKD are common comorbidities that serve as independent risk factors for each other, though uncertainty remains regarding the role of hyperuricemia in the development and progression of renal disease. An extensive body of literature supports safe and effective urate management practices for patients with gout and CKD. However, there remains an overall paucity of data guiding the use of anti-inflammatory therapies in this population.

REFERENCES

1. Lawrence RC, et al. Estimates of the prevalence of arthritis and other rheumatic conditions in the United States. Part II. Arthritis Rheum. 2008;58(1):26–35.
2. Singh G, et al. Gout and hyperuricaemia in the USA: Prevalence and trends. Rheumatology. 2019;58(12):2177–80.
3. Zhu Y, et al. Prevalence of gout and hyperuricemia in the US general population: The National Health and Nutrition Examination Survey 2007–2008. Arthritis Rheum. 2011;63(10):3136–41.

4. 2020 USRDS Annual Data Report: Epidemiology of Kidney Disease in the United States. *National Institutes of Health, National Institute of Diabetes and Digestive and Kidney Diseases.* Bethesda, MD; 2020. Available from: https://usrds-adr.niddk.nih.gov/2020/chronic-kidney-disease/1-ckd-in-the-general-population.

5. Bikbov B, et al. Global, regional, and national burden of chronic kidney disease, 1990–2017: A systematic analysis for the Global Burden of Disease Study 2017. Lancet. 2020;395(10225):709–33.

6. Fryar CD, et al. Hypertension prevalence and control among adults: United States, 2015–2016. NCHS Data Brief. 2017;289:1–8. Available from: www.cdc.gov/nchs/data/databriefs/db289_table.pdf#2

7. Murphy D, et al. Trends in prevalence of chronic kidney disease in the United States. Ann Intern Med. 2016;165(7):473–81.

8. Roughley MJ, et al. Gout and risk of chronic kidney disease and nephrolithiasis: Meta-analysis of observational studies. Arthritis Res Ther. 2015;17(1).

9. Zhu Y, et al. Comorbidities of gout and hyperuricemia in the US general population: NHANES 2007–2008. Am J Med. 2012;125(7):679–87.e1.

10. Krishnan E. Reduced glomerular function and prevalence of gout: NHANES 2009–10. PLoS ONE. 2012;7(11):1–9.

11. Singh JA, et al. Gout is associated with a higher risk of chronic renal disease in older adults: A retrospective cohort study of U.S. Medicare population. BMC Nephrol. 2019;20(1):5–11.

12. Gonçalves DLN, et al. A systematic review and meta-analysis of the association between uric acid levels and chronic kidney disease. Sci Rep. 2022;12(1):1–13.

13. Goldberg A, et al. Mini review: Reappraisal of uric acid in chronic kidney disease. Am J Nephrol. 2021;52(10–11):837–44.

14. Krishnan E, et al. Serum urate and incidence of kidney disease among veterans with gout. J Rheumatol. 2013;40(7):1166–72.

15. Rosolowsky ET, et al. High-normal serum uric acid is associated with impaired glomerular filtration rate in nonproteinuric patients with type 1 diabetes. Clin J Am Soc Nephrol. 2008;3(3):706–13.

16. Singh JA, et al. Are allopurinol dose and duration of use nephroprotective in the elderly? A Medicare claims study of allopurinol use and incident renal failure. Ann Rheum Dis. 2017;76(1):133–9.

17. Badve SV, et al. Effects of allopurinol on the progression of chronic kidney disease. N Engl J Med. 2020;382(26):2504–13.

18. Doria A, et al. Serum urate lowering with allopurinol and kidney function in type 1 diabetes. N Engl J Med. 2020;382(26):2493–503.

19. McCormick N, et al. Racial and sex disparities in gout prevalence among US adults. JAMA Netw Open. 2022;5(8):E2226804.

20. Coresh J, et al. Prevalence of chronic kidney disease and decreased kidney function in the adult US population: Third National Health and Nutrition Examination Survey. Am J Kidney Dis. 2003;41(1):1–12.

21. Yokose C, et al. Trends in prevalence of gout among US Asian adults, 2011–2018. JAMA Netw Open. 2023;6(4):E239501.

22. Sorensen LB. Role of the intestinal tract in the elimination of uric acid. Arthritis Rheum. 1965;8(4):694–706.

23. Mandal AK, et al. The molecular physiology of uric acid homeostasis. Annu Rev Physiol. 2015;77:323–45.

24. Keenan RT. The biology of urate. Semin Arthritis Rheum. 2020;50(3):S2–10.

25. Ohashi Y, et al. Evaluation of ABCG2-mediated extra-renal urate excretion in hemodialysis patients. Sci Rep. 2023;13(1):1–11.

26. Matsuo H, et al. Common defects of ABCG2, a high-capacity urate exporter, cause gout: A function-based genetic analysis in a Japanese population. Sci Transl Med. 2009;1(5):1–9.

27. Hoque KM, et al. The ABCG2 Q141K hyperuricemia and gout associated variant illuminates the physiology of human urate excretion. Nat Commun. 2020;11(1):1–15.

28. Jing J, et al. Genetics of serum urate concentrations and gout in a high-risk population, patients with chronic kidney disease. Sci Rep. 2018;8(1):1–9.

29. Devuyst O, et al. Uromodulin: From physiology to rare and complex kidney disorders. Nat Rev Nephrol. 2017;13(9):525–44.

30. Arenas M-D, et al. Serum Urate Levels of Hemodialyzed Renal Patients Revisited. JCR J Clin Rheumatol. 2021;27(8):e362–6.
31. Murea M, et al. The physiology of uric acid and the impact of end-stage kidney disease and dialysis. Semin Dial. 2019;32:47–57.
32. Sombolos K, et al. Clinical evaluation of four different high-flux hemodialyzers under conventional conditions in vivo. Am J Nephrol. 1997;17(5):406–12.
33. Eloot S, et al. Removal of different classes of uremic toxins in APD vs CAPD: A randomized cross-over study. Perit Dial Int. 2015;35(4):436–42.
34. Yeo E, et al. Serum urate levels and therapy in adults treated with long-term dialysis: A retrospective cross-sectional study. Intern Med J. 2019;49(7):838–42.
35. Hsu SP, et al. Serum uric acid levels show a "J-shaped" association with all-cause mortality in haemodialysis patients. Nephrol Dial Transplan. 2004;19(2):457–62.
36. Zawada AM, et al. Serum uric acid and mortality risk among hemodialysis patients. Kidney Int Reports. 2020;5(8):1196–206.
37. Rohn B, et al. Association of hyperuricemia and serum uric acid lowering therapy with mortality in hemodialysis patients. Ren Fail. 2020;42(1):1067–75.
38. Iwata N, et al. Urgent hemodialysis induced an acute gout attack in a patient with multiple tophi: Report of a rare case. CEN Case Reports. 2012;1(2):130–1.
39. Zhang Y, et al. Gout among patients with dialysis: Prevalence, associated factors, treatment patterns, and outcomes- population-based retrospective cohort study. Kidney360. 2023;4(2):177–87.
40. Hande KR, et al. Severe allopurinol toxicity. Description and guidelines for prevention in patients with renal insufficiency. Am J Med. 1984;76(1):47–56.
41. Dalbeth N, et al. Dose adjustment of allopurinol according to creatinine clearance does not provide adequate control of hyperuricemia in patients with gout. J Rheumatol. 2006;33(8):1646–50.
42. Stamp LK, et al. Using allopurinol above the dose based on creatinine clearance is effective and safe in patients with chronic gout, including those with renal impairment. Arthritis Rheum. 2011;63(2):412–21.
43. Stamp LK, et al. Starting dose is a risk factor for allopurinol hypersensitivity syndrome: A proposed safe starting dose of allopurinol. Arthritis Rheum. 2012;64(8):2529–36.
44. Mazzali M, et al. Hyperuricemia induces a primary renal arteriolopathy in rats by a blood pressure-independent mechanism. Am J Physiol—Ren Physiol. 2002;282(6 51–6):F991–7.
45. Leoncini G, et al. Uric acid lowering for slowing CKD progression after the CKD-FIX trial: A solved question or still a dilemma? Clin Kidney J. 2022;15(9):1666–74.
46. Sellmayr M, et al. Only hyperuricemia with crystalluria, but not asymptomatic hyperuricemia, drives progression of chronic kidney disease. J Am Soc Nephrol. 2020;31(12):2773–92.
47. Chonchol M, et al. Relationship of uric acid with progression of kidney disease. Am J Kidney Dis. 2007;50(2):239–47.
48. Su X, et al. Effects of uric acid-lowering therapy in patients with chronic kidney disease: A meta-analysis. Seguro AC, editor. PLoS ONE. 2017;12(11):e0187550.
49. Kimura K, et al. Febuxostat therapy for patients with stage 3 CKD and asymptomatic hyperuricemia: A randomized trial. Am J Kidney Dis. 2018;72(6):798–810.
50. Wanner C, et al. Empagliflozin and progression of kidney disease in type 2 diabetes. N Engl J Med. 2016;375(4):323–34.
51. Neal B, et al. Canagliflozin and cardiovascular and renal events in type 2 diabetes. N Engl J Med. 2017;377(7):644–57.
52. Perkovic V, et al. Canagliflozin and renal outcomes in type 2 diabetes and nephropathy. N Engl J Med. 2019;380(24):2295–306.
53. Heerspink HJL, et al. Dapagliflozin in patients with chronic kidney disease. N Engl J Med. 2020;383(15):1436–46.
54. The EMPA-KIDNEY Collaborative Group, Herrington WG, et al. Empagliflozin in patients with chronic kidney disease. N Engl J Med. 2023;388(2):117–27.
55. de Boer IH, et al. Diabetes management in chronic kidney disease: A consensus report by the American diabetes association (ADA) and kidney disease: Improving global outcomes (KDIGO). Diabetes Care. 2022;45(12):3075–90.
56. Li JW, B et al. The effects of canagliflozin on gout in type 2 diabetes: A post-hoc analysis of the CANVAS program. Lancet Rheumatol. 2019;1(4):e220–8.

57. Doehner W, et al. Sodium–glucose cotransporter 2 inhibitor treatment lowers serum uric acid in patients with heart failure with reduced ejection fraction—lessons from clinical trials. Letter regarding the article 'Dapagliflozin reduces uric acid concentration, an indepen. Eur J Heart Fail. 2022;24(10):1993–4.

58. Ferreira JP, et al. Empagliflozin and uric acid metabolism in diabetes: A post hoc analysis of the EMPA-REG OUTCOME trial. Diabetes, Obes Metab. 2022;24(1):135–41.

59. Banerjee M, et al. Can SGLT2 inhibitors prevent incident gout? A systematic review and meta-analysis. Acta Diabetol. 2022;59(6):783–91.

60. Fralick M, et al. Assessing the risk for gout with sodium–glucose cotransporter-2 inhibitors in patients with type 2 diabetes a population-based cohort study. Ann Intern Med. 2020;172(3):186–94.

61. Lund LC, et al. Sodium-glucose cotransporter-2 inhibitors and the risk of gout: A Danish population based cohort study and symmetry analysis. Pharmacoepidemiol Drug Saf. 2021;30(10):1391–5.

62. Chung MC, et al. Association of sodium-glucose transport protein 2 inhibitor use for type 2 diabetes and incidence of gout in Taiwan. JAMA Netw Open. 2021;4(11):e2135353.

63. Wright DFB, et. al. The development and evaluation of dose-prediction tools for allopurinol therapy (Easy Allo tools). Br J Clin Pharmacol. 2024 May;90(5):1268–79.

64. Stamp LK, et al. A randomised controlled trial of the efficacy and safety of allopurinol dose escalation to achieve target serum urate in people with gout. Ann Rheum Dis. 2017;76(9):1522–8.

65. FitzGerald JD, et al. 2020 American college of rheumatology guideline for the management of gout. Arthritis Care Res. 2020;72(6):744–60.

66. Gooch K, Culleton BF, Manns BJ, et al. NSAID use and progression of chronic kidney disease. Am J Med. 2007;120(3):1–7.

67. Sriperumbuduri S, et alS. The case for cautious consumption: NSAIDs in chronic kidney disease. Curr Opin Nephrol Hypertens. 2019;28(2):163–70.

68. Perneger TV, et al. Risk of kidney failure associated with the use of acetaminophen, aspirin, and nonsteroidal antiinflammatory drugs. N Engl J Med. 1994;331(25):1675–9.

69. Chang YK, et al. Increased risk of End-Stage Renal Disease (ESRD) requiring chronic dialysis is associated with use of Nonsteroidal Anti-Inflammatory Drugs (NSAIDs): Nationwide case-crossover study. Med (United States). 2015;94(38):1–7.

70. Becker MA, et al. Treatment of gout flares. UpToDate. 2019;1–20. Available from: www.uptodate.com/contents/treatment-of-gout-flares.

71. Tang KS, et al. Nonsteroidal anti-inflammatory drugs in end-stage kidney disease: Dangerous or underutilized? Expert Opin Pharmacother. 2021;22(6):769–77.

72. Pisaniello HL, et al. Efficacy and safety of gout flare prophylaxis and therapy use in people with chronic kidney disease: A gout, hyperuricemia and crystal-associated disease network (G-CAN)-initiated literature review. Arthritis Res Ther. 2021;23(1):1–18.

73. Terkeltaub RA. Colchicine update: 2008. Semin Arthritis Rheum. 2009;38(6):411–19.

74. Wallace SL, et al. Renal function predicts colchicine toxicity: Guidelines for the prophylactic use of colchicine in gout. J Rheumatol. 1991;18(2):264–9.

75. Kuncl RW, et al. Colchicine myopathy and neuropathy. N Engl J Med. 1987;316(25):1562–8.

76. Colchicine and other drugs for gout. Vol. 51, The Medical Letter on Drugs and Therapeutics, 2009, pp. 93–4.

77. Wason S, et al. Single-Dose, open-label study of the differences in pharmacokinetics of colchicine in subjects with renal impairment, including end-stage renal disease. Clin Drug Investig. 2014;34(12):845–55.

78. Richette P, et al. 2016 updated EULAR evidence-based recommendations for the management of gout. Ann Rheum Dis. 2017;76(1):29–42.

79. Bardin T, et al. Impact of comorbidities on gout and hyperuricaemia: An update on prevalence and treatment options. BMC Med. 2017;15(1):1–10.

80. Kannuthurai V, et al. Management of patients with gout and kidney disease: A review of available therapies and common missteps. Kidney360. 2023;4:1332–40.

81. Janssen CA, et al. Anakinra for the treatment of acute gout flares: A randomized, double-blind, placebo-controlled, active-comparator, non-inferiority trial. Rheumatol (United Kingdom). 2019;58(8):1344–52.

82. Schlesinger N, et al. Canakinumab for acute gouty arthritis in patients with limited treatment options: Results from two randomised, multicentre, active-controlled, double-blind trials and their initial extensions. Ann Rheum Dis. 2012;71(11):1839–48.

83. Saag KG, et al. A randomized, Phase II study evaluating the efficacy and safety of anakinra in the treatment of gout flares. Arthritis Rheumatol. 2021;73(8):1533–42.
84. Yang BB, et al. Pharmacokinetics of anakinra in subjects with different levels of renal function. Clin Pharmacol Ther. 2003;74(1):85–94.
85. Anakinra. Lexi-Drugs. UpToDate Lexidrug. UpToDate Inc. Available from: https://online.lexi.com. Accessed December 19, 2023.
86. Chakraborty A, et al. Pharmacokinetic and pharmacodynamic properties of canakinumab, a human anti-interleukin-1β monoclonal antibody. Clin Pharmacokinet. 2012;51(6):e1–18.

PART III
SPECIAL CONSIDERATIONS

13 Bone Health in Rheumatology Patients with Renal Disease

S. Bobo Tanner, Cinduja Nathan, and Sergio Infante

13.1 INTRODUCTION

Inflammatory rheumatic diseases have long been associated with bone loss and increased rates of fracture. Degradation in bone health has been noted in a variety of rheumatic conditions, including rheumatoid arthritis (RA), lupus, Sjögren's syndrome, systemic sclerosis, vasculitis, and polymyalgia rheumatica, as well as other autoimmune diseases (1–10). Indeed, rheumatoid arthritis has been established as an independent risk factor for fractures and is included as an element in the Fracture Risk Assessment Tool (FRAX®) or fracture risk calculator (11). Proposed causal factors have included the effects of inflammation, medications such as glucocorticoids, gait and balance disturbances, increased risk of falls, nutritional deficiencies, and hypogonadism. Another risk factor for fractures and CKD is diabetes mellitus, and it has been estimated that approximately 20% of patients with RA have diabetes mellitus (12). The exact mechanisms for increased fractures in the rheumatology population is not completely understood, and as a result, a prospective cohort of patients with inflammatory rheumatic diseases (Rh-GIOP) has been established to further investigate bone health in these patients (13–15). The American College of Rheumatology (ACR) has continued to refine guidelines for glucocorticoid-induced osteoporosis (GIOP) to assist the clinician in the management of fracture risk in patients treated with glucocorticoids (16).

Renal disease is common in patients with rheumatic disease. The occurrence of renal disease brings another risk factor for poor bone health to these patients due to the existence of the syndrome that came to be known in 2006 as chronic kidney disease–metabolic bone disease (CKD-MBD) (17). Patients with CKD have an increased fracture risk compared with the general population (18–25). The systemic disorder of bone structure, metabolism, and cellular function leading to compromised bone strength in these patients with CKD is known as renal osteodystrophy (ROD).

The focus of this chapter is on the bone health evaluation and management of patients with concomitant inflammatory rheumatic disease and CKD-MBD. Traditional bone health assessment tools are often used, including dual-energy x-ray absorptiometry (DXA), fracture risk assessment, serum bone turnover biomarkers, and other laboratory evaluations to investigate secondary causes of poor bone health.

Currently available osteoporosis medications are also used to treat patients with CKD-MBD with the goal of reducing fracture risk. However, the process of evaluating and treating poor bone health and increased risk of fracture is difficult in the CKD-MBD population due to limited data. There are no FDA-approved medications for reducing the risk of fracture in CKD-MBD patients, and there are no randomized control trials proving that bone-targeted agents can prevent fractures in patients with CKD-MBD.

Nevertheless, there have been clinical trials of bone-targeted treatments that have included a small number of patients with CKD, leading to the retrospective analysis and extrapolation of data to generate information for patients with CKD-MBD. Furthermore, there are guidelines, including those promulgated by Kidney Disease Improving Global Outcomes (KDIGO) and the European Renal Osteodystrophy workgroup (EUROD), that can assist the clinician in managing such patients (26, 27). Many questions remain, however, including the specific value of DXA imaging in this population as well as the efficacy and safety of currently available bone-targeted treatments in CKD-MBD.

13.2 ASSESSING BONE HEALTH IN THE RHEUMATOLOGY PATIENT WITH CKD

Assessing bone health requires the utilization of various tools in order to obtain a complete picture of the risk for fracture for each patient. Such tools assist in driving management decisions to ensure that a wholistic approach to treatment is adopted.

13.3 LABORATORY EVALUATION

The Bone Health and Osteoporosis Foundation and others have recommended baseline laboratory testing to evaluate patients for secondary causes of osteoporosis (28, 29). CKD-MBD represents complex metabolic disturbances in the bone, including disorders of calcium and phosphate metabolism, calcitriol deficiency, and secondary hyperparathyroidism. Many of the recommended tests

DOI: 10.1201/9781003438373-16

are part of standard chemistry profiles, as well as endocrine functions such as those of thyroid, parathyroid, and gonadal hormones and nutritional parameters such as vitamin D deficiency, and thus can help assess the CKD-MBD as well as screen for other skeletal diseases such as multiple myeloma.

Another group of laboratory evaluations can provide a window into the metabolic activity of bone. These bone metabolism assays are collectively known as bone turnover markers and are subdivided into those that primarily reflect osteoclastic or resorptive activity in bone, including C-telopeptide, N-telopeptide, and TRAP5b, or those that reflect osteoblastic or anabolic activity, such as bone-specific alkaline phosphatase (BSAP), osteocalcin, and procollagen 1 N- terminal peptide (30). Several of these serum bone turnover markers are cleared through the kidney and therefore less reliable tools in evaluating bone metabolism in patients with CKD (31). However, the 2017 KDIGO guidelines note that BSAP and the biomarker intact parathyroid hormone (PTH) can be used to evaluate bone disease because markedly high or low values predict underlying bone turnover (26). Thus, BSAP and PTH are important lab tests for the profile of patients with CKD-MBD.

13.4 BONE BIOPSY

ROD refers to the changes in bone that are seen in patients with CKD. These changes are the result of a complex pathophysiology involving disturbances in a variety of factors, including calcium, phosphate, parathyroid hormone, and vitamin D, that occur in the presence of declining renal function.

Types of ROD can be established with tetracycline double-labeled bone biopsy. The class of tetracycline antibiotics has the property of being deposited along the border of bone, where active calcification and bone formation are taking place. The specimens must be processed with alcohol preservative and not decalcified. Using fluorescent microscopy, the production of bone can be visualized, and histomorphometric patterns can be seen.

These histomorphometric patterns can demonstrate dynamic and static properties of the bone, including either low turnover or high turnover bone activity, mineralization, and bone volume. The turnover, mineralization, and volume (TMV) classification system is used to define the type of ROD (32–34). The relatively low number of pathology labs that can process and analyze these specimens has limited the widespread use of this procedure in clinical practice, but the yield can be quite valuable in clarifying the specific nature of renal osteodystrophy.

In patients with CKD, the assessment of cortical bone structure is important because cortical bone is associated with peripheral fractures and CKD can affect cortical porosity and bone loss (35).

Up until 2017, tetracycline-labeled bone biopsies were a significant part of the KDIGO guidelines for evaluating patients with CKD-MBD, but the role of this biopsy procedure has been largely supplanted by the use of bone turnover markers in the new guidelines (26, 36). In patients with CKD 3a–5, it is still reasonable to perform a tetracycline double-labeled bone biopsy if the results will impact treatment and in situations where adynamic bone disease needs to be excluded prior to antiresorptive treatment. Many have advocated for the more widespread use of labeled bone biopsies in CKD-MBD because it is the only technique that can provide comprehensive information on all bone parameters (37).

13.5 IMPACT MICROINDENTATION

A novel clinical tool has been developed for the *in vivo* determination of mechanical bone properties using a hand-held device that measures the impact microindentation of cortical bone, the OsteoProbe®. By measuring the indentation depth, the bone material strength index (BMSi) can be calculated. Cortical bone is an important determinant of bone strength in CKD-MBD patients, and this device appears to identify cortical material composition such as the mineral-to-matrix ratio and the content of water or advanced glycation in products rather than microarchitecture or porosity in determining bone strength. Limited studies indicate that BMSi is associated with BMD and fractures in patients with CKD, and its role in the CKD-MBD patient population requires further exploration (38, 39).

13.6 IMAGING

Radiographic findings in patients with CKD can mimic those of underlying rheumatologic conditions, including rheumatoid arthritis and spondyloarthropathies. These findings include demineralization at joint margins and subligamentous areas (40, 41). Additionally, subchondral resorption around the sacroiliac joints may suggest ankylosing spondylitis, and resorption in the region of the retrocalcaneal bursa or insertion of the patella aponeurosis may be confused with reactive arthritis, formerly known as Reiter's syndrome. Clinical correlation and further imaging may be required to distinguish these findings as due to renal osteodystrophy rather than an underlying rheumatologic condition.

13.7 DXA BONE DENSITY TESTING

DXA bone density testing is the mainstay of bone health assessment in the adult population. However, in patients with CKD, the results from DXA testing may be affected by soft tissue calcifications and furthermore do not distinguish types of ROD. Nevertheless, prospective cohort studies have shown value in DXA BMD measurements for predicting peripheral fractures and hip fractures in patients with CKD 3–5D, especially those with CKD 3 (24, 42–45).

As a result, the 2017 KDIGO guidelines recommend that patients with CKD 3A-G5D and evidence of CKD-MBD and/or risk factors for osteoporosis undergo bone mineral density (BMD) testing to assess fracture risk if the results will impact treatment decisions (26).

The European guidelines recommend obtaining hip and lumbar spine (and forearm if it can be correctly performed) DXA bone density measurement in patients with CKD 4–5D if the patient is a postmenopausal woman or a man over the age of 50. Repeat DXA measurements are noted to be important if results will influence clinical management or in changes in the BMD are expected to exceed the least significant change (LSC) for DXA testing done at that facility (46).

It is important to recognize that although DXA is the method of choice for the clinical measurement bone mineral density, the performance and interpretation of DXA requires training and skill to produce reliable and accurate results. It has been reported that up to 90% of BMD reports contain at least one error. These errors can lead to inaccurate diagnosis and inappropriate treatment decisions (47).

13.8 VERTEBRAL FRACTURE ASSESSMENT

Vertebral fractures are common in patients with CKD but often unrecognized. The presence of vertebral fractures can predict future fractures, but their presence may not come to the attention of the clinician. Therefore, the European guidelines recommend that all CKD patients undergoing a DXA should also receive an assessment for the presence of vertebral fractures using either lateral spine imaging or the ability of DXA equipment to generate a morphometric lateral vertebral image and thus a vertebral fracture assessment (VFA) (46). In addition, these guidelines recommend that patients undergo VFA if risk factors are present, including a > 4 cm height loss, kyphosis, or recent long-term glucocorticoid therapy. The ACR guidelines also recommend imaging of the spine for possible vertebral fracture at the time of starting GC treatment and every 1–2 years thereafter while on GC therapy (16). VFA imaging can also indicate the presence of abdominal aortic calcification, which can be useful in stratifying cardiovascular risk (48).

13.9 TRABECULAR BONE SCORE

One of the concerns with DXA bone density measurement is its sole focus on bone quantity, which is but one aspect of bone quality and strength. In patients with CKD, bone quantity may be falsely elevated due to the presence of vascular and joint calcifications that are falsely included as bone with the DXA BMD measurement. This inclusion of calcified tissue as bone may, in turn, underestimate the fracture risk in CKD patients when the risk is solely based on DXA BMD measurement.

To overcome this shortcoming of DXA BMD measurement, an additional aspect of bone strength, microarchitecture, can be estimated non-invasively with the use of data collected at the time of the DXA measurement. Additional software is now available for DXA bone density testing devices that allows for the calculation of a trabecular bone score (TBS). The TBS software analyzes the spatial organization of pixel intensity from the DXA images and generates a gray-level textural index or score. The score correlates with the apparent microstructure of the bone and is a DXA-independent risk factor for fractures that can be applied to the FRAX® calculator (49). There is conflicting evidence about the usefulness of TBS as an independent prediction tool for fracture risk over the full range of patients with CKD 3–5D as well as post renal transplantation (50–55). Thus, the use of TBS in CKD is an area that requires further clarification.

13.10 FRACTURE RISK ASSESSMENT TOOLS IN PATIENTS WITH CKD

The FRAX® was developed at the University of Sheffield and made available for international public use in 2008. This tool was designed to predict fracture risk in the general population and relies on entering a series of risk factors for an individual patient, which are then weighted, and then an estimate of the individual patient's 10-year major osteoporosis fracture risk and hip fracture risk are generated. National thresholds have been established for guiding decisions about treatment to reduce the fracture risk. This tool has been applied to patients with various stages of CKD and appears to be valuable in predicting fracture risk (56). Whitlock et al. concluded that the relationship between FRAX® in nondialysis CKD patients and major osteoporotic fracture is stronger than that relationship in patients with preserved renal function (56).

Other fracture risk prediction tools have been studied for value in the CKD population, including Qfracture and Garvan, although they were developed with country-specific data from Britain and Australia, respectively. The conclusion was that Garvan tended to underestimate fractures in CKD 3, where Qfracture was adequately calibrated in all CKD strata (57).

13.11 TREATMENT APPROACH TO REDUCE FRACTURE RISK IN THE RHEUMATOLOGY PATIENT WITH CKD-MBD

Reducing fracture risk begins with the basics of treatment for osteoporosis: exercise, fall prevention, and appropriate nutritional support (28). Patients with CKD-MBD require collaboration among rheumatologists, nephrologists, and primary care physicians. Addressing metabolic bone disease in this patient population requires specific knowledge of calcium, phosphorus, vitamin D, PTH, and bone turnover marker parameters to maximize bone health prior to osteoporosis medication.

Calcium and vitamin D intake are routine issues in patients with CKD, especially those with secondary hyperparathyroidism (58). Adequate calcium intake can often be achieved through the diet, but vitamin D deficiency may require significant supplementation. Although vitamin D deficiency is common in CKD patients and associated with fractures, the optimal target level of 25-hydroxy vitamin D in these patients is not certain, and fracture risk reduction has not been established. Elevated parathyroid hormone levels have been noted to be an independent risk factor for fractures, vascular events, and death in patients with CKD 3–4 (59). Hyperphosphatemia occurs early in CKD and promotes PTH release, and it is critical to control hyperphosphatemia with dietary modification and phosphate binders.

As many of these patients have been on or are maintained on glucocorticoids, it is important to consult the guidelines offered by the ACR (16). In 2022, the ACR updated its guidelines for glucocorticoid-induced osteoporosis (GIOP) prevention and treatment, which include risk stratifying patients as being at low, moderate, or high risk of fracture. Treatment recommendations are based on the risk strata.

Importantly, the ACR 2022 GIOP guidelines include a statement for patients with CKD or renal transplant and an eGFR < 35mL/minute and recommend a consultation with a "metabolic bone disease expert evaluation for chronic kidney disease-mineral and bone disorder".

There are no FDA-approved medications for the CKD-MBD patient population, and there are no randomized controlled trials proving that bone targeted agents can prevent fractures in patients with CKD-MBD. Some of the clinical trials with bone-targeted treatments have included a small number of patients with CKD, leading to the retrospective analysis and extrapolation of data to generate information for patients with CKD-MBD. Despite the limited data, there are guidelines that have embraced the use of osteoporosis medications in patients with CKD-MBD considered at risk for fracture (26).

13.12 ANTIRESORPTIVE AGENTS

Bisphosphonates are the most prescribed osteoporosis medications, and most clinicians who treat osteoporosis are very familiar with their use. However, there is concern about using these medications in CKD patients because of their clearance by the kidneys. Furthermore, the benefit tends to accrue within 3 to 5 years of treatment, and prolonged treatment may not be helpful (60, 61). Thus, the dose and duration of treatment are topics of concern in patients with CKD. When using bisphosphonates to treat patients with CKD, be aware that there are conflicting reports from analysis in various administrative databases on the effect of bisphosphonates on bone density, fracture rates, mortality, and the progression of CKD. These datasets contain confounding variables that may challenge study conclusions but offer an opportunity for further research (62–68).

Denosumab is a potent antiresorptive medication approved for postmenopausal osteoporosis, glucocorticoid-induced osteoporosis, and male osteoporosis. There has been extrapolated data that indicates its value in CKD 3A patients (69). More recent data also indicates this medication can be helpful in patients receiving hemodialysis, including improving bone density and microarchitecture. One of the drawbacks of this therapy remains the possibility of hypocalcemia. The medication is typically given as a subcutaneous injection every 6 months, and in the days and weeks following there is the possibility of hypocalcemia. The incidence of post-injection hypocalcemia was 7% in the dialysis group, which may require urgent calcium supplementation as well as changes in the calcium content of the dialysate bath (70, 71).

13.13 ANABOLIC AGENTS

Teriparatide and abaloparatide are fragments of human parathyroid hormone and parathyroid hormone-related peptide, respectively. They are administered as a self-injection daily and have shown a significant ability to increase bone density and reduce fracture risk. A post-hoc analysis of the pivotal trials demonstrated improvement in BMD and fracture risk reduction in patients with normal PTH levels and CKD 1–3 versus normal renal function (72, 73). CKD patients were more likely to have hypercalcemia or hyperuricemia but no reported kidney stones or gout episodes. In Japan, there have been small studies of CKD 4–5 and hemodialysis patients who were thought to have adynamic bone disease and treated with daily or weekly doses of teriparatide that were generally well-tolerated (74–76). One of the studies indicated an improvement in lumbar spine BMD (77).

The KDIGO guidelines rely heavily on the use of biomarkers, including PTH and bone-specific alkaline phosphatase levels, for guidance and selecting an anabolic therapy for a patient (26).

Romosozumab is a potent monthly injectable osteoporotic medication that has properties of both anabolic activity and antiresorptive activity. It is a monoclonal antibody that inhibits sclerostin, and it has been suggested that serum sclerostin levels may confirm the diagnosis of high bone turnover in CKD 5D patients (78). In the registration trials for this medication, bone density improvements were equivalent in patients with normal renal function compared to those with decreased renal function. Furthermore, the fracture data revealed equivalent decreases in fracture risk between patients with normal renal function and those with lower eGFRs (79).

The concern with romosozumab has been the possible increased risk of cardiovascular (CV) events that was noted in one of the clinical trials in which alendronate was the control treatment. CV events were not seen in the registration trials that used a placebo control. Additionally, there is data from a placebo-controlled study in Japan using romosozumab in patients undergoing hemodialysis with baseline low cardiovascular risk that showed an effect of improving bone density at the spine and femoral neck while altering bone turnover markers in a pattern consistent with anabolic activity (80). Importantly, there were no increases in cardiovascular events. Thus, there may be a role for this medication in carefully selected patients with CKD undergoing hemodialysis.

13.14 CONCLUSION

The evaluation and management of patients with concomitant rheumatic disease and CKD-MBD involves typical bone health assessment tools such as laboratory evaluation, DXA, and fracture risk assessment. The results of these investigations need to be interpreted considering CKD, and the focus of treatment begins with typical efforts to reduce fracture, including exercise, fall prevention, and adequate nutrition. The use of bone-targeted medication in these patients is somewhat more difficult in view of the lack of large-scale randomized prospective clinical trials dedicated to this patient population. Thus, the management of these patients requires interactive participation among the patients, the primary care physicians, the rheumatologists, and the nephrologists.

REFERENCES

1. Ceccarelli F, et al. Fragility fractures in lupus patients: Associated factors and comparison of four fracture risk assessment tools. Lupus. 2023;32(11):1320–7.
2. Chen J, et al. A meta-analysis of fracture risk and bone mineral density in patients with systemic sclerosis. Clin Rheumatol. 2020;39(4):1181–9.
3. Coury F, et al. Osteoimmunology of bone loss in inflammatory rheumatic diseases. Front Immunol. 2019;10:679.
4. Epsley S, et al. The effect of inflammation on bone. Front Physiol. 2020;11:511799.
5. Raterman HG, et al. Pharmacological management of osteoporosis in rheumatoid arthritis patients: A review of the literature and practical guide. Drugs Aging. 2019;36(12):1061–72.
6. Rogers B, et al. Clinical features associated with rate of fractures in patients with systemic sclerosis: A US cohort study. Arthritis Care Res (Hoboken). 2023 Nov;75(11):2379–88.
7. Rotta D, et al. Osteoporosis in inflammatory arthritides: New perspective on pathogenesis and treatment. Front Med (Lausanne). 2020;7:613720.

8. Tu X, et al. High prevalence and risk factors for osteoporosis in 1839 patients with systemic sclerosis: A systematic review and meta-analysis. Clin Rheumatol. 2023;42(4):1087–99.
9. Wu S, Ye Z, et al. The causal relationship between autoimmune diseases and osteoporosis: A study based on Mendelian randomization. Front Endocrinol (Lausanne). 2023;14:1196269.
10. Zerbini CAF, et al. Biologic therapies and bone loss in rheumatoid arthritis. Osteoporos Int. 2017;28(2):429–46.
11. Broy SB, et al. Official positions for FRAX® clinical regarding rheumatoid arthritis from joint official positions development conference of the international society for clinical densitometry and international osteoporosis foundation on FRAX®. J Clin Densitom. 2011;14(3):184–9.
12. Albrecht K, et al. High prevalence of diabetes in patients with rheumatoid arthritis: Results from a questionnaire survey linked to claims data. Rheumatology (Oxford). 2018;57(2):329–36.
13. Palmowski A, et al. No association between methotrexate and impaired bone mineral density in a cohort of patients with polymyalgia rheumatica, giant cell arteritis, granulomatosis with polyangiitis and other vasculitides-a cross-sectional analysis with dose-response analyses. Rheumatol Int. 2023;43(5):903–9.
14. Palmowski A, et al. Glucocorticoids are not associated with bone mineral density in patients with polymyalgia rheumatica, giant cell arteritis and other vasculitides-cross-sectional baseline analysis of the prospective Rh-GIOP cohort. Cells. 2022;11(3).
15. Wiebe E, et al. Optimising both disease control and glucocorticoid dosing is essential for bone protection in patients with rheumatic disease. Ann Rheum Dis. 2022;81(9):1313–22.
16. Humphrey MB, et al. 2022 American college of rheumatology guideline for the prevention and treatment of glucocorticoid-induced osteoporosis. Arthritis Rheumatol. 2023 Dec;75(12):2088–102.
17. Moe S, et al. Definition, evaluation, and classification of renal osteodystrophy: A position statement from kidney disease: Improving global outcomes (KDIGO). Kidney Int. 2006;69(11):1945–53.
18. Lindberg JS, et al. Osteoporosis in end-state renal disease. Semin Nephrol. 1999;19(2):115–22.
19. Alem AM, et al. Increased risk of hip fracture among patients with end-stage renal disease. Kidney Int. 2000;58(1):396–9.
20. Dukas L, et al. In elderly men and women treated for osteoporosis a low creatinine clearance of <65 ml/min is a risk factor for falls and fractures. Osteoporos Int. 2005;16(12):1683–90.
21. Nickolas TL, et al. Relationship between moderate to severe kidney disease and hip fracture in the United States. J Am Soc Nephrol. 2006;17(11):3223–32.
22. Ensrud KE, et al. Renal function and risk of hip and vertebral fractures in older women. Arch Intern Med. 2007;167(2):133–9.
23. Fried LF, et al. Association of kidney function with incident hip fracture in older adults. J Am Soc Nephrol. 2007;18(1):282–6.
24. Dooley AC, et al. Increased risk of hip fracture among men with CKD. Am J Kidney Dis. 2008;51(1):38–44.
25. Naylor KL, et al. The three-year incidence of fracture in chronic kidney disease. Kidney Int. 2014;86(4):810–18.
26. Ketteler M, et al. Executive summary of the 2017 KDIGO chronic kidney disease-mineral and bone disorder (CKD-MBD) guideline update: What's changed and why it matters. Kidney Int. 2017;92(1):26–36.
27. Evenepoel P, et al. European Consensus Statement on the diagnosis and management of osteoporosis in chronic kidney disease stages G4-G5D. Nephrol Dial Transplant. 2021;36(1):42–59.
28. LeBoff MS, et al. The clinician's guide to prevention and treatment of osteoporosis. Osteoporos Int. 2022;33(10):2049–102.
29. Lewiecki EM. Evaluating patients for secondary causes of osteoporosis. Curr Osteoporos Rep. 2022;20(1):1–12.
30. Sprague SM, et al. Diagnostic accuracy of bone turnover markers and bone histology in patients with CKD treated by dialysis. Am J Kidney Dis. 2016;67(4):559–66.
31. Greenblatt MB, et al. Bone turnover markers in the diagnosis and monitoring of metabolic bone disease. Clin Chem. 2017;63(2):464–74.
32. Dalle Carbonare L, et al. [Histologic diagnosis of metabolic bone diseases: Bone histomorphometry]. Reumatismo. 2004;56(1):15–23.

33. Dalle Carbonare L, et al. Bone biopsy for histomorphometry in chronic kidney disease (CKD): State-of-the-art and new perspectives. J Clin Med. 2021;10(19).
34. Malluche HH, et al. Renal osteodystrophy: What's in a name? Presentation of a clinically useful new model to interpret bone histologic findings. Clin Nephrol. 2006;65(4):235–42.
35. Nickolas TL, et al. Rapid cortical bone loss in patients with chronic kidney disease. J Bone Miner Res. 2013;28(8):1811–20.
36. Evenepoel P, et al. Update on the role of bone biopsy in the management of patients with CKD-MBD. J Nephrol. 2017;30(5):645–52.
37. Fusaro M, et al. Time for revival of bone biopsy with histomorphometric analysis in chronic kidney disease (CKD): Moving from skepticism to pragmatism. Nutrients. 2022;14(9).
38. Holloway-Kew KL, et al. Bone material strength index is associated with prior fracture in men with and without moderate chronic kidney disease. Bone. 2020;133:115241.
39. Rufus-Membere P, et al. Associations between bone material strength index, calcaneal quantitative ultrasound, and bone mineral density in men. J Endocr Soc. 2021;5(4):bvaa179.
40. Sundaram M, et al. Erosive azotemic osteodystrophy. AJR Am J Roentgenol. 1981;136(2):363–7.
41. Tigges S, et al. Renal osteodystrophy: Imaging findings that mimic those of other diseases. AJR Am J Roentgenol. 1995;165(1):143–8.
42. Iimori S, et al. Diagnostic usefulness of bone mineral density and biochemical markers of bone turnover in predicting fracture in CKD stage 5D patients—a single-center cohort study. Nephrol Dial Transplant. 2012;27(1):345–51.
43. Yenchek RH, et al. Bone mineral density and fracture risk in older individuals with CKD. Clin J Am Soc Nephrol. 2012;7(7):1130–6.
44. Bucur RC, et al. Low bone mineral density and fractures in stages 3–5 CKD: An updated systematic review and meta-analysis. Osteoporos Int. 2015;26(2):449–58.
45. West SL, et al. Bone mineral density predicts fractures in chronic kidney disease. J Bone Miner Res. 2015;30(5):913–19.
46. Evenepoel P, et al. Diagnosis and management of osteoporosis in chronic kidney disease stages 4 to 5D: A call for a shift from nihilism to pragmatism. Osteoporos Int. 2021;32(12):2397–405.
47. Martineau P, et al. Bone mineral densitometry reporting: Pearls and pitfalls. Can Assoc Radiol J. 2021;72(3):490–504.
48. Toussaint ND, et al. Determination and validation of aortic calcification measurement from lateral bone densitometry in dialysis patients. Clin J Am Soc Nephrol. 2009;4(1):119–27.
49. McCloskey EV, et al. A meta-analysis of trabecular bone score in fracture risk prediction and its relationship to FRAX®. J Bone Miner Res. 2016;31(5):940–8.
50. Naylor KL, et al. Trabecular bone score in kidney transplant recipients. Osteoporos Int. 2016;27(3):1115–21.
51. Naylor KL, et al. Trabecular bone score and incident fragility fracture risk in adults with reduced kidney function. Clin J Am Soc Nephrol. 2016;11(11):2032–40.
52. Yun HJ, et al. Trabecular bone score may indicate chronic kidney disease-mineral and bone disorder (CKD-MBD) phenotypes in hemodialysis patients: A prospective observational study. BMC Nephrol. 2020;21(1):299.
53. Poiana C, et al. Utility of trabecular bone score (TBS) in bone quality and fracture risk assessment in patients on maintenance dialysis. Front Med (Lausanne). 2021;8:782837.
54. Shevroja E, et al. Review on the utility of trabecular bone score, a surrogate of bone micro-architecture, in the chronic kidney disease spectrum and in kidney transplant recipients. Front Endocrinol (Lausanne). 2018;9:561.
55. Rampersad C, et al. Trabecular bone score in patients with chronic kidney disease. Osteoporos Int. 2020;31(10):1905–12.
56. Whitlock RH, et al. The fracture risk assessment tool (FRAX®) predicts fracture risk in patients with chronic kidney disease. Kidney Int. 2019;95(2):447–54.
57. Desbiens LC, et al. Comparison of fracture prediction tools in individuals without and with early chronic kidney disease: A population-based analysis of CARTaGENE. J Bone Miner Res. 2020;35(6):1048–57.
58. Levin A, et al. Prevalence of abnormal serum vitamin D, PTH, calcium, and phosphorus in patients with chronic kidney disease: Results of the study to evaluate early kidney disease. Kidney Int. 2007;71(1):31–8.

59. Geng S, et al. Parathyroid hormone independently predicts fracture, vascular events, and death in patients with stage 3 and 4 chronic kidney disease. Osteoporos Int. 2019;30(10):2019–25.
60. Eriksen EF, et al. Update on long-term treatment with bisphosphonates for postmeno-pausal osteoporosis: A systematic review. Bone. 2014;58:126–35.
61. Seeman E, et al. Antiresorptive and anabolic agents in the prevention and reversal of bone fragility. Nat Rev Rheumatol. 2019;15(4):225–36.
62. Rodd C. Bisphosphonates in dialysis and transplantation patients: Efficacy and safety issues. Perit Dial Int. 2001;21(Suppl 3):S256–60.
63. Wilson LM, et al. Benefits and harms of osteoporosis medications in patients with chronic kidney disease: A systematic review and meta-analysis. Ann Intern Med. 2017;166(9):649–58.
64. Abrahamsen B, et al. The association between renal function and BMD response to bisphosphonate treatment: Real-world cohort study using linked national registers. Bone. 2020;137:115371.
65. Robinson DE, et al. Safety of oral bisphosphonates in moderate-to-severe chronic kidney disease: A binational cohort analysis. J Bone Miner Res. 2021;36(5):820–32.
66. Robinson DE, et al. Bisphosphonates to reduce bone fractures in stage 3B+ chronic kidney disease: A propensity score-matched cohort study. Health Technol Assess. 2021;25(17):1–106.
67. Hara T, et al. Effectiveness of pharmacological interventions versus placebo or no treat-ment for osteoporosis in patients with CKD stages 3–5D: Editorial summary of a cochrane review. Am J Kidney Dis. 2022;80(6):794–6.
68. Ali MS, et al. Alendronate use and bone mineral density gains in women with moderate-severe (stages 3B-5) chronic kidney disease: An open cohort multivariable and propensity score analysis from Funen, Denmark. Arch Osteoporos. 2020;15(1):81.
69. Jamal SA, et al. Effects of denosumab on fracture and bone mineral density by level of kidney function. J Bone Miner Res. 2011;26(8):1829–35.
70. Iseri K, et al. Long-term effect of denosumab on bone disease in patients with CKD. Clin J Am Soc Nephrol. 2023;18(9):1195–203.
71. Nickolas TL. Treating osteoporosis with denosumab in patients on hemodialysis: the good, the bad, and the ugly. Clinical Journal of the American Society of Nephrology. 2023;18(9):1116–18.
72. Miller PD, et al. Teriparatide in postmenopausal women with osteoporosis and mild or moderate renal impairment. Osteoporos Int. 2007;18(1):59–68.
73. Bilezikian JP, et al. Abaloparatide in patients with mild or moderate renal impairment: Results from the ACTIVE phase 3 trial. Curr Med Res Opin. 2019;35(12):2097–102.
74. Nishikawa A, et al. Safety and effectiveness of daily teriparatide for osteoporosis in patients with severe stages of chronic kidney disease: Post hoc analysis of a postmarketing observational study. Clin Interv Aging. 2016;11:1653–9.
75. Sumida K, et al. Once-weekly teriparatide in hemodialysis patients with hypoparathy-roidism and low bone mass: A prospective study. Osteoporos Int. 2016;27(4):1441–50.
76. Yamamoto J, et al. Impact of weekly teriparatide on the bone and mineral metabolism in hemodialysis patients with relatively low serum parathyroid hormone: A pilot study. Ther Apher Dial. 2020;24(2):146–53.
77. Cejka D, et al. Treatment of hemodialysis-associated adynamic bone disease with teripa-ratide (PTH1–34): A pilot study. Kidney Blood Press Res. 2010;33(3):221–6.
78. Cejka D, et al. Sclerostin and Dickkopf-1 in renal osteodystrophy. Clin J Am Soc Nephrol. 2011;6(4):877–82.
79. Miller PD, et al. Efficacy and safety of romosozumab among postmenopausal women With osteoporosis and mild-to-moderate chronic kidney disease. J Bone Miner Res. 2022;37(8):1437–45.
80. Sato M, et al. Efficacy of romosozumab in patients with osteoporosis on maintenance hemodialysis in Japan; an observational study. J Bone Miner Metab. 2021;39(6):1082–90.

14 Dialysis and Kidney Transplantation Outcomes in Rheumatic Disease Patients

Manal Alotaibi[†], Karina D. Torralba[†], Vaneet K. Sandhu[‡], and Sam Kant[‡]
[†]These are co-first authors.
[‡]These are co-senior authors.

14.1 INTRODUCTION

End-stage kidney failure or disease (ESKD) is considered when kidneys lose function, requiring kidney replacement therapy (KRT) in the form of dialysis or even organ transplantation. ESKD may manifest in patients with systemic rheumatic diseases either as a direct outcome of the diseases themselves or because of treatment-related toxicities. This chapter is dedicated to the former. The most common autoimmune inflammatory rheumatic diseases (AIRDs) that develop ESKD include systemic lupus erythematosus (SLE), systemic sclerosis (SSc), and antineutrophil cytoplasmic antibody (ANCA)-associated vasculitides (AAVs) like granulomatosis with polyangiitis (GPA) and microscopic polyangiitis (MPA). Among metabolic arthropathies, ESKD is most prevalent in gout.

14.2 CONSIDERATIONS FOR STARTING DIALYSIS

There are no specific guidelines for patients with rheumatic disease with chronic kidney disease (CKD) as to the initiation of kidney replacement therapy, whether via hemodialysis (HD) or peritoneal dialysis (PD); decision-making processes are often complex. KRT should be considered when any of the following are present: Symptoms or signs attributable to ESKD, e.g., neurological features due to uremia, pericarditis, anorexia, refractory acid–base or electrolyte abnormalities, reduced energy level, unexplained weight loss, intractable pruritus, or bleeding; uncontrollable volume status or blood pressure; or progressive nutritional deterioration (1). The mean estimated glomerular filtration rate (eGFR) value at which dialysis is initiated based on registry data varies per country; in the USA, the value is about $11mL/minute/1.73m^2$. Risk equations can help assist in predicting a time frame when KRT may be necessary (1).

Urgent dialysis is associated with lower survival rates and higher morbidity, contributed to by lack of patient preparedness (1). The patient's perception of autonomy and quality of life should equally be given credence; in general, home HD and PD have been successful due to the patient's perception of autonomy (1).

14.2.1 Outcomes in Rheumatic Disease Patients on Dialysis

Much of the information on outcomes of rheumatic disease patients on dialysis are based on single-center experiences or registry data from integrated health systems. This section focuses on major rheumatic diseases where renal disease occurs in ≥20% of cases.

SLE

Approximately 30% of SLE patients with lupus nephritis (LN) will progress to needing KRT (2). Resoundingly contrary to prior notions that lupus "burns out" once RRT is started, flares can still occur, as shown in nine of 24 studies (3). Black female patients have higher rates of flare (4). At a median follow up of 45 months, 32 (26%) experienced flares with hematologic manifestations (40%) most prevalent (31% thrombocytopenia; 21% leucopenia); corticosteroids were mostly used to treat flares, but cyclophosphamide and mycophenolate mofetil (MMF) were also used (5). Worse outcomes were noted in patients with histopathologic cellular crescents and a higher chronicity index, high dsDNA autoantibody levels, and low eGFR (6). There is limited information on the management of LN patients on dialysis. In a small study (n = 7), the addition of belimumab was associated with improvements in serum creatinine, urine output, and immunologic parameters (7).

SSc

SSc can present with distinct phenotypes based on histopathological studies; rapidly progressive kidney failure is most associated with scleroderma renal crisis (SRC), overlap with ANCA-associated vasculitis in a minority, and nephrotic syndrome (8). SRC, typified by acute renal failure and severe hypertension in a diffuse-type SSc patient with anti-RNA polymerase III antibodies, can progress to ESKD despite angiotensin-converting enzyme inhibitor usage and require transplantation despite blood pressure normalization (9). The adjusted annual incidence and prevalence for RRT in SSC-ESRD is estimated to be 0.11–0.26 and 0.73–0.95 per million population,

 DOI: 10.1201/9781003438373-17

respectively. The 5-year survival probability for patients on >90 days of KRT is 38.9% (10); this poor prognosis has been replicated in a French registry (11).

GPA/MPA

An ERA-EDTA study of 12 AAV registries with 2511 patients (1755 with GPA, 756 MPA) showed an incidence of 1.05 per million population for GPA and 0.45 per million population with MPA, with 558 (22.2%) undergoing kidney transplant (12). The 10-year probability of survival after >90 KRT days was 32.5% (12). A 9-year French registry study of 425 AAV patients (165 MPA, 259 GPA) on KRT showed that 14% required transplant while 4% recovered function (13). Survival rates were comparable to those in other patients without AAV: 96%, 85%, 68%, and 53% at 3 months and 1, 3, and 5 years, respectively, with median survival on dialysis being 5.35 years. Independent risk factors associated with mortality included age, peripheral artery disease, and frailty. +PR3 ANCA patients have a higher likelihood of having a disease relapse post-transplant (14). A United States Renal System study showed an improvement in mortality from 1995–2014, with cardiovascular disease (CVD) and infections being leading causes (15).

Gout

A British registry study of 68,897 gout patients and 554,964 matched controls showed that gout is associated with increased CKD and ESKD risk compared to controls (16). Gout itself can lead to CKD, including nephrolithiasis. The pooled prevalence of CKD stage 3 is 24%, whereas the prevalence of self-reported nephrolithiasis is 14% (17). However, the relationship between gout and renal disease is complicated by the fact that CKD itself is associated with higher rates of gout (25%) and hyperuricemia (60%) (18). This makes it challenging to clarify KRT outcomes in this population.

Other AIRDs

Kidney disease is much less common in other AIRDs; therefore, there is limited data on outcomes related to dialysis. Less than 10% of individuals with Sjögren's syndrome develop kidney disease (19). Renal amyloidosis resulting in rheumatoid arthritis (RA) is extremely rare.

14.2.2 Treatment Considerations for Rheumatic Disease Patients on Dialysis

Rheumatic disease patients are at risk for morbidity and mortality related to infections, cardiovascular disease (CVD), and fractures. These problems are further exacerbated with the onset of CKD or ESKD. The ensuing section focuses on these issues as they relate to rheumatic disease patients on dialysis.

Bone Health

CKD leading to dialysis is associated with complex and profound alterations in bone and mineral metabolism that increase fracture risks (20). Collectively attributed to mineral and bone disorders associated with CKD (CKD-MBD), factors related to menopausal status, age, and genetics should also be considered. KDIGO highlights renal osteodystrophy (ROD) as a key issue; adynamic bone disease (ABD), a variant of ROD, is marked by reduced osteoblasts and osteoclasts, thin osteoid seams, and low bone turnover (21). Dialysis patients have reduced bone mass due to secondary hyperparathyroidism and increased bone turnover, as well as decreased bone quality due to abnormal chemical composition and microarchitecture.

Dual-energy x-ray absorptiometry (DXA), used to evaluate bone mass and predict fracture risk, is included in management guidelines for dialysis patients (22). However, its ability to predict fracture is less efficient in dialysis populations, as the fracture risk in these populations is more related to low bone quality. The trabecular bone score (TBS), an index of bone microarchitecture correlating with the trabecular organization of cancellous bone independent of total amount of osseous tissue and determined by a DXA-derived algorithm, has fracture prediction value (23). TBS augments the ability of the fracture risk assessment (FRAX) score to predict fracture. There is low TBS in AIRDs, e.g., SLE, SSc, ankylosing spondylitis, polymyalgia rheumatica, and RA (24). TBS better reflects glucocorticoid effects on bone quality as compared to DXA alone (25).

Evidence for osteoporosis treatment in dialysis patients is limited. Bisphosphonates should be with caution given the ABD risks in more advanced CKD; an extensive review has been provided by Nitta et al. (26) and by Tanner et al. as published elsewhere in this book. 1Weekly teriparatide, a parathyroid hormone (PTH) analog, in patients on HD with low PTH sans parathyroidectomy can increase trabecular bone mass (27). Romosozumab, a sclerostin inhibitor, can increase BMD among HD patients without increasing their risk of CVD from romosozumab use (28). Fall risk assessments are essential, as hospitalization (67.6%), skilled nursing facility admission (30.7%), and death

(26.1%) can result after dialysis initiation, as noted among 3.6% of 81,653 patients in a US Medicare cohort who had a serious fall injury pre-dialysis (29).

Infections

Based on ERA-EDTA registry data (1993–2007; 168,156 dialysis patients), dialysis was associated with an 82-fold risk of death from an infection (30). A single-center retrospective study of LN patients in Taiwan, when compared to age- and sex-matched controls, showed a higher infection risk related to peritonitis (31); this is consistent with a study that showed that patients on PD had increased rates of peritonitis, while HD patients tended to have sepsis (32). Recommendations for the management of chronic and opportunistic infections have been formulated by the European Alliance of Associations for Rheumatology (33). There is limited data on infection risks for AIRD patients on KRT.

Immuno-dysregulatory mechanisms that drive autoimmunity often coexist with immunodeficiency; an evaluation for immunodeficiency should be considered in patients with recurrent infections (34). The risk of infection must be balanced against the risk of disease relapse when considering continuing immunosuppression in patients with lupus and ANCA-associated vasculitis. Evidence related to dysbiosis separately related to autoimmunity and CKD also theoretically may increase infection risks (35, 36).

CVD

Dialysis patients have a 25-fold increased risk of sudden cardiac death compared to the general population; 29% of these cases are caused by arrhythmias and occur most commonly on the first dialysis day after the long interdialytic gap, suggesting that abrupt changes in electrolytes, uremic toxins, and fluid are contributory (37). CVD is a known cause of death in SLE, with immune dysregulation driving the process (38). Medicaid databases show that SLE patients have a 27% higher risk of CVD when compared to diabetes patients and a two-fold higher risk when compared to the general population, with the highest relative risk in the 18–39 year age group (39). Among GPA patients, heart failure and arrhythmias are also prevalent (40). AAV patients have a three-fold higher risk of CVD compared to non-AAV comparators (41).

CVD management guidelines in rheumatic disease populations (e.g., gout, SLE, and AAV) have been outlined (42). More research is needed addressing CVD risk among AIRD patients on dialysis.

Health-Related Quality of Life (HRQoL)

Perceived physical health among 2693 patients with moderate–severe CKD is lower compared to that in the general population (43). HRQoL necessitates the consideration of patient-reported outcomes and social determinants of health. Increased body swelling or electrolyte fluctuations can exacerbate pain, fatigue, and impaired physical functioning, which are already manifestations of rheumatic diseases. LN patients, often younger and with greater disease activity, report difficulty with self-care, mobility, pain, and mood (44, 45). Polypharmacy, medication side effects, and frequent medical visits all contribute to this challenge.

Medication Management in Dialysis

Multiple medications used to treat AIRDs are eliminated through the kidneys and require modified dosing for CKD patients or may need to be given after dialysis (Table 14.1). While poor knowledge about dose adjustments of medications for kidney dysfunction exists, this can be countered through contextualized hands-on education (46).

14.3 RENAL TRANSPLANTATION IN RHEUMATIC DISEASE PATIENTS

This section will focus mainly on providing an overview of transplantation considerations and outcomes in SLE and the AAVs MPA and GPA. There is limited data on other rheumatic diseases, and these are explained in other chapters in this book.

14.3.1 Eligibility Criteria for Renal Transplantation

SLE

Although kidney transplantation is a viable option for most LN patients, HD is usually initiated for those progressing to ESKD or those with RPGN (93), with the aim to facilitate the disease into a quiescent state. Achieving remission is crucial before advancing to transplantation (93–96). Additionally, it has been shown that 3 to 6 months of dialysis is often adequate for functional recovery before considering transplantation (93–95). Alternatively, individuals in complete

Table 14.1: Renal Dose Adjustment Recommendations for Commonly Used Medications for Rheumatic Diseases

Non-Biologic/Non-Targeted Synthetic Medications

Allopurinol	50mg/day starting dose in CKD and gout eGFR: >30–60mL/minute/1.73m², 50mg daily; >15–30, 50mg every other day; 5–15, 50mg twice weekly; <5, 50mg daily (47)
Colchicine	Not recommended when CrCL < 30mL/minute (48) *CrCl < 30mL/minute*: No more than once every 2 weeks (49)
Hydroxychloroquine	Risk of toxic reactions may be greater in kidney impairment, use with caution in elderly patients (50) Use of HCQ in all patients with SLE and LN, with dose adjustments according to body weight and GFR (51)
Methotrexate	Avoid in dialysis (52) or dose after dialysis (53). *CrCl > 50 mL/minute*: No dose adjustment necessary *10–50*: 50% of dose *<10*: Avoid use (54)
Sulfasalazine	Use with caution at lowest effective dose in CKD. Maximum dose 1000mg/day in hemodialysis (55)
Leflunomide	Not adequately studied for in CKD or ESKD (56)
Azathioprine (AZA)	*CrCl < 30mL/minute*: 50–100% of dose On day of dialysis, dose post-dialysis (57)
Mycophenolate mofetil Mycophenolic acid	If eGFR < 25, avoid doses greater than 1gm BID (58) No dose adjustments for patients experiencing delayed renal graft function postoperatively *eGFR ≤ 30 mL/minute/1.73m²*: Use with caution (59)
Cyclophosphamide	Dose reduction 20–30% in severe kidney impairment Dialyze at least 12 hours after intravenous infusion (60).
Cyclosporine	Not recommended in kidney impairment (61)
Tacrolimus	Consider dosing at the lower end of the therapeutic dosing range with kidney impairment (62).
Voclosporin	*eGFR ≤ 45mL/minute/1.73m²*: Not recommended unless benefit exceeds the risk *eGFR ≤ 30mL/minute/1.73m²*: Dose reduction (63)

Biologics

TNF inhibitors	Inadequate data in patients with kidney impairment (64)
Tocilizumab	*Mild–moderate kidney impairment*: No adjustment required
Sarilumab	*Severe kidney impairment*: Has not been studied (65, 66)
Secukinumab	Use for patients with renal impairment not described in FDA-PI (67–76).
Ustekinumab	
Ixekizumab	
Risankizumab	
Bimekizumab	
Guselkumab	
Abatacept	
Mepolizumab	
Benralizumab	
Anifrolumab	
Canakinumab	*Kidney impairment*: No formal studies have been done (77, 78).
Rilonacept	
Anakinra	Substantially renally excreted; drug toxicity may be greater with renal impairment (79)
Pegloticase	No dose adjustment in kidney impairment (80, 81)
Belimumab	

(Continued)

Table 14.1: (Continued)

Rituximab	Renal toxicity reported in the setting of NHL (tumor lysis syndrome) or with drug interactions, not formally studied in rheumatic diseases (82)

Pooled Antibody + Biological Agent

Human immunoglobulin (subcutaneous or intravenous)	Screen all patients for kidney disease. Product selection (sucrose containing IVIG can cause kidney impairment), volume, route of administration, dose (high doses 1000 to 2400mg/kg) and rate of infusion can cause impairment; acute impairment occurs usually within 1–10 days of administration and resolves within 4 weeks. In 40% of cases, HD is needed with recovery within 2 weeks. Notably, high-dose IVIG has been used successfully for panel-reactive antibody suppression in highly sensitized late-stage CKD patients on dialysis awaiting transplantation (83).

Small-Molecule Drugs/Targeted Synthetic Anti-Rheumatic Disease Drugs

Apremilast	*CrCl < 30mL/minute*: Dose reduction to 30mg daily (84)
Tofacitinib	*Moderate–severe kidney impairment*: Dose adjustment recommended (85)
Upadacitinib	No adjustment in RA, PsA, AS, Nr-AxSpA *eGFR < 15mL/minute/1.73m²*: Not recommended (86)
Baricitinib	*eGFR 30–60mL/minute/1.73m²*: 50% dose reduction *eGFR <30mL/minute/1.73m²*: Not recommended (87)
Nintedanib	Mild–moderate kidney impairment: no dose adjustment required; has not been studied in severe impairment (88)

Medications for Osteoporosis/Fracture Prevention

Bisphosphonates	*CrCl < 35mL/minute and dialysis*: not recommended (26)
Teriparatide Abaloparatide	No dosage adjustment for kidney impairment (89, 90)
Denosumab	No dose adjustment for kidney impairment
Romosozumab	*CrCl < 30 mL/minute or dialysis*: High risk of hypocalcemia. Monitor calcium, phosphorus and magnesium. Properly supplement calcium and vitamin D (91, 92).

Abbreviations: AS, ankylosing spondylitis; AIRDs, autoimmune rheumatic diseases; CrCl, creatinine clearance; eGFR, estimated glomerular filtration rate; FDA, Food and Drug Administration; NHL, non-Hodgkin's lymphoma; Nr-AxSpA, non-radiographic axial spondylarthritis; PI, package insert; PsA, psoriatic arthritis; RA, rheumatoid arthritis; SLE, systemic lupus erythematosus

Note: Stages of CKD: Stage 1: kidney damage (e.g., albuminuria) with normal or increased GFR (>90mL/minute/1.73m²); Stage 2: kidney damage (e.g., albuminuria) with mild reduction in GFR (60–89mL/minute/1.73m²); Stage 3a: mild to moderate reduction in GFR (45–59mL/minute/1.73m²); Stage 3b: moderate reduction in GFR (30–44mL/minute/1.73m²); Stage 4: severe reduction in GFR (15–29mL/minute/1.73m²); Stage 5: kidney failure (GFR <15mL/minute/1.73m² or dialysis)

*These are summarized recommendations from medical literature including FDA-PIs; please refer to published recommendations by the pharmaceutical company and the FDA for complete information.

remission for a substantial period of time before reaching ESKD may proceed with preemptive renal transplant, especially if a suitable living donor is available (95).

GPA/MPA

Kidney transplantation is increasingly becoming a treatment option for these patients, and outcomes have shown gradual improvements over the years. The clinical remission of vasculitis should be sustained for 12 months before considering transplantation (97–99). KDIGO recommends 6 months of remission before considering renal transplantation; persistent ANCA should not delay transplantation (100).

14.3.2 Pre-Transplant Assessment of Rheumatic Disease Activity and Organ Involvement

SLE

SLE patients may experience premature CVD, which is known to be the leading cause of morbidity and mortality in SLE (101); a thorough evaluation for CVD is recommended pre-transplantation (102), although traditional risk factors may not apply. Additionally, screening for the presence of antiphospholipid antibodies is important, as these contribute to early graft thrombosis (103, 104).

AAV

The definition of remission in GPA/MPA generally entails the absence of clinical symptoms indicative of active AAV. While circulating ANCAs may not reliably indicate active disease, consistently elevated levels, particularly of PR3-ANCA, are a significant risk factor for relapse (14, 105). The association between ANCA positivity and AAV recurrence post-transplant is not clear. Some studies suggest that ANCAs are not linked to post-transplant AAV relapses. However, patients with positive ANCAs at the time of transplant were more prone to relapse (17%) compared to those with normal ANCA levels (5%) (106). Post-transplant relapse risk appears to be highest among recipients with PR3-ANCA positivity (14).

14.3.3 Balancing Rheumatic Disease Control and Organ Transplantation Outcomes in Rheumatic Disease Transplant Recipients

SLE

Post-transplant immunosuppression (IS) typically follows routine practices. Post-transplant recipients experiencing recurrent LN generally maintain their existing IS for transplant maintenance. However, those with clinically evident disease and severe histopathologic lesions, corresponding to WHO class III or IV in the graft, may necessitate additional IS (93).

AAV

The choice of IS post-transplant has traditionally been at the discretion of transplant centers. Until the early 1980s, standard therapy consisted of AZA and corticosteroids, with the routine adoption of cyclosporine from that point onward (107). Current post-transplant protocols commonly involve induction IS (often with antithymocyte globulin) and a combination of oral tacrolimus, MMF, and corticosteroids (108). MMF was less effective than AZA in maintaining disease remission in non-transplanted patients with AAV (109). In a comparative analysis of 69 non-transplant GPA/MPA patients who received cyclophosphamide followed by either AZA, MMF, or MMF after AZA, it was observed that patients with higher disease activity at the time of diagnosis who received MMF had a lower cumulative ESKD-free survival rate compared to those who used AZA (110). However, recent studies on post-transplant AAV patients on MMF, tacrolimus, and corticosteroids reported favorable patient outcomes, including low relapse rates (106, 111, 112).

14.3.4 Graft Survival and Function, and Recurrence of Autoimmune Disease Post-Transplant

SLE

The risk of recurrent LN (RLN) post-transplantation varies between 2 and 30% and can occur as early as 6–16 years post-transplant (93, 113). Clinically apparent RLN is mostly characterized by mild histologic lesions (93, 114). The largest cohort study suggests that RLN in the graft is uncommon (32, 93, 114). It is very important to differentiate clinically apparent recurrent LN in the allograft from incident histopathological findings in the graft without symptoms. Post-transplant RLN manifests as kidney dysfunction, either as an acute increase in serum creatinine or a gradual rise or as the onset of new proteinuria or glomerular hematuria, or both. When histologic RLN in the graft coincides with rapid renal deterioration, other causes of acute renal dysfunction such as acute rejection, chronic allograft nephropathy, and calcineurin inhibitor toxicity should be considered (32, 93, 114). Any transplanted LN patient showing new-onset or worsening proteinuria and/or hematuria and severe proliferative histopathologic lesions may require the modification of IS. Higher doses of MMF (2–3gm per day) or initiating cyclophosphamide intravenously and discontinuing the current IS are options. Usually, corticosteroids are started, usually methylprednisolone 500–1000mg/day for 3 consecutive days, followed by a taper. Cyclophosphamide is particularly considered in cases featuring rapid renal deterioration with a histopathologic crescentic pattern and in situations involving severe extrarenal disease, such as pulmonary hemorrhage, cerebritis, or other life-threatening SLE-related phenomena. Although there is limited data, these approaches for post-transplant RLN are informed by studies on LN affecting the native kidney (93)

GPA/MPA

Relapse rates of AAV post-transplant are low, around 0.003 to 0.076 per patient per year (99). The average time from transplant to recurrence is 30.9 months. GPA patients are more prone to relapse over those with MPA; recurrence rates are higher in patients with +ANCA at time of transplant (99). The duration of disease, circulating ANCA pattern, previous cyclosporine treatments, KRT length, and donor type do not seem to influence relapse risks post-transplant. Approximately 60% of recurrent AAVs involve the transplanted kidney, either alone or in combination with other organs, while isolated extrarenal involvement occurs in 40% of cases (99, 115). Microscopic hematuria and proteinuria are early indicators of graft relapse, typically associated with or shortly followed by renal impairment. Histologic features closely resemble those observed in the native kidney, depicting a focal or diffuse pauci-immune extra-capillary necrotizing glomerulonephritis in acute phases. IS for post-transplant AAV relapse is similar to what is used for non-transplanted patients, ranging from increased corticosteroids to cyclophosphamide, with plasma exchange therapy used in selected patients. Cyclophosphamide remains the gold standard in the induction treatment of generalized AAV and AAV glomerulonephritis and has demonstrated success in post-transplant relapses in numerous studies. Rituximab is considered a standard post-transplant therapy used for antibody-mediated rejection or in cases of ABO-blood-group- or human-leukocyte-antigen-incompatible transplantation. However, the efficacy of rituximab for recurrent post-transplant AAV is limited to case reports. Further studies are needed (112).

14.3.5 Infections Post-Transplant

Infections have been identified as factors contributing to morbidity and mortality after kidney transplantation in cases involving lupus nephritis. Extended exposure to IS both pre-ESKD and post-ESKD and transplant may theoretically increase susceptibility to infections. However, this is not consistent with published literature, as the prevalence of serious infections is not significantly higher in recipients with SLE compared to non-SLE patients (93).

14.3.6 Long-Term Management and Optimizing Outcomes
SLE

A retrospective multicenter study unequivocally demonstrated superior survival and lower complication rates associated with transplants in LN patients compared to those on dialysis (116). LN recurrence in the graft can result in poorer outcomes compared to those in other kidney transplant recipients. Despite initial reservations, in 1975 the American College of Surgeons/National Institute of Health Transplant Registry allowed for renal transplants in lupus patients by revealing outcomes comparable to non-lupus patients (117). Subsequent studies consistently show similar 5- and 10-year graft survival rates between lupus and non-lupus patients (93, 114, 118). Those with antiphospholipid autoantibodies who have received kidneys from living donors face a higher recurrence risk (103). African American ethnicity is independently associated with recurrent LN in the allograft and is linked to reduced survival (119). Death is primarily attributed to cardiovascular disease. Delayed complications, including malignancies, avascular necrosis, and osteoporosis, have been infrequently reported (93).

AAV

The long-term impact of GPA/MPA recurrence after renal transplant is still uncertain (112). The Australia and New Zealand Dialysis and Transplant Registry revealed that recurrent AAVs after transplantation were associated with a 10-year graft loss rate of 7.7% (120). While the survival advantages of transplantation are clear in AAV with ESRD (97, 99), it should be noted that transplant recipients are generally younger than those undergoing dialysis, with potentially fewer comorbidities. Transplanted patients experience lower relapse rates compared to dialysis patients and those with CKD not on dialysis (97, 99).

14.4 Conclusion

The management of ESKD in AIRDs requires individualized and holistic treatment approaches and the complex coordination of care. Although more research is needed, providing the best information possible to patients will facilitate shared decision-making processes. Patients' perception of autonomy and quality of life should equally be given credence.

REFERENCES

1. Chan CT, et al. Conference participants. Dialysis initiation, modality choice, access, and prescription: Conclusions from a kidney disease: Improving global outcomes (KDIGO) controversies conference. Kidney Int. 2019;96(1):37–47.

2. Anders HJ, et al. A pathophysiology-based approach to the diagnosis and treatment of lupus nephritis. Kidney Int. 2016;90:493–501.
3. Mattos P, et al. Disease activity in systemic lupus erythematosus patients with end-stage renal disease: Systematic review of the literature. Clin Rheumatol. 2012;31(6):897–905.
4. Krane NK, et al. Persistent lupus activity in end-stage renal disease. Am J Kidney Dis. 1999;33(5):872–9.
5. Kim YE, et al. Disease flare of systemic lupus erythematosus in patients with endstage renal disease on dialysis. J Rheumatol. 2022;49(10):1131–7.
6. Krassanairawiwong K, et al. Revised ISN/RPS 2018 classification of lupus renal pathology predict clinical remission. Int Urol Nephrol. 2021;53:1391–8.
7. Liu D, et al. Efficacy and safety of belimumab in systemic lupus erythematosus patients with severe lupus nephritis requiring renal replacement therapy. Lupus. 2022;31(12):1456–67.
8. Tonsawan P, et al. Renal pathology and clinical associations in systemic sclerosis: A historical cohort study. Int J Gen Med. 2019;12:323–31.
9. Maritati F, et al. Kidney transplantation in systemic sclerosis: Advances in graft, disease, and patient outcome. Front Immunol. 2022;13:878736.
10. Hruskova Z, et al. Characteristics and outcomes of patients with systemic sclerosis (Scleroderma) requiring renal replacement therapy in Europe: Results from the ERA-EDTA registry. Am J Kidney Dis. 2019;73(2):184–93.
11. Lavergne A, et al. Systemic sclerosis and end-stage renal disease: Study of patient characteristics, follow-up and outcomes in France. J Nephrol. 2021;34(2):617–25.
12. Hruskova Z, et al. Characteristics and outcomes of granulomatosis with polyangiitis (Wegener) and microscopic polyangiitis requiring renal replacement therapy: Results from the European renal association-European dialysis and transplant association registry. Am J Kidney Dis. 2015;66(4):613–20.
13. Romeu M, et al. Survival of patients with ANCA-associated vasculitis on chronic dialysis: Data from the French REIN registry from 2002 to 2011. QJM. 2014;107(7):545–55.
14. Geetha D, et al. Relevance of ANCA positivity at the time of renal transplantation in ANCA associated vasculitis. J Nephrol. 2017;30(1):147–53.
15. Wallace ZS, et al. Improving mortality in end-stage renal disease due to granulomatosis with polyangiitis (Wegener's) from 1995 to 2014: Data from the United States renal data system. Arthritis Care Res (Hoboken). 2018;70(10):1495–500.
16. Stack AG, Johnson ME, Blak B, et al. Gout and the risk of advanced chronic kidney disease in the UK health system: A national cohort study. BMJ Open. 2019;9:e031550.
17. Roughley MJ, et al. Gout and risk of chronic kidney disease and nephrolithiasis: Meta-analysis of observational studies. Arthritis Res Ther. 2015;17(1):90.
18. Johnson RJ, et al. Uric acid and chronic kidney disease: Still more to do. Kidney Int Rep. 2022;8(2):229–39.
19. François H, et al. Renal involvement in primary Sjögren syndrome. Nat Rev Nephrol. 2016;12(2):82–93.
20. Evenepoel P, et al. European Renal Osteodystrophy (EUROD) workgroup, an initiative of the CKD-MBD working group of the ERA-EDTA, and the committee of Scientific Advisors and National Societies of the IOF. European Consensus Statement on the diagnosis and management of osteoporosis in chronic kidney disease stages G4-G5D. Nephrol Dial Transplant. 2021;36(1):42–59.
21. Moe S, et al. Kidney disease: Improving global outcomes (KDIGO). Definition, evaluation, and classification of renal osteodystrophy: A position statement from kidney disease: Improving global outcomes (KDIGO). Kidney Int. 2006;69(11):1945–53.
22. Ketteler M, et al. Diagnosis, evaluation, prevention, and treatment of chronic kidney disease-mineral and bone disorder: Synopsis of the kidney disease: Improving global outcomes 2017 clinical practice guideline update. Ann Intern Med. 2018;168(6):422–30.
23. Poiana C, et al. Utility of trabecular bone score (TBS) in bone quality and fracture risk assessment in patients on maintenance dialysis. Front Med (Lausanne). 2022;8:782837.
24. Ruaro B, et al. What role does trabecular bone score play in chronic inflammatory rheumatic diseases? Front Med (Lausanne). 2020;7:600697.
25. Nowakowska-Płaza A, et al. Clinical utility of trabecular bone score (TBS) in fracture risk assessment of patients with rheumatic diseases treated with Glucocorticoids. Horm Metab Res. 2021;53(8):499–503.

26. Nitta K, et al. Management of osteoporosis in chronic kidney disease. Intern Med. 2017;56(24):3271–6.
27. Yamamoto J, et al. Impact of weekly teriparatide on the bone and mineral metabolism in hemodialysis patients with relatively low serum parathyroid hormone: A pilot study. Ther Apher Dial. 2020;24(2):146–53.
28. Sato M, et al. Efficacy of romosozumab in patients with osteoporosis on maintenance hemodialysis in Japan; an observational study. J Bone Miner Metab. 2021;39(6):1082–90.
29. Bowling CB, et al. Serious fall injury history and adverse health outcomes after initiating hemodialysis among older U.S. adults. J Gerontol A Biol Sci Med Sci. 2018;73(9):1216–21.
30. Vogelzang JL, et al. Mortality from infections and malignancies in patients treated with renal replacement therapy: Data from the ERA-EDTA registry. Nephrol Dial Transplant. 2015;30(6):1028–37.
31. Huang JW, et al. Systemic lupus erythematosus and peritoneal dialysis: Outcomes and infectious complications. Perit Dial Int. 2001;21(2):143–7.
32. Tsai WT, et al. Long-term outcomes in lupus patients receiving different renal replacement therapy. J Microbiol Immunol Infect. 2019;52(4):648–53.
33. Fragoulis GE, et al. 2022 EULAR recommendations for screening and prophylaxis of chronic and opportunistic infections in adults with autoimmune inflammatory rheumatic diseases. Ann Rheum Dis. 2023;82(6):742–53.
34. Schmidt RE, et al. Autoimmunity and primary immunodeficiency: Two sides of the same coin? Nat Rev Rheumatol. 2017;14(1):7–18.
35. Yang T, et al. The gut microbiota and the brain-gut-kidney axis in hypertension and chronic kidney disease. Nat Rev Nephrol. 2018;14(7):442–56.
36. Wang Y, et al. Gut dysbiosis in rheumatic diseases: A systematic review and meta-analysis of 92 observational studies. EBioMedicine. 2022;80:104055.
37. Rhee CM, et al. Dialysis prescription and sudden death. Semin Nephrol. 2018;38(6):570–81.
38. Oliveira CB, et al. Cardiovascular disease risk and pathogenesis in systemic lupus erythematosus. Semin Immunopathol. 2022;44(3):309–24.
39. Barbhaiya M, et al. Comparative risks of cardiovascular disease in patients with systemic lupus erythematosus, diabetes mellitus, and in general medicaid recipients. Arthritis Care Res (Hoboken). 2020;72(10):1431–9.
40. Sun G, et al. Long-term risk of heart failure and other adverse cardiovascular outcomes in granulomatosis with polyangiitis: A nationwide cohort study. J Rheumatol. 2022;49(3):291–8.
41. Berti A, et al. Risk of cardiovascular disease and venous thromboembolism among patients with incident ANCA-associated vasculitis: A 20-year population-based cohort study. Mayo Clin Proc. 2018;93(5):597–606.
42. Drosos GC, et al. EULAR recommendations for cardiovascular risk management in rheumatic and musculoskeletal diseases, including systemic lupus erythematosus and antiphospholipid syndrome. Ann Rheum Dis. 2022;81(6):768–79.
43. Legrand K, et al. Perceived health and quality of life in patients with CKD, including those with kidney failure: findings from national surveys in france. Am J Kidney Dis. 2020;75(6):868–78.
44. Muhammed H, et al. Neuropsychiatric manifestations are not uncommon in Indian lupus patients and negatively affect quality of life. Lupus 2018;27:688–93.
45. Sumanathissa M, et al. Prevalence of major depressive episode among patients with pre-dialysis chronic kidney disease. Int J Psychiatry Med. 2011;41:47–56.
46. Loiodice JM, et al. Dose adjustment of rheumatology and allergy/immunology medications in chronic kidney disease: Awareness and knowledge among internal medicine housestaff. Proc (Bayl Univ Med Cent). 2023;36(5):627–34.
47. FitzGerald JD, et al. 2020 American college of rheumatology guideline for the management of gout. Arthritis Care Res (Hoboken). 2020;72(6):744–60.
48. Wallace SL, et al. Renal function predicts colchicine toxicity: Guidelines for prophylactic use of colchicine in gout. J Rheumatol. 1991;18:264–9.
49. Colcrys [package insert]. Deerfield, IL: Takeda Pharamaceuticals America, Inc; 2012.
50. Plaquenil [package insert]. St Michael, Barbados: Concordia Pharmaceuticals Inc.; 2015.
51. Fanouriakis A, et al. 2019 update of the joint European League against rheumatism and European renal Association-European dialysis and transplant association (EULAR/ERA-EDTA) recommendations for the management of lupus nephritis. Ann Rheum Dis. 2020;79:713–23.

52. Al-Hasani H, et al. Methotrexate for rheumatoid arthritis patients who are on hemodialysis. Rheumatol Int. 2011;31(12):1545–7.
53. Huffman DH, et al. Pharmacokinetics of methotrexate. Clin Pharmacol Ther. 1973;14:572–9.
54. Aronoff GR, et al. *Drug Prescribing in Renal Failure: Dosing Guidelines for Adults and Children.* 5th ed. Philadelphia, PA: American College of Physicians; 2007, p. 101.
55. Akiyama Y, et al. Retrospective study of salazosulfapyridine in eight patients with rheumatoid arthritis on hemodialysis. Mod Rheumatol. 2014;24(2):285–90.
56. Williams JW, et al. Experiences with leflunomide in solid organ transplantation. Transplantation. 2002;73(3):358–66.
57. Schusziarra V, Ziekursch V, Schlamp R, Siemensen HC. Pharmacokinetics of azathioprine under haemodialysis. Int J Clin Pharmacol Biopharm. 1976;14(4):298–302.
58. Cellcept [package insert]. South San Francisco, CA: Genentech USA, Inc.; 2018.
59. Myfortic [package insert]. Stein, Switzerland: Novartis Pharma Stein AG; 2009.
60. Haubitz M, et al. Cyclophosphamide pharmacokinetics and dose requirements in patients with renal insufficiency. Kidney Int. 2002;61(4):1495–501.
61. Neoral [package insert]. East Hanover, NJ: Novartis Pharmaceuticals Corporation; 2023.
62. Prograf [package insert]. Northbrook, IL: Astellas Pharma US, Inc.; 2022.
63. Lupkynis [package insert]. Victoria, BC Canada; 2021.
64. Hueber AJ, et al. Anti-tumour necrosis factor alpha therapy in patients with impaired renal function. Ann Rheum Dis. 2007;66(7):981–2.
65. Actemra [package insert]. South San Francisco, CA: Genentech, Inc.; 2017.
66. Kevsara [package insert]. Bridgewater, NJ: Sanofi-Aventis U.S. LLC; 2017.
67. Cosentyx [package insert]. East Hanover, NJ: Novartis Pharmaceuticals Corporation; 2023.
68. Stelara [package insert]. Horsham, PA: Janssen Biotech, Inc.; 2012.
69. Taltz [package insert]. Indianapolis, IN: Eli Lilly and Company; 2022.
70. Skyrizi [package insert]. North Chicago, IL: AbbVie Inc.; 2022.
71. Tremfya [package insert]. Horsham, PA: Janssen Biotech, Inc.; 2019.
72. Bimzelx [package insert]. Smyrna, GA: UCB, Inc.; 2023.
73. Orencia [package insert]. Princeton, NJ: Bristol-Myers Squibb Company; 2013.
74. Nucala [package insert]. Philadelphia, PA: GlaxoSmithKline LLC; 2023.
75. Fasenra [package insert]. Södertälje, Sweden: AstraZeneca AB; 2019.
76. Saphnelo [package insert]. Södertälje, Sweden SE: AstraZeneca AB;2023.
77. Ilaris [package insert]. East Hanover, NJ: Novartis Pharmaceuticals Corporation; 2016.
78. Arcalyst [product insert]. London, UK: Kiniksa Pharmaceuticals (UK), Ltd; 2021.
79. Kineret [package insert]. Stockholm, Sweden: Swedish Orphan Biovitrum AB (publ); 2020.
80. Krystexxa [package insert]. Glendale, WI: Crealta Pharmaceuticals LLC.; 2014.
81. Benlysta [package insert]. Philadelphia, PA: GlaxoSmithKline LLC; 2022.
82. Rituxan [package insert]. South San Francisco, CA: Genentech, Inc.; 2010.
83. Kobayashi RH, et al. Immune globulin therapy and kidney disease: Overview and screening, monitoring, and management recommendations. Am J Health Syst Pharm. 2022;79(17):1415–23.
84. Otezla [package insert]. Thousand Oaks, CA: Amgen Inc.; 2023.
85. Xeljanz [package insert]. New York, NY: Pfizer Inc.; 2018.
86. Rinvoq [package insert]. North Chicago, IL: AbbVie Inc.; 2023.
87. Olumiant [package insert]. Indianapolis, IN: Eli Lilly and Company; 2022.
88. Ofev [package insert]. Ridgefield, CT: Boehringer Ingelheim Pharmaceuticals, Inc.; 2020.
89. Forteo [package insert]. Indianapolis, IN: Eli Lilly and Company; 2021.
90. Tymlos [package insert]. Boston, MA: Radius Health, Inc. 2023.
91. Prolia [package insert]. Thousand Oaks, CA: Amgen Inc.; 2010.
92. Evenity [package insert]. Thousand Oaks, CA: Amgen Inc.; 2019.
93. Lionaki S, et al. Kidney transplantation in patients with systemic lupus erythematosus. World J Transplant. 2014;4(3):176–82.
94. Fries JF, et al. Late-stage lupus nephropathy. J Rheumatol. 1974;1(2):166–75.
95. Naveed A, et al. Preemptive kidney transplantation in systemic lupus erythematosus. Transplant Proc. 2011;43(10):3713–14.
96. Cairoli E, et al. Renal transplantation in systemic lupus erythematosus: Outcome and prognostic factors in 50 cases from a single centre. Biomed Res Int. 2014;2014:746192.

97. Wallace ZS, et al. Improved survival with renal transplantation for end-stage renal disease due to granulomatosis with polyangiitis: Data from the United States Renal Data System. Ann Rheum Dis. 2018;77(9):1333–8.

98. Geetha D, et al. Renal transplantation in anti-neutrophil cytoplasmic antibody vasculitis. Expert Rev Clin Immunol. 2018;14(3):235–40.

99. Binda V, et al. Anti-neutrophil cytoplasmic antibody-associated vasculitis in kidney transplantation. Medicina (Kaunas). 2021;57(12):1325.

100. Kidney Disease: Improving Global Outcomes (KDIGO) Glomerular Diseases Work Group. KDIGO 2021 clinical practice guideline for the management of glomerular diseases. Kidney Int. 2021;100(4S):S1–S276.

101. McMahon M, et al. Systemic lupus erythematosus and cardiovascular disease: Prediction and potential for therapeutic intervention. Expert Rev Clin Immunol. 2011;7(2):227–41.

102. Palepu S, et al. Screening for cardiovascular disease before kidney transplantation. World J Transplant. 2015;5(4):276–86.

103. Choi JY, et al. Living donor renal transplantation in patients with antiphospholipid syndrome: A case report. Medicine (Baltimore). 2016;95(46):e5419.

104. Ames PR, et al. Antiphospholipid antibodies and renal transplant: A systematic review and meta-analysis. Semin Arthritis Rheum. 2019;48(6):1041–52.

105. Ahn SS, et al. Management of antineutrophil cytoplasmic antibody-associated vasculitis: A review of recent guidelines. J Rheum Dis. 2023;30(2):72–87.

106. Marco H, et al. Catalan study group of glomerular diseases (GLOMCAT). Long-term outcome of antineutrophil cytoplasmic antibody-associated small vessel vasculitis after renal transplantation. Clin Transplant. 2013;27(3):338–47.

107. Ekberg H, et al. ELITE-symphony study. Reduced exposure to calcineurin inhibitors in renal transplantation. N Engl J Med. 2007;357(25):2562–75.

108. Lentine KL, et al. OPTN/SRTR 2021 annual data report: Kidney. Am J Transplant. 2023;23(Suppl 2):S21–S120.

109. Hiemstra TF, et al. Mycophenolate mofetil vs azathioprine for remission maintenance in anti-neutrophil cytoplasmic antibody-associated vasculitis: A randomized controlled trial. JAMA. 2010;304:2381–8.

110. Pyo JY, et al. The efficacy of mycophenolate mofetil in remission maintenance therapy for microscopic polyangiitis and granulomatosis with polyangiitis. Yonsei Med J. 2021;62(6):494–502.

111. Tang W, et al. The outcomes of patients with ESRD and ANCA-associated vasculitis in Australia and New Zealand. Clin J Am Soc Nephrol. 2013;8:773–80.

112. Hruskova Z, et al. Renal transplantation in anti-neutrophil cytoplasmic antibody-associated vasculitis. Nephrol Dial Transplant. 2015;30(Suppl 1):i159–63.

113. Ciszek M, et al. Kidney transplant recipients with rheumatic diseases: Epidemiological data from the polish transplant registries 1998–2015. Transplant Proc. 2018;50(6):1654–7.

114. Horta-Baas G, et al. Renal transplantation in systemic lupus erythematosus: Comparison of graft survival with other causes of end-stage renal disease. Reumatol Clin (Engl Ed). 2019;15(3):140–5.

115. Infante B, et al. Recurrent glomerulonephritis after renal transplantation: The clinical problem. Int J Mol Sci. 2020;21(17):5954.

116. Kang SH, et al. Comparison of clinical outcomes by different renal replacement therapy in patients with end-stage renal disease secondary to lupus nephritis. Korean J Intern Med. 2011;26:60–7.

117. Renal transplantation in congenital and metabolic diseases. A report from the ASC/NIH renal transplant registry. JAMA. 1975;232(2):148–536.

118. Contreras G, et al. Recurrence of lupus nephritis after kidney transplantation. J Am Soc Nephrol. 2010;21(7):1200–7.

119. Contreras G, et al. Kidney allograft survival of African American and Caucasian American recipients with lupus. Lupus. 2014;23(2):151–8.

120. Briganti E, et al. Risk of renal allograft loss from recurrent glomerulonephritis. N Engl J Med. 2002;11:347(2):103–9.

15 Musculoskeletal Complications in Dialysis Patients

Ana Valle and Shereen N. Mahmood

15.1 INTRODUCTION

End-stage renal disease (ESRD) is irreversible renal failure requiring routine dialysis (1). The types of renal replacement therapy available are hemodialysis (HD) and peritoneal dialysis (PD), with a significant majority of ESRD patients in the United States using HD (2). Many rheumatic conditions affect the kidneys and lead to ESRD. This may occur directly, such as when systemic lupus erythematosus (SLE) or ANCA-assoc-iated vasculitis (AAV) disease activity in the kidneys causes glomerulonephritis. Indirectly, ESRD can occur due to the treatment of rheumatic diseases. For instance, non-steroidal anti-inflammatory agents can lead to ESRD through acute renal failure or nephrotic syndrome (3). Chronic glucocorticoid use is associated with type 2 diabetes mellitus, which can lead to ESRD via diabetic nephropathy.

While the prevalence of rheumatic conditions in chronic kidney disease has been reported more frequently, the prevalence of comorbid ESRD and rheumatic conditions is less reported, although rheumatologic disease-specific data is increasing (3). Costenbader et al. reported that 10–30% of SLE patients progress to ESRD (4). Others report that 20–30% of AAV patients will have ESRD within 3–7 years of diagnosis (5).

There have been reports that rheumatic conditions may be quiescent during renal failure (5). However, Broder et al. showed that SLE patients on dialysis with at least two or more rheumatology visits yearly had an increased 4-year survival rate when compared to patients who had two or fewer visits yearly. A meta-analysis by Pope et al. found that rates of AAV relapse in AAV patients with ESRD were lower than in AAV patients without ESRD. However, the rate of infection and mortality in AAV patients with comorbid ESRD was high (6). Thus, while flare frequency may decrease after ESRD onset, flares are still possible and likely undertreated, which impacts patient survival (7). An astute clinician must continue to monitor for rheumatic disease activity and treat flares in ESRD patients, which restricts the use of specific medications.

In addition, ESRD has its own musculoskeletal (MSK) disorders. Some estimate that ~63–78% of the ESRD population has MSK complications ranging from non-specific pain to pathologic fractures (8–10). As patients live longer due to renal replacement and its prevalence rises, we can only expect that these MSK disorders will continue to impact patients (8). It is necessary for rheumatologists to consider MSK conditions unique and secondary to ESRD as we evaluate autoimmune disease activity in this population. Thus, here we review the soft tissue, bone, and joint manifestations associated with ESRD.

15.2 GENERALIZED PAIN AND FATIGUE

Similar to the rheumatic population, generalized MSK pain and fatigue are prevalent in the ESRD community. Between 45% and 94% of dialysis patients report fatigue (10–13). The estimates of body aches and pain are similarly high, with a prevalence of 76% (12). Others have found that 51% of their dialysis cohort has a coexisting chronic pain syndrome (13). These symptoms are likely multifactorial due to anemia and inflammation from renal failure, metabolic derangements including secondary hyperparathyroidism, concomitant mood and sleep disorders, and a lack of physical activity. Given this complexity, a targeted intervention for chronic pain or fatigue has been difficult to find (11–12). Like the rheumatic population, non-specific symptoms are often not fully addressed by the medical community and lead to patient frustration (10, 12). In fact, Davison et al. prospectively found that pain management in their ESRD population was suboptimal 74.8% of the time (10). A renally modified adaptation of the World Health Organization's three-step analgesic ladder has been suggested (Table 15.1) (13). However, these treatments are symptomatic. Knowledge and treatment gaps continue to be present, and calls to address the pain of the ESRD community are growing (10–12).

15.3 MUSCLE DISORDERS

Muscle cramps, aches, and pains are among the most common, and often unaddressed, complaints in ESRD (10–12). A cross-sectional study found that about one-third of HD patients experienced both myalgias and muscle cramps (14). HD focus groups based in the United States revealed an even higher prevalence. Flythe et al. found that most HD patients have these symptoms, which decrease quality of life and require treatment prioritization (12).

DOI: 10.1201/9781003438373-18

Table 15.1: Comparison of the World Health Organization's Three-Step Analgesic Ladder and Santoro et al.'s Renal Adaptation of the Analgesic Ladder

Steps	Conventional Analgesic Ladder	Renally Modified Analgesic Ladder
Step 1: Mild pain *Pain scale 1–3*	Acetaminophen NSAIDs COX-2 inhibitors	Acetaminophen
Step 2: Moderate pain *Pain scale 4–6*	Tramadol Hydrocodone Oxycodone (+/– acetaminophen) Codeine	Tramadol Hydrocodone Oxycodone (+/– acetaminophen)
Step 3: Severe pain *Pain scale 7–10*	Fentanyl Methadone Hydromorphone Oxycodone (+/– acetaminophen) Morphine	Fentanyl Methadone Hydromorphone Oxycodone (+/– acetaminophen)

Muscle cramps may arise during dialysis or at nighttime, leading to sleep disturbances (15). Osmotic shifts, excessive volume removal, inadequate oxygen delivery, carnitine deficiency, and uremia have all been implicated and highlight many knowledge gaps (11, 16–17). A time-dependent association between muscle cramps and pain with HD vintage has been established (10, 18). Administering vitamins C and E to combat these symptoms has shown promise (11). As we determine how to best address these MSK conditions, their consequences, including early dialysis cessation and continued hypervolemia, are well-documented (16).

These MSK complaints, along with muscle weakness, are likely manifestations of the metabolic derangements and inflammatory state caused by kidney failure and renal replacement. Wyngaert et al. found 86.7% of their HD cohort had impaired quadriceps strength and 92% had an abnormal 6-minute walking test. In the same cohort, most patients reported decreased mobility and difficulty with daily activities (19). Others found that 64% of patients > 65 years of age had generalized weakness and significantly worse physical abilities; depression was a frequent comorbidity (20). In ESRD, muscle weakness is prominent in the lower extremities, and most patients have an increased fall risk (19). A generalized pattern of weakness with significant muscle atrophy has also been described and attributed to the homeostatic and hormonal changes caused by renal replacement (20). This weakness impacts patients' quality of life and function (19). Isoyama et al. reports that 26% of HD patients regularly exercised, 58% could complete daily activities but not exercise, and 16% could not complete daily activities (21).

A severe presentation seen in ESRD is sarcopenia. This geriatric condition is marked by a progressive decline in skeletal muscle mass and strength, which leads to a decrease in muscle function (22–23). The estimates in the elderly HD population vary, but it is known that older age, lower body mass index, elevated c-reactive protein, and the presence of beta-2-microglobulin suggestive of dialysis-associated amyloid are risk factors for sarcopenia (21–24). The inflammation and metabolic derangements found in ESRD likely contribute to its presence (24). HD access can have local effects on muscle function. A deficiency of erythropoietin, vitamin D, androgen, and carnitine predisposes ESRD patients to muscle weakness and sarcopenia. In comparison to the general elderly population, those with sarcopenia had more fractures and an increased risk of physical disability and cognitive decline (21, 23). Isoyama et al. found that 29% of sarcopenic individuals expired within 29 months. Measures of muscle strength and mass were inversely associated with mortality (21).

15.4 OTHER SOFT TISSUE INVOLVEMENT

MSK developments in ESRD may overlap with the presentation and/or sequelae of rheumatic conditions. Thus, it is prudent to consider the underlying mechanism leading to soft tissue manifestations.

About 22.5% of ESRD patients report tendon pathologies, most often of the quadriceps, patella, or Achilles (8, 18). Others report a similar prevalence of flexor tenosynovitis (29%), and trigger finger (stenosing tenosynovitis) are also common (14, 25). When tendon rupture occurs, it is due to calcifications. The risk of tendon rupture in the ESRD population must be considered when rheumatic patients with ESRD are prescribed glucocorticoids or hydroxychloroquine, which carry independent risks of tendon rupture (17).

Nerve entrapment may occur as well, and it is hypothesized to occur due to ischemia from an underlying vasculopathy or amyloid deposition (9). Carpal tunnel syndrome is a frequent complaint, with reports ranging from 14–24% in the ESRD population (14, 18, 25). Some have shown that dialysis vintage is associated with a higher risk of carpal tunnel syndrome, although there does not seem to be an association with older age (8). Tarsal tunnel syndrome is also common.

Bursal inflammation is also frequently present in ESRD. A cross-sectional study found that greater trochanteric pain syndrome was the second most reported etiology of hip pain in ESRD patients (26).

15.5 SKIN MANIFESTATIONS

The major skin manifestations of ESRD are calcifications, which occur due to renal osteodystrophy (17). Calcium deposits can occur throughout the body, including the skin, soft tissue, and joints. Skin calcifications may be physically and aesthetically bothersome. Haroon et al. found a quarter of their cohort had such calcifications (14).

An extreme presentation of skin calcium deposition is calcific uremic arteriolopathy (CUA), previously known as calciphylaxis. These severely painful and pruritic calcium plaques lead to ulceration, eschars, and skin necrosis (17). One study found CUA was more frequent in PD. Once it is present, CUA is a harbinger of advanced ESRD and associated with a mortality rate of 33–80% within 6 months (27).

Nephrogenic systemic fibrosis was another devastating skin manifestation of ESRD without effective therapy. Pruritic, painful lesions developed after ESRD individuals were exposed to gadolinium contrast. Rapid government action across multiple countries has minimized this exposure, and it is now a rare disease (13).

PD has its own soft tissue challenges, predominantly the formation of hernias, which ~10–25% of PD patients have. These may be complicated by genital edema in men or abdominal wall edema (28).

15.6 JOINT DISORDERS

Joint pain is often reported in cohorts (25–37%) and is usually asymmetric, oligoarticular pain of the larger joints (14, 25). The presence of arthralgias does not always correlate with radiologic evidence of joint damage (26). Joint disorders, including arthralgias, in the ESRD population have been associated with poor disability and functional outcomes (25).

Osteoarthritis (OA) develops ~6 years after the initiation of HD (9). Although OA is a common manifestation of advanced age, it is found in the ESRD population in higher frequencies than in individuals of similar age without renal failure (8–9). In fact, dialysis-dependent individuals undergo total hip arthroplasties at a rate six times greater than that in the general population, and OA is the most common indication (29).

Recent small studies reveal that calcium pyrophosphate is the most common crystal arthropathy in ESRD (8). Previously, basic calcium phosphate deposition was more prevalent, but it has decreased as hyperphosphatemia is treated. Calcium oxalate deposition must be discussed, given these crystals cannot be removed through dialysis. Chondrocalcinosis on radiograph could be caused by any of these crystals (30). Few have studied the prevalence of these crystal arthropathies or differentiated their diagnoses in recent years.

Gout differs from the aforementioned crystalline disease. It is an independent risk factor for ESRD development; gouty nephropathy accounts for 0.02% of the United States Renal Data System (USRDS) (31–32). However, its disease activity may change after ESRD onset. Ifudu et al. reported 70% of patients in a small sample did not have a recurrence of gout after 25 months of dialysis. Of the remaining 30% who had a flare, the frequency decreased by 50% (33). Yet Cohen et al.'s population-level study of the USRDS found that the incidence of gout attacks within the first and second year of HD initiation were similar to that in the general public, at 5% and 15%, respectively (32). In vitro models that expose monocytes from ESRD individuals to monosodium urate crystals found significantly fewer proinflammatory cytokines, suggesting a mechanism for the decreased gout activity in ESRD (34). The prevalence of other inflammatory joint disease, including rheumatoid arthritis (RA) and psoriatic arthritis, is similar to that in the general population (8).

Avascular necrosis (AVN) is uncommon in comparison to the aforementioned articular diseases. When it does occur, it often leads to hip fracture. Glucocorticoids increase the risk of AVN as observed in the renal transplant population (30). Abbot et al. found AVN to be the most common reason for total hip arthroplasties specifically in ESRD patients with SLE (29).

A significant cause of joint damage in ESRD is dialysis-associated amyloidosis, which occurs when β2-microglobulin (B2M) deposition causes a destructive arthropathy (3). In dialysis, B2M misfolds into amyloid fibrils that accumulate in the small joints of the hands, shoulders, and spine (30, 35). The classic triad of B2M amyloidosis consists of shoulder arthritis, carpal tunnel syndrome, and hand flexor tenosynovitis (14, 30). The risk of B2M amyloid increases with dialysis vintage; by ~12 years of dialysis, almost all patients have amyloid deposition (9, 30). Past studies revealed 18–35.5% of dialysis patients were impacted by B2M amyloidosis (9, 35). This number has decreased as the use of high-flux dialyzers have declined (3, 35).

B2M amyloidosis causes significant shoulder joint and rotator cuff dysfunction. Deposition between and inside the muscles and tendons of the rotator cuff increases their thickness, giving the illusion of shoulder pads and increasing the risk of tissue rupture. Non-inflammatory and hemorrhagic effusions may occur, and there is a progressive loss of motion (30). This can also be seen in the hand joints, with radiographic evidence distinctive from that of OA (30, 35). Amyloid deposition may be missed on radiographs, but it can be detected by computed tomography (CT) or magnetic resonance imaging (MRI) (30).

Of note, dialysis-associated amyloidosis differs from RA-associated amyloidosis, which is due to the deposition of amyloid A (AA). When ESRD occurs due to RA-associated AA, outcomes are worse. In 22 cases with AA due to RA leading to ESRD, 41% died within 2 months of dialysis initiation, most often due to sepsis (36). Reassuringly, when Immonen et al. reviewed the Finnish Registry for Kidney Diseases for amyloidosis associated with inflammatory arthritis, they found a decline in cases that required renal replacement, suggesting that the use of rheumatic medications may prevent the development of AA (37).

15.7 BONE DISORDERS

A major ESRD complication is renal osteodystrophy from secondary hyperparathyroidism, also called chronic kidney disease–metabolic bone disease (CKD-MBD) (13, 18, 38).

Renal osteodystrophies are classified based on their underlying mechanism. High bone turnover is a hallmark of osteitis fibrosa cystica (OFC), in which there is an increase in osteoid with less mineralization, leading to bone resorption (18, 38, 39). Classically, OFC is asymptomatic or causes mild bone pain (13). On occasion, it may present as destructive, painful osteolytic lesions that can fracture (40). These are also known as brown tumors due to a brown appearance from microfractures, hemorrhage, and bone collapse (18, 38). Due to treatment with phosphate binders, calcimimetics, and vitamin D, OFC has decreased (39). A study with American and European patients found that 24% of dialysis patients had OFC (40).

On the contrary, adynamic bone disease has low bone turnover due to excessive calcium and vitamin D, which suppress parathyroid hormone (17). Given that most ESRD patients receive these treatments, adynamic bone disease is now more frequent, with estimates between 50% and 58% (8, 39). Rarely, ESRD patients develop osteosclerosis, or increased bone density, due to increased osteoid from secondary hyperparathyroidism (41).

Osteomalacia occurs in vitamin D deficiency and decreases bone mineralization. Common symptoms include weakness; bone pain, often worse with palpation; and skeletal deformities (39). In the past, vitamin D deficiencies were frequently uncorrected, and dialysate contained aluminum, both of which predisposed patients to osteomalacia (39–40).

CKD-MDB may present as a mixed uremic osteodystrophy with features of both OFC and osteomalacia: both high bone formation and abnormal mineralization. Clinical findings are non-specific, and its prevalence and mechanism require further evaluation (42).

CKD-MDB can progress to osteoporosis. Only one-third of ESRD patients have normal bone mineral density, while another third have osteopenia, and the last third have osteoporosis (43). Most ESRD patients with osteoporosis also have sarcopenia. This combination is associated with frequent fractures and higher mortality (23). ESRD has been reported as an independent risk factor for hip fragility fracture by 3.2–4.4 folds (44). Thus, it is imperative to decrease modifiable risk factors when possible, such as glucocorticoid use.

15.8 MUSCULOSKELETAL INFECTIONS

The ESRD population has an increased risk of infection, including osteomyelitis and septic arthritis. HD access with a tunneled catheter or AV graft allows for the hematogenous spread of pathogens (45). Uremia in ESRD leads to both humoral and cellular immune dysfunction. One study revealed that 12% of all HD deaths in the United States were due to infection (45). Thus, intra-articular glucocorticoid injections must be carefully considered in ESRD (30). New emerging data reveals that chronic joint damage, regardless of the source, may be a risk factor for joint infection (9, 45).

15.9 CONCLUSION

Dialysis can sustain life for many years after renal failure. Yet ESRD and renal replacement have distinct MSK clinical manifestations. Many of the findings discussed in this chapter occur on a spectrum: from arthralgias to joint erosion, from hip pain to hip replacement, from muscular pain to sarcopenia; the majority are secondary to hyperparathyroidism. Vigilance for the MSK disorders that occur in ESRD may preserve patients' function and survival.

REFERENCES

1. Levey AS, et al. Nomenclature for kidney function and disease: Executive summary and glossary from a kidney disease: Improving global outcomes consensus conference. Perit Dial Int. 2021;41(1):5–14.
2. Johansen KL, et al. US renal data system 2022 annual data report: Epidemiology of kidney disease in the United States. Am J Kidney Dis. 2023;81(3 Suppl 1):A8–11.
3. Anders HJ, et al. Renal co-morbidity in patients with rheumatic diseases. Arthritis Res Ther. 2011;13(3):222.
4. Costenbader KH, et al. Trends in the incidence, demographics, and outcomes of end-stage renal disease due to lupus nephritis in the US from 1995 to 2006. Arthritis Rheum. 2011;63(6):1681–8.
5. Honda S, et al. Management of end-stage renal disease associated with systemic rheumatic diseases. JMA J. 2020;3(1):20–8.
6. Broder A, et al. Undertreatment of disease activity in systemic lupus erythematosus patients with endstage renal failure is associated with increased all-cause mortality. J Rheumatol. 2011;38(11):2382–9.
7. Pope V, et al. Outcomes in ANCA-associated vasculitis patients with end-stage kidney disease on renal replacement therapy-A meta-analysis. Semin Arthritis Rheum. 2023;60:152189.
8. Hage S, et al. Musculoskeletal disorders in hemodialysis patients: Different disease clustering according to age and dialysis vintage. Clin Rheumatol. 2020;39(2):533–9.
9. Akasbi N, et al. Rheumatic complications of long term treatment with hemodialysis. Rheumatol Int. 2012;32(5):1161–3.
10. Davison SN. Pain in hemodialysis patients: Prevalence, cause, severity, and management. Am J Kidney Dis. 2003;42(6):1239–47.
11. Moledina DG, et al. Pharmacologic treatment of common symptoms in dialysis patients: A narrative review. Semin Dial. 2015;28(4):377–83.
12. Flythe JE, et al. Symptom prioritization among adults receiving in-center hemodialysis: A mixed methods study. Clin J Am Soc Nephrol. 2018;13(5):735–45.
13. Santoro D, et al. Pain in end-stage renal disease: A frequent and neglected clinical problem. Clin Nephrol. 2013;79(Suppl 1):S2–11.
14. Haroon MM, et al. Rheumatic and musculoskeletal manifestations in renal hemodialysis patients. Int J Clin Rheumatol. 2018;13(5):264–9.
15. Khajehdehi P, et al. A randomized, double-blind, placebo-controlled trial of supplementary vitamins E, C and their combination for treatment of haemodialysis cramps. Nephrol Dial Transplant. 2001;16(7):1448–51.
16. Flythe JE, et al. Fostering innovation in symptom management among hemodialysis patients: Paths forward for insomnia, muscle cramps, and fatigue. Clin J Am Soc Nephrol. 2019;14(1):150–60.
17. Bardin T. Musculoskeletal manifestations of chronic renal failure. Current Opin Rheumatol. 2003;15(1):48–54.
18. Afifi WM, et al. Musculoskeletal manifestations in end-stage renal disease patients on hemodialysis and relation to parathyroid dysfunction. Saudi J Kidney Dis Transpl. 2019;30(1):68–82.
19. Vanden Wyngaert K, et al. Associations between the measures of physical function, risk of falls and the quality of life in haemodialysis patients: A cross-sectional study. BMC Nephrol. 2020;21(1):7.

20. Fidan F, et al. Quality of life and correlation with musculoskeletal problems, hand disability and depression in patients with hemodialysis. Int J Rheum Dis. 2016;19(2):159–66.

21. Isoyama N, et al. Comparative associations of muscle mass and muscle strength with mortality in dialysis patients. Clin J Am Soc Nephrol. 2014;9(10):1720–8.

22. Kim JK, et al. Prevalence of and factors associated with sarcopenia in elderly patients with end-stage renal disease. Clin Nutr. 2014;33(1):64–8.

23. Xiang T, et al. Sarcopenia and osteosarcopenia among patients undergoing hemodialysis. Front Endocrinol (Lausanne). 2023;14:1181139.

24. Shu X, et al. Diagnosis, prevalence, and mortality of sarcopenia in dialysis patients: A systematic review and meta-analysis. J Cachexia Sarcopenia Muscle. 2022;13(1):145–58.

25. El-Najjar AR, et al. Musculoskeletal disorders in hemodialysis patients and its impact on physical function. Egypt Rheumatol Rehabil. 2014;41:152–9.

26. Şenlikci HB, et al. Factors associated with hip pain in end-stage renal disease patients on prevalent hemodialysis: A cross-sectional study. Egypt Rheumatol Rehabil. 2021;48(27).

27. Fine A, et al. Calciphylaxis is usually non-ulcerating: Risk factors, outcome and therapy. Kidney Int. 2002;61(6):2210–17.

28. Bargman JM. Complications of peritoneal dialysis related to increased intraabdominal pressure. Kidney Int Suppl. 1993;40:S75–80.

29. Abbott KC, et al. Total hip arthroplasty in chronic dialysis patients in the United States. J Nephrol. 2003;16(1):34–9.

30. Kay J, et al. Osteoarticular disorders of renal origin: Disease-related and iatrogenic. Baillieres Best Pract Res Clin Rheumatol. 2000;14(2):285–305.

31. Yu KH, et al. Risk of end-stage renal disease associated with gout: A nationwide population study. Arthritis Res Ther. 2012;14(2):R83.

32. Cohen SD, et al. Association of incident gout and mortality in dialysis patients. J Am Soc Nephrol. 2008;19(11):2204–10.

33. Ifudu O, et al. Gouty arthritis in end-stage renal disease: Clinical course and rarity of new cases. Am J Kidney Dis. 1994;23(3):347–51.

34. Schreiner O, et al. Reduced secretion of proinflammatory cytokines of monosodium urate crystal-stimulated monocytes in chronic renal failure: An explanation for infrequent gout episodes in chronic renal failure patients? Nephrol Dial Transplant. 2000;15(5):644–9.

35. Tagami A, et al. Epidemiological survey and risk factor analysis of dialysis-related amyloidosis including destructive spondyloarthropathy, dialysis amyloid arthropathy, and carpal tunnel syndrome. J Bone Miner Metab. 2020;38(1):78–85.

36. Sanai T, et al. Role of amyloidosis in determining the prognosis of dialyzed patients with rheumatoid arthritis. Rheumatol Int. 2007;27(4):363–7.

37. Immonen K, et al. A marked decline in the incidence of renal replacement therapy for amyloidosis associated with inflammatory rheumatic diseases—data from nationwide registries in Finland. Amyloid. 2011;18(1):25–8.

38. Wiederkehr M. Brown tumor complicating end-stage kidney disease. Clin Nephrol Case Stud. 2020;8:72–9.

39. Hruska KA, et al. Renal osteodystrophy. N Engl J Med. 1995;333(3):166–74.

40. Malluche HH, et al. Renal osteodystrophy in the first decade of the new millennium: Analysis of 630 bone biopsies in black and white patients. J Bone Miner Res. 2011;26(6):1368–76.

41. Murphey MD, et al. Musculoskeletal manifestations of chronic renal insufficiency. Radiographics. 1993;13(2):357–79.

42. Elkhouli E, et al. Mixed uremic osteodystrophy: An ill-described common bone pathology in patients with chronic kidney disease. Osteoporos Int. 2023;34(12):2003–12.

43. Brunerová L, et al. Osteoporosis and impaired trabecular bone score in hemodialysis patients. Kidney Blood Press Res. 2016;41(3):345–54.

44. Peterkin-McCalman R, et al. Fractures in patients with rheumatoid arthritis and end-stage renal disease. Arch Osteoporos. 2020;15(1):146.

45. Aitkens L, et al. Septic arthritis in the end-stage renal disease population. J Investig Med. 2022;70(2):383–90.

Index

Note: Page numbers in *italics* indicate a figure and page numbers in **bold** indicate a table on the corresponding page.

A

ACE inhibitors (ACE-I), 40, 92, 95, 99, 102–104, 112
acute interstitial nephritis (AIN), 20, 24, 41, *118*
   NSAID-induced, 111
acute kidney injury (AKI), 2, 5–6, 20, 22, 72, 101, **109–110**
   manifestation of LN, 51
   NSAIDs, 18
   rhabdomyolysis-induced, 112
   sarcoidosis, 116
adynamic bone disease (ABD), 135, 138, 143, 156
allopurinol hypersensitivity syndrome (AHS), 24, 126
American College of Rheumatology (ACR)
   EULAR, 76, 99
   IgG4-RD classification criteria, 119
   management of SLE, 59
   proliferative nephritis, 59
amyloid, 9, 111, 154–156
ANCA-associated vasculitis (AAV), 33, 40–41, 153
   B-cell depleting therapies, 72
   efficacy of rituximab, 148
   glomerulonephritis, 11, 153
   kidney biopsy, 73, 74
angiotensin-converting enzyme (ACE), 91
angiotensin-converting enzyme inhibitors (ACEis)
   acute kidney injury (AKI), 51
   anti-RNA polymerase III antibodies, 142
anifrolumab, **30**, 40, 59, **145**
anti-neutrophil cytoplasmic antibodies (ANCAs)
   assessing treatment response, 77
   cyclophosphamide, 75, **76**
   EGPA, 77
   epidemiology, 72
   glucocorticoid-sparing strategies, 76–77
   granulomatosis, 70, **71**
   kidney involvement, 72–74, *73*, *74*
   maintenance, 76
   pathogenesis, 72
   rituximab, 75
   treatment of special populations, 75, **75**
antiphospholipid syndrome (APS), 11, 26, 31, 32
apremilast, 24
Aspreva Lupus Management Study (ALMS), 56
autoantibodies, 55
autoimmune inflammatory rheumatic diseases (AIRDs), 142–144, 146, 148
avascular necrosis (AVN), 155–156
azathioprine (AZA), 20, 39, 40, 75, 145, 147

B

Behcet's disease, 24, 32
belimumab, 39, 40, 57–60, 142
Biologics, 25, **29**, 33, 92, 108, 111, **145**
β2-microglobulin (B2M), 156
   uveitis, 41

bone health

bone health
   anabolic agents, 138
   antiresorptive agents, 137–138
   biopsy, 135
   CKD, 136–137
   CKD-MBD, 137
   DXA bone density testing, 136
   imaging, 135–136
   impact microindentation, 135
   inflammatory rheumatic diseases, 134
   laboratory evaluation, 134–135
   rheumatology patient with CKD, 134
   trabecular bone score, 136
   variety of rheumatic conditions, 134
   vertebral fractures, 136

C

calcific uremic arteriolopathy (CUA), 155
calcineurin inhibitors (CNIs), 21, 39, 40, 57–58
cardiovascular (CV) events, 138
catastrophic APS (CAPS), 32
Childhood Arthritis and Rheumatology Research Alliance (CARRA), 39
chronic kidney disease (CKD), 124, 26
   anti-inflammatory medications, 127
   colchicine, 127, 128
   cortical bone structure, 135
   ESKD and kidney transplantation, 42
   fracture risk prediction tools, 137
   glucocorticoids, 128
   hypercalcemia/hyperuricemia, 138
   IL-1 inhibitors, 128
   methotrexate, 24
   nephrolithiasis, 143
   NSAIDs, 127
   risk factor, 134
   urate management, 126–127
chronic kidney disease epidemiology collaboration (CKD-EPI), 2
chronic kidney disease–metabolic bone disease (CKD-MBD), 134–138, 156, 143
colchicine, 22–24, **23**, 34, 86, 127, 128, 145
complete renal response (CRR), 50, 57, 59
computerized tomography angiography (CTA), 91, 94
C-reactive protein (CRP), 82, 92
cryoglobulins
   chronic immune stimulation, 81
   clinical features, 81, **83–84**
   immunoglobulins (Igs), 81
   nerve biopsy, 82
   renal biopsy, 82
   steroids, 84
   treatment, 82
   types, 81, **82**
cyclophosphamide (CYC), 20, 39, 57
cytokines, 52, 57, 90, 92, 104, 110, 155

D

deficiency of adenosine deaminase 2 (DADA2), 93, 94
dendritic cells (DCs), 52
dialysis and kidney transplantation outcomes
    AIRDs, 143
    bone health, 143–144
    challenges, 147–148
    CVD, 144
    eligibility criteria for renal transplantation, 144,
        146
    ESKD, 142
    gout, 143
    GPA/MPA, 143
    HRQoL, 144
    infections, 144
    long-term management and optimizing outcomes,
        148
    outcomes, 147–148
    pre-transplant assessment, 146–147
    rheumatic disease control and organ
        transplantation outcomes, 147
    symptoms/signs, 142
    systemic lupus erythematosus (SLE), 142
    systemic sclerosis (SSc), 142–143
disease-modifying anti-rheumatic drugs (DMARDs)
    gold and penicillamine, 109
    landscape of kidney disease, 108
    methotrexate, 117
    renal injury, 33

E

endothelin-1 (ET-1), 101, 103
end-stage kidney failure/disease (ESKD)
    chronic renal disease, 59
    immunosuppression, 8, 119
    kidney transplantation, 42
    management, 148
    risk of progression, 50
    systemic rheumatic diseases, 142
end-stage renal disease (ESRD), 33, 125, 153
    bursal inflammation, 155
    dialysis-associated amyloidosis, 156
    intra-articular glucocorticoid injections, 157
    microhematuria/proteinuria, 87
    muscle disorders, 153
    nephrogenic systemic fibrosis, 155
    NSAIDs, 127
    treatment of rheumatic diseases, 153
eosinophilic granulomatosis with polyangiitis
    (EGPA), 8, 70, 77
estimated glomerular filtration rate (eGFR), 2, 18, 74, 142
    chronic kidney disease (CKD), 124
    belimumab, 57
    endogenous plasma markers, 43
    measurement of GFR (mGFR), 2
European League Against Rheumatism (EULAR)
    ACR guidelines, 59
    management of SD, 118
    SRC treatment, 102
European Renal Osteodystrophy workgroup
    (EUROD), 134
European Respiratory Society (ERS), 117

F

five-factor score (FFS), 94
fracture risk assessment (FRAX), 134, 136, 137, 143
Fracture Risk Assessment Tool (FRAX®), 134, 136, 137

G

glomerular disease
    nephritic syndrome, *see* nephritic syndrome
    nephrotic syndrome, 9
    tubulointerstitial nephritis, *see* tubulo-interstitial
        nephritis (TIN)
glomerular filtration rate (GFR), 2, 72, 26
glomerulonephritis, 53, 91
glucocorticoid-induced osteoporosis (GIOP), 137
glucocorticoids (GCs), 92
GnRH agonists (GnRHAs), 42
Gout, 22–24, 34, 124–128, 138, 142–144, 155
granulomatosis with polyangiitis (GPA), 8, 32, 70

H

health-related quality of life (HRQoL), 70, 120, 144
hydroxychloroquine, 20, 32, 40, 57, 59, 86, **109**, 117, 118,
    145, 155
Hyperparathyroidism, 134, 137, 143, 153, 156, 157
hypertension, 91
hypocomplementemic urticarial vasculitis syndrome
    (HUVS), 85–86

I

idiopathic inflammatory myopathies (IIMs),
    112–113
IgA nephropathy, 112
IgA vasculitis (IgAV), 41, 81, 83, 84, 85
IgG4-related disease (IgG4-RD), 119–120
immune complex (IC) vasculitis
    anti-GBM, 85
    common features, 81, **82**
    cryoglobulins, *see* cryoglobulins
    drug-induced, 86, 87
    HUVS, 85–86
    IGA, 84–85
    monoclonal gammopathy, 87
immunoglobulin and complement components
    (ICs), 81
International Society of Nephrology/Renal
    Pathology Society (ISN/RPS), 54
intravenous immunoglobulin (IVIG), 86, 118, 146, 18, 20–21

J

Janus Kinase (JAK) inhibitors, 21–22, **22**
juvenile idiopathic arthritis (JIA), 33

K

kidney disease
    IgG4-related disease (IgG4-RD), 119–120
    manifestations and evaluation, 120, **121**
    sarcoidosis, *116*, 116–117
    Sjogren's disease (SD), **117**, 117–119

Kidney Disease–Improving Global Outcomes (KDIGO) guidelines, 59, 101, 134
kidney replacement therapy (KRT), 72, 142–144, 148

L

leflunomide, 20
leukocytoclastic vasculitis (LCV), 81, 86, 87
lupus anticoagulant (LAC), 32
lupus nephritis (LN)
    biomarkers, 54–56
    biopsy classification and histopathology, 53–54
    endoplasmic reticulum (ER), 52–53
    epidemiology and risk factors, 5, 50–51
    genetics, 51–52
    guidelines, 59–60
    ianalumab, 59
    immune cells, 52
    immune complex deposition, 53
    immune complexes, 53
    obinutuzumab, 58, 59
    treatment, 56–59
lymphocytes, 52
lymphoma, 12, 81, 82, 120

M

macroalbuminuria, 5
magnetic resonance angiography (MRA), 91, 92
measurement of GFR (mGFR), 2, 43
medications, dosing and monitoring
    biologic DMARDs, 21, **22**
    myriad medications, 18
    NSAIDs, 18
    rheumatologic drug classes, 18
    dual-energy x-ray absorptiometry (DXA), 134, 136, 138, 143
methotrexate (MTX), 18, 20
microalbuminuria, 3, 5, 108, 124
microangiopathic hemolytic anemia (MAHA), 101, 102
microscopic polyangiitis (MPA)
    cyclophosphamide (CYC), 75
    eosinophil-targeted therapies, 70
    glomerulonephritis, 70
    granulomatosis with polyangiitis (GPA), 70
    kidney involvement, 8, 72
    renal transplant, 148
mixed connective tissue disease (MCTD), 34, 107, 113
musculoskeletal complications in dialysis patients
    bone disorders, 156
    chronic kidney disease, 153
    ESRD, 153
    generalized pain and fatigue, 153, **154**
    infections, 156–157
    joint disorders, 155–156
    muscle disorders, 153, 154
    skin manifestations, 155
    soft tissue involvement, 154–155
mycophenolate mofetil (MMF), 20, 39, 56
myeloid cells, 52

N

nephritic syndrome
    anti-GBM disease, 8–9
    antineutrophilic cytoplasmic antibody (ANCA)-associated glomerulonephritis, 8
    cryoglobulinemic glomerulonephritis, 8
    glomerular inflammation, 7
    IgA vasculitis, 8
    lupus nephritis (LN), 7–8
    tissue disease syndromes, 7–8
noncoding RNA (ncRNA), 52
non-steroidal anti-inflammatory drugs (NSAIDs), 86, **86**, **18**
normal anion gap metabolic acidosis (NAGMA), 118

O

osteitis fibrosa cystica (OFC), 156
osteoarthritis (OA), 155
Osteomalacia, 156
osteoporosis, 42, 134, 136, 137, 143, **146**, 148, 156

P

parathyroid hormone (PTH), 135, 137, 138, 143
pediatric rheumatologic disease
    ANCA-associated vasculitis (AAV), 40–41
    anti-GBM disease, 41
    cyclophosphamide, 42
    glucocorticoids (GCs), 42
    guidelines, 39
    IgA vasculitis (IgAV), 41
    kidney transplant, 42–43
    LUNAR trial, 40
    measurement of kidney function, 39, 43
    pediatric-centered to adult-centered care, 44, 45
    systemic lupus erythematosus (SLE), 39–40
    TINU, 41
    vaccinations, 43–44, **44**
pegloticase, 24
percutaneous renal artery angioplasty (PTRA), 92
point-of-care ultrasound (POCUS), 5
polyarteritis nodosa (PAN), 10
    clinical manifestations, 93–94
    definition, 92
    diagnosis, 94
    epidemiology, 92, **92**
    pathogenesis, 92, 93, *93*
    treatment, 94–95
pregnant patient with rheumatic disease
    APS/catastrophic APS, 32
    causes of proteinuria, 27, **27**
    connective tissue diseases, 34
    fetal complications, 27
    gestational proteinuria, 26
    glomerular diseases, 26
    inflammatory arthritides, 33
    kidney disease, 35
    nephrology, 26
    renal biopsies, 26
    renovascular changes, 26
    rheumatic medications, 34–35
    systemic lupus erythematosus (SLE), 27, **28–31**, 32
    vasculitis, 32–33
Preventing Early Renal Loss in Diabetes (PERL) trial, 126
probenecid, 24
proteinuria, 55

R

rapidly progressive glomerulonephritis (RPGN), 72, 82–84, 102, 144
renal artery stenosis (RAS), 90–92
renal disease
    dialysis and urate excretion, 125–126
    prevalence of gout, 124
    urate transporters, 124, *125*
renal-limited vasculitis (RLV), 70, 72, 73, 75, 76
renal manifestations
    idiopathic inflammatory myopathies (IIMs), 112–113
    rheumatoid arthritis, *see* rheumatoid arthritis
    spondyloarthropathies (SpAs), 111–112
renal osteodystrophy (ROD), 134, 135, 143
renovascular hypertension (RVH), 91, *91*, 92, 94
rheumatic disease
    clinical features, 11, **11–13**
    GFR, 2
    glomerular disease, *see* glomerular disease
    kidney biopsy, 6, **6**
    non-rheumatologic diagnostic workup, 13
    rheumatologic and kidney diseases, 2
    rheumatologic diagnostic workup, 13, *14*
    ultrasound, 5–6
    urine diagnostics, *see* urine diagnostics
    vascular renal injury, 10–11
rheumatoid arthritis
    chronic inflammation, 108
    glomerulonephritis (GN), 108–110, **109–110**
    prevalence of kidney disease, 108
    renal involvement, 111
    renal manifestations, 107, **107–108**
    secondary amyloidosis, 111
risk evaluation and mitigation strategy (REMS), 34
rituximab, 8, 40, 41, 53, 58, 59, 75, 76, 82, 84, 85, 111, 113, 117–120, 148

S

Sarcoidosis, 9–10, 81, 116–121
Scleroderma Clinical Trials Consortium Scleroderma Renal Crisis Working Group, 101
scleroderma renal crisis (SRC), 10–11, 34
    ACE inhibitors, 102–103
    alpha-blockers, 102–103
    angiotensin receptor blockers, 102–103
    calcium channel blockers, 102–103
    diagnosis, 101
    epidemiology, 99
    histopathology, 101, *101*
    other treatments, 103–104
    outcomes, 99
    pathophysiology, 99, 101
    prevention, 102
    renal replacement therapy, 103
    renal transplant, 103
    risk factors, 99
    systemic sclerosis (SSc), 99, *101*
Single Hub and Access point for pediatric Rheumatology in Europe (SHARE), 39, 41
Sjogren's disease (SD), **117**, 117–119, 33–34

small-for-gestational-age (SGA), 33
small-vessel vasculitis (SVV), 81, 85
Spondyloarthropathies (SpAs), 111–112
sterile pyuria, 4, 41
sulfasalazine, 10, 19, 20, 29, 109, 145
systemic lupus erythematosus (SLE)
    anifrolumab, 59
    belimumab, 57
    biological agents, 40
    CVD management guidelines, 144
    cyclosporine, 21
    dendritic cells (DCs), 52
    hydroxychloroquine, 20
    lupus nephritis, 7, 50
    mortality, 50
    nephrotic syndrome, 7
    renal involvement, 50
    urine sediment, 55
systemic sclerosis (SSc), 99, *101*, 142–143

T

Takayasu arteritis (TAK)
    clinical manifestations, 90–91
    definition, 90
    diagnosis, 91, 92
    epidemiology, 90
    pathogenesis, 90
    treatment, 92
thrombotic thrombocytopenic purpura (TTP), 102
tubulointerstitial inflammation, 53
tubulo-interstitial nephritis (TIN), 118, 119, 121
    drug induced, 10
    IgG4-related kidney disease, 10
    non-rheumatologic entities, 9
    sarcoidosis, 9–10
    Sjogren's disease, 9
tubulo-interstitial nephritis with uveitis (TINU) syndrome, 41
turnover, mineralization, and volume (TMV), 135

U

United States Renal Data System (USRDS), 155
urine albumin-to-creatinine ratio (uACR), 3, 5, 9
urine diagnostics
    dipstick, 3, **3**
    evaluation of proteinuria, 4, 5
    evolving urinary biomarkers, 5
    sediment examination, 4, *4*
urine protein-to-creatinine ratio (uPCR), 3, 5, 6, 9, 58

V

vascular cell adhesion molecule (VCAM), 56
vertebral fracture assessment (VFA), 136
vitamin D, 42, 135, 137, 154, 156
voclosporin (VOC), 40

X

xanthine oxidase inhibitors, 24